patient care®

PROCEDURES FOR YOUR PRACTICE

AF710573

patient care®
PROCEDURES FOR YOUR PRACTICE

Edited by

Charles E. Driscoll, M.D.
Professor and Head
Department of Family Practice
The University of Iowa
Iowa City, Iowa

Robert E. Rakel, M.D.
Associate Dean for Academic and Clinical Affairs
Professor and Chairman
Department of Family Medicine
Baylor College of Medicine
Houston, Texas

Practice Management Information Corporation
Los Angeles, California 90010

Library of Congress Cataloging-in-Publication Data

Patient care procedures for your practice / edited by Charles E.
Driscoll, Robert E. Rakel.—2nd ed.
p. cm.
Articles reprinted from Patient care.
Includes bibliographical references.
Includes index.
ISBN 1-878487-29-9
1. Family medicine. I. Driscoll, Charles E. II. Rakel, Robert
E. III. Patient care.
[DNLM: 1. Family Practice—methods—collected works. WB 110
P298]
RC46.P293 1991
616—dc20
DNLM/DLC
for Library of Congress 90-13257
CIP

Practice Management Information Corporation
Los Angeles, California 90010

Printed in the United States of America

Copyright © 1991 by Practice Management Information Corporation, Los Angeles, CA 90010. All rights reserved. None of the content of this publication may be reproduced, stored in a retrieval system, or transmitted in any form or by any means (electronic, mechanical, photocopying, recording, or otherwise) without the prior written permission of the publisher.

The authors and publisher have exerted every effort to ensure that drug selection, dosage, and therapeutic modalities set forth in this text are in accord with current recommendations and practice at the time of publication. However, in view of ongoing research, changes in government regulations, and the constant flow of information relating to drug therapy and drug reactions, the reader is urged to check the package insert for each drug for any change in indications and dosage and for added warnings and precautions. This is particularly important when the recommended agent is a new or infrequently employed drug.

Contents

Contributors vii

Foreword ix

Preface xi

Acknowledgments xiii

PART I CARDIOVASCULAR PROCEDURES 1

1. Starting an IV Line in an Adult 3
2. Starting an IV Line in a Newborn 9
3. Emergency Intraosseous Infusion 15
4. Emergency Cannulation of the Femoral Vein 21
5. Cardiopulmonary Resuscitation in Adults 27
6. Cardiopulmonary Resuscitation in Infants and Children 33
7. Managing Airway Obstruction in Children 41
8. Internal Jugular Vein Catheterization 45
9. Emergency Defibrillation and Cardioversion 51
10. Exercise Treadmill Testing 57

PART II PULMONARY PROCEDURES 65

11. Thoracentesis for Fluid Removal 67
12. Endotracheal Intubation 73
13. Emergency Cricothyroidotomy 79
14. Spirometry 85
15. Chest Tube Insertion 89
16. Tactile Orotracheal Intubation 99
17. Arterial Puncture for Blood Gas Specimens 103

PART III GASTROINTESTINAL PROCEDURES 109

18. Emergency Gastric Intubation 111
19. Flexible Fiberoptic Sigmoidoscopy 119
20. Rubber Band Ligation of Hemorrhoids 127
21. Paracentesis and Peritoneal Lavage 133
22. Digital Removal of Fecal Impaction 141
23. Skinfold Measurements 145

PART IV MUSCULOSKELETAL/CONNECTIVE TISSUE PROCEDURES 155

24. Aspiration and Injection of Joints 157
25. Trigger Point Injection 167
26. Management of TMJ Dislocation 175
27. Compressive Ankle Splinting 181
28. Immobilizing Clavicular Fractures 185

PART V GENITOURINARY PROCEDURES 195
29. Suprapubic Bladder Tap in Infants and Children 197
30. Newborn Circumcision with the Gomco Clamp 201
31. Passing a Urinary Catheter 211
32. Emergency Treatment of Priapism: Intracorporeal Aspiration and Irrigation 219
33. Examining a Male Patient for Genital Warts 223

PART VI OBSTETRICS AND GYNECOLOGY PROCEDURES 227
34. Inserting an Intrauterine Device 229
35. Fine-Needle Aspiration of the Breast 237
36. Endometrial Biopsy 243
37. Biopsy of the Uterine Cervix 249
38. Culdocentesis 253
39. Delivery without an Episiotomy 257
40. Minimally Invasive Endometrial Sampling 261

PART VII DERMATOLOGY PROCEDURES 267
41. Administering Local Anesthesia 269
42. Punch Biopsy of the Skin 283
43. Removing a Skin Cyst 287
44. Cryotherapy for Skin Lesions 291
45. Repair of Simple Lacerations 299
46. Incision and Drainage of Cutaneous Abscesses 307
47. Paronychia: Incision and Drainage 313
48. Treatment of Ingrown Toenail 319
49. Removing a Ring from a Swollen Finger 327
50. Removing Fishhooks 331
51. Electrocoagulation 337
52. Wood's Light Examination 345

PART VIII EAR, NOSE, THROAT PROCEDURES 351
53. Laryngoscopy 353
54. Removing Impacted Cerumen from the Ear 361
55. Tympanometry 367
56. Controlling Posterior Epistaxis 373

PART IX EYE PROCEDURES 379
57. Removing a Foreign Body from the Eye 381

PART X NEUROLOGY PROCEDURES 387
58. Lumbar Puncture in Adults 389
59. Lumbar Puncture in Infants and Children 395
60. Patient-Controlled Analgesia 401

PART XI BEHAVIORAL MEDICINE PROCEDURES 405
61. Progressive Muscle Relaxation 407
62. Hypnosis in Office Practice 415

INDEX 421

Contributors

A. Timothy Appenheimer, M.D.
USB Hospital
Dixon, Illinois

Martin Bartolac, M.D.
Dean Clinic-East Madison Office
Madison, Wisconsin

Elizabeth A. Burns, M.D.
Associate Professor
Department of Family Practice
The University of Iowa
Iowa City, Iowa

Carol Buss, R.D.
Private Practitioner
Coralville, Iowa

Rollo J. Coble, M.D.
Associate (retired)
Department of Family Practice
University of Iowa College of Medicine
Iowa City, Iowa

Phillip Couchman, M.D.
Clinical Associate Professor (retired)
Department of Family Practice
University of Iowa
Iowa City, Iowa

Nancy Cwach, M.D.
Private Practitioner
Iowa City, Iowa

Keith E. Davis, M.D.
Private Practitioner
Shoshone, Idaho

Richard C. Dobyns, M.D.
Associate
Department of Family Practice
The University of Iowa
Iowa City, Iowa

Thomas A. Francis, M.D.
Private Practitioner
Los Arlos Family Practice
Scottsdale, Arizona

Holly Hendrickson, M.D.
Geriatrics Fellow
Department of Family Practice
The University of Iowa
Iowa City, Iowa

Dan Heslinga, M.D.
Emergency Department Physician
Castle Medical Center
Kailua, Hawaii

Georgianna S. Hoffman, R.N., M.A., C.S.
Psychotherapist
Center for Marital and Sexual Counceling
1016 E. College St.
Iowa City, Iowa 52240

Charles D. Huss, M.D.
Directory
Emergency Care Unit
Mercy Hospital
500 Market St.
Iowa City, Iowa 52245

Rafael Ivan Iriarte, M.D.
Department of Family Practice
University of Puerto Rico
School of Medicine
San Juan, Puerto Rico

Ralph Knudson, M.D.
Assistant Professor
Department of Family Practice
The University of Iowa
Iowa City, Iowa

John Littler, M.D.
Staff Physician
Emergency Department
Covenant Medical Center
Waterloo, Iowa

Elizabeth M. Loeb, M.D.
Private Practitioner
Iowa City Family Practice Clinic
Iowa City, Iowa

Ronald B. Low, M.D.
Associate Professor
Emergency Medicine
East Carolina University
Pitt County Memorial Hospital
Greenville, NC 27835-6028

Gerald J. McGowan, M.D.
Director, Family Practice Residency
Siouxland Medical Education Foundation, Inc.
Sioux City, Iowa

Richard E. Munns, M.D.
Clinical Associate Professor (retired)
Department of Family Practice
University of Iowa
Iowa City, Iowa

Timothy J. Nagel, M.D.
Private Practitioner
Decorah, Iowa

Gayle Nelson, R.N.
Coordinator, Family Physicians Learning Laboratory
Department of Family Practice
The University of Iowa
Iowa City, Iowa

Richard W. Niska, M.D.
Department Director
Emergency Medicine
Hastings Indian Hospital
100 South Bliss Ave.
Tahlequah, Oklahoma 74464

Darrell Randle, M.D.
Resident in Anesthesiology
Department of Anesthesiology
Letterman Army Medical Center
Presidio of San Francisco
San Francisco, California

Leroy R. Schlesselman, M.D.
Private Practitioner
Cedar Rapids, Iowa

Elliott D. Schmerler, M.D.
Private Practitioner
Incline Village, Nevada

Ann Stein, M.D.
Associate
Department of Family Practice
The University of Iowa
Iowa City, Iowa

Lawrence Steinkraus, M.D.
Private Practitioner
Iowa City, Iowa

Bev True, M.D.
Family Practice Resident
Department of Family Medicine
University of Washington
Seattle, Washington

Leslie E. Weber, M.D.
Associate
Department of Family Practice
The University of Iowa
Iowa City, Iowa

Glenys O. Williams, M.D.
Professor
Department of Family Practice
The University of Iowa
Iowa City, Iowa

Paul S. Williamson, M.D.
Private Practitioner
Associates in Family Care
Olathe, Kansas

Foreword

Too often, in the haste to transmit new information, textbooks emphasize the new and uncommon techniques. Standard and common, or only occasionally performed, procedures are ignored or at least not given the detailed attention needed to perform the procedure well.

This book is designed to provide concise, practical information on procedures usually performed in family practice. The information in each chapter is organized into the materials needed, the technique for performing the procedure, follow-up, complications, and suggested readings. Perhaps the most valuable feature is the quality of the hand drawn illustrations. My favorites are in the chapters "Newborn Circumcision with the Gomco Clamp" and "Injection of Joints." Where else can you find illustrated descriptions on removing impacted cerumen, starting an IV, or passing a urinary catheter?

This second edition is considerably expanded and includes many new and useful procedures in such diverse areas as removing fecal impaction, the emergency treatment of priapism, hypnosis, and muscle relaxation exercises. This book will be of greatest value to the medical student and resident performing a procedure for the first or second time. It will be equally valuable to the experienced clinician who may not have performed the procedure recently and desires a quick, timely, and concise refresher. The procedures are described in a step-by-step manner with illustrations amplifying key points.

It is the variety of experiences and challenges in family practice that makes our discipline so exciting and rewarding. Ours is a pragmatic discipline and the procedures we do must be done efficiently, quickly, and safely.

This book is written by experienced family physicians who know the details that are important when performing a procedure in the office. It is intended to help family physicians provide up-to-date care of high quality for their patients. I am proud to have been able to play a small part in its development.

Robert E. Rakel, M.D.

Preface

We are pleased to present to our readers the second edition of *Procedures for Your Practice.* We hope it will serve many interests ranging from those of the medical student who is learning a new procedure for the first time to those of the experienced clinician who wants to brush up on the anatomic landmarks and steps of an infrequently used procedure. Many times in a busy primary care practice, a technical procedure will aid in the diagnosis or management of a patient's condition; having an available reference to review should add to the quality of care at each encounter.

This second edition presents an expanded number of procedures reorganized by organ system. Previously written procedures have all been reviewed and updated to ensure that they have kept pace with new developments in equipment, technique, and acceptance in the community of medicine.

These "Procedures for Your Practice" have all appeared in the journal. *Patient Care.* Having newly updated them for this book, we hope it will serve as a clear reference for appropriate indications, contraindications, and methods for performing the procedures most often needed in your practice. Please feel free to give us your feedback about this new volume's usefulness and any new ideas that we can include in future editions. We hope you find it a useful addition to your library.

Charles E. Driscoll, MD

Acknowledgments

These procedures for your practice are drawn from *Patient Care* magazine. The authors are hands-on practitioners who know and do what they are talking about, and show you how to do it simply and safely. The coeditors of the book have been the coordinators of the magazine series: Dr. Rakel introduced the first procedure in 1983; Dr. Driscoll began in 1985 and continues to produce the series.

Charles E. Driscoll, M.D., is professor and head of the Department of Family Practice at the University of Iowa College of Medicine in Iowa City, coauthor of *The Handbook of Family Practice,* and Family Practice Desk References.

Robert E. Rakel, M.D., is chairman of the Department of Family Medicine at Baylor College of Medicine in Houston, author of *Principles of Family Medicine,* and editor of *Textbook of Family Practice* and *Conn's Current Therapy.*

Illustrators for the magazine series and the book were: **Paul Singh-Roy, Kevin Somerville, Marcia Hartsock, Michael Leonard, Kathryn Born, Charles Boyter, Floyd Hosmer, and David Factor.**

We especially want to acknowledge the efforts of the following people: **Robert L. Edsall**, editor of *Patient Care,* who was there at each step from conception to completion of the book; **Richard F. Graber**, who edited the original manuscripts; **Jane Monaghan**, who supervised compilation of the procedures; **Karen Clements**, for her editorial assistance; **Jean Palmay** and **Joan C. Shamlian**, for their secretarial and clerical support on this publication; and **Caroline Mast**, who was an invaluable assistant to Drs. Driscoll and Rakel, and all of us in pulling and keeping all the contributions together.

I

Cardiovascular Procedures

1

Starting an IV Line in an Adult

Phillip Couchman, MD
Keith E. Davis, MD

An IV infusion serves numerous purposes, from administering medication and anesthesia, to parenteral nutrition, restoration of blood volume, and measurement of central venous pressure and blood gases. Peripheral venipuncture is the most common infusion technique, and the cannula-over-needle IV catheter procedure described here is preferable to the conventional rigid needle for an adult. When the catheter is inserted and secured, it is much more trouble free than a rigid needle and usually allows the patient some movement at the site.

Materials

- IV stand
- IV solution
- IV tubing, connected to the bottle or bag of solution and flushed with solution to remove air bubbles
- Antiseptic for skin prep: povidone-iodine solution (Betadine) or alcohol
- Rubber gloves
- Gauze pads
- Lidocaine HCl (Xylocaine) (optional)
- 26- or 30-gauge intradermal needle (optional)
- 19- or 20-gauge venipuncture needle (optional)
- Adhesive tape (cloth or paper)
- Sterile gauze dressing
- Tourniquet or blood pressure cuff
- IV catheter of appropriate size (may come in a kit also containing tourniquet, prepping swabs, and tape)
- Cotton or gauze
- Padded arm board or splint

Site Selection

The choice of a site for an IV insertion should be based on several factors: the general condition of the patient's veins, the existence of inflammation and tenderness at previous sites of infusion, and the anticipated amount of patient activity and movement after the catheter is in place. One general rule is to choose a site that is as distal as possible. In the event that an optimum site is ruined, possibly from a previous infusion, you may still be able to use the more proximal part of the vein. In a life-threatening situation, use the most accessible vein.

An important consideration is the amount of time that the catheter must remain in place.

Short-term IV access is associated with quick surgical procedures and diagnostic tests. In patients whose veins are difficult to visualize, the dorsum of the hand is a good insertion site. Look for a vein that branches distally, and enter the vein at the junction of the branches. This minimizes rolling of the vein being entered—a problem often encountered in patients with tough vein walls. Other major insertion sites include the large vein on the radial side of the wrist (or as distal on the forearm as possible), and, when clearly visible, a vein on the volar aspect of the forearm.

Long-term IV access, for such things as parenteral nutrition or medication delivery, has different site requirements than short-term IVs. In this case, it is advisable to avoid placement at the wrist or elbow, as these sites often require the addition of an uncomfortable splint or arm board to prevent displacement of the catheter and infiltration of the IV solution when the patient moves.

Keeping these facts in mind will facilitate preparation for the procedure and ensure a calmer, more comfortable experience for the patient.

Preparation

1. Hang the bottle or bag of IV solution from the IV stand, ready for use.
2. Tear or cut off sections of adhesive tape and place them within convenient reach.
3. Thoroughly wash your hands, and don rubber gloves if protection against potentially contaminated blood or body fluids is required.
4. Apply a tourniquet or blood pressure cuff proximal to the site selected. If you use a blood pressure cuff, set the pressure midway between the patient's diastolic and systolic pressures. In an emergency, 100 mmHg is a reasonable estimate for the patient with a palpable pulse. If cuff pressure is too high, blood will not enter the extremity, the patient will become uncomfortable, and veins will not distend. If cuff pressure is too low, blood flow will not be obstructed, and venous distention will not occur.
5. If you have difficulty locating a favorable point of entry, let the patient's arm hang over the edge of the bed briefly to improve venous distention, place a heating pad or warm towel over the site for a few

minutes, or gently tap the skin over the vein. If you must palpate for a deep vein, apply antiseptic to your fingertips first.

6. Cleanse the site thoroughly with povidone-iodine solution or alcohol on gauze pads.

Note: A local anesthetic such as lidocaine can facilitate painless venipuncture, especially with larger cannula insertion. Use a 26- or 30-gauge intradermal needle and infiltrate carefully and slowly to avoid distortion of the venous structure.

PROCEDURE

1. With your nondominant hand, apply traction to the skin distal to the entry site.

2. With your dominant hand, hold the catheter, with the needle bevel side up, at a 20-degree angle to the vein (Figure 1-1).

3. Insert the needle with steady pressure until you see a blood return in the needle hub. If you are introducing a large cannula, consider first puncturing the dermis with a sharp, 19- or 20-gauge venipuncture needle to facilitate entry. Elevate the skin with the needle to avoid injury to the vein you will subsequently cannulate.

4. With your nondominant hand, advance the catheter alone into the vein while holding the needle immobile with your dominant hand (Figure 1-2). Once the catheter is in the vein, remove the needle and advance the catheter to the desired position. (If advancement is difficult, attaching the IV tubing to the catheter hub and running the infusion at a slow rate may make it easier.)

5. Remove the tourniquet or blood pressure cuff, attach the IV tubing to the catheter hub, and start the infusion. Should a valve in a

Figure 1-1 Proper angle for needle insertion.

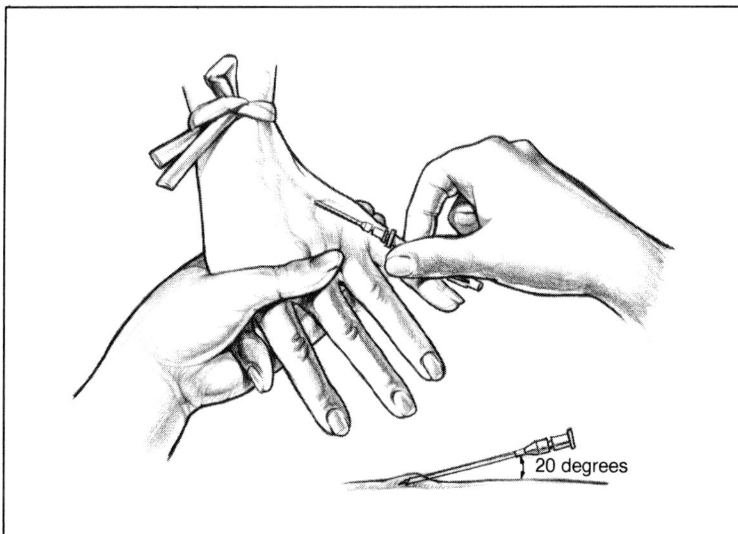

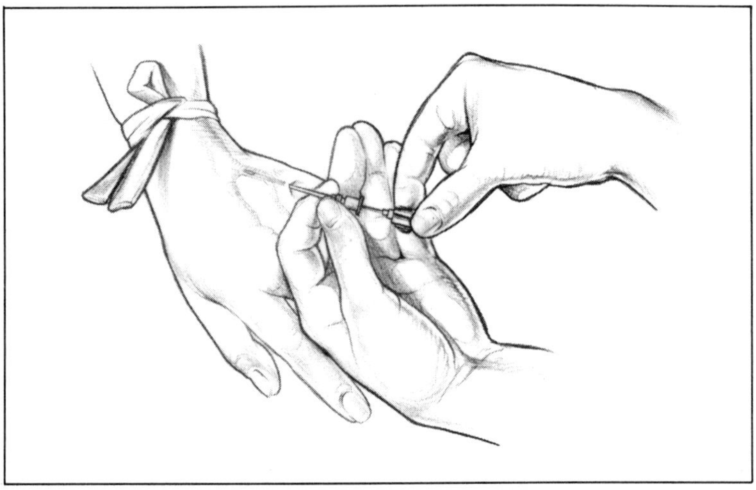

Figure 1-2 Immobilize needle while advancing catheter into the vein.

large vein obstruct flow, withdraw the catheter slightly or advance it to a different position until the solution flows. If a hematoma or swelling occurs at the entry site, remove the catheter, and apply pressure over the site of bleeding, using a gauze pad. Select a new site, and enter the vein without applying a tourniquet or blood pressure cuff.

6. If the infusion flows smoothly, use cotton or gauze to remove any blood or spilled solution; then apply a sterile gauze dressing over the site. Secure the catheter to the skin with tape (Figure 1-3); also secure the patient's arm to a board, if necessary.

Complications

Local complications, largely avoidable with careful site selection and technique, include, in order of frequency:

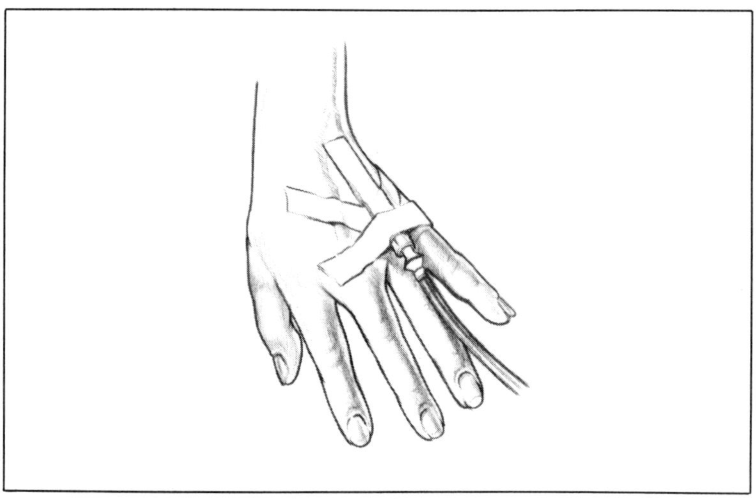

Figure 1-3 Secure catheter in place with tape.

- Hematoma
- Phlebitis
- Thrombosis
- Cellulitis

Systemic complications include:

- Air embolism
- Pulmonary thromboembolism
- Sepsis

An uncommon complication in cannula-over-needle IV catheter placement is catheter fragment embolism. This will not happen if you do not attempt to reintroduce the needle into the catheter. If you need to try a second site, for example, use a new catheter set rather than run the risk of this complication.

Suggested Readings

Kaye W: Intravenous techniques, in McIntyre KM, Lewis AJ (eds): *Textbook of Advanced Cardiac Life Support.* Dallas, American Heart Association, 1981, pp xii-1-xii-12.

Ludbrook J, Jamieson GG: Disorders of veins, in Sabiston DC Jr (ed): *Davis-Christopher Textbook of Surgery: The Biological Basis of Modern Surgical Practice,* ed 12. Philadelphia, WB Saunders Co, 1981, pp 1808-1827.

2

Starting an IV Line in a Newborn

Paul S. Williamson, MD
Richard C. Dobyns, MD

Successful insertion of peripheral IV lines in the neonate is a psychomotor skill that improves only with practice. Once a successful technique is mastered, it must be performed frequently in order to maintain a competent level of skill. The procedure for inserting an IV line in a newborn infant can be modified and adapted for implementation in the older infant, 12–18 months of age. The older, stronger infant does not require more postinsertion restraint.

Indications for an IV insertion include infusion of fluids or delivery of IV medications through an indwelling line, though this same basic cannulation technique is also recommended for rapid entry and removal, such as obtaining blood samples with a steel needle on a syringe.

The average duration of peripheral IV access at one site is approximately 24–48 hours in the neonate receiving antibiotic therapy and 48–72 hours in the neonate receiving only crystalloid infusion.

Materials

- A worktable—preferably a neonatal intensive care bed with movable side rails, overhead light, and radiant warmer
- IV tubing set, IV pole, heparin lock, and bottle of IV fluid
- IV catheter—22-gauge Abbocath or 24-gauge Jelco; catheter should be preflushed with sterile saline; a 23- or 25-gauge butterfly may be used as a temporary line
- 4 × 4-in. gauze pad and clear adhesive tape (½ in. wide, 1½ in. long) to cover and protect needle site after insertion
- Four ½ × 3-in. strips of tape and four 1 × 3-in. strips of double-backed tape to secure the catheter and arm board, precut and stuck within easy reach; double-backed tape prevents skin damage, especially in premature infants; to prepare a strip of double-backed tape, stick together two pieces of adhesive tape, one shorter than the other, so that the only adhesive exposed is at the ends of the longer piece

- Alcohol prep pads
- Arm board, which can be fashioned from a tongue blade covered with gauze padding
- Antibiotic ointment

Site Selection

The choices of location for an IV insertion in an infant are very different from those in an adult. In order of decreasing desirability, they are as follows:

- The superficial veins on the dorsum of the hand
- The greater saphenous vein at the medial aspect of the ankle, just anterior to the medial malleolus
- The veins in the antecubital area, which may be visible, but more often only palpable
- A scalp vein, clearly visible after shaving off a patch of the hair, but this is often unpopular with parents.

Positioning the Infant

Place the infant supine on the work surface, and have your assistant immobilize the access site and control all other extremities by wrapping the infant in a towel, papoose style, if need be. Careful restraint is essential: A kicking foot can quickly undo a lot of work.

- *For insertion into veins on the dorsum of the hand,* have your assistant grasp the upper arm so that his or her thumb and index finger serve as a tourniquet. With one hand, palmar flex the infant's wrist, applying skin traction with your thumb to facilitate needle insertion (Figure 2-1). **Warning:** Too much flexion of the wrist can flatten the vein you are trying to cannulate.
- *For insertion into the saphenous vein,* hold the infant's foot in extension with a slight varus angle. Have your assistant's hand proximal on the leg, out of your way, grasping the calf as a tourniquet. Have him use his other hand and forearm to restrain the infant's arms and body.
- *For insertion into veins in the antecubital area,* have your assistant stabilize the infant's shoulder with the palm of one hand, which also serves as a tourniquet around the upper arm. Have him use the other hand to hold the infant's elbow in extension.

Note: Once cannulated, the antecubital vein works well, but insertion is sometimes difficult because the vein traverses a joint, valves hinder the return of blood, and the vein is difficult to see.

- *For insertion into a scalp vein,* place the infant with his head at the edge of the table and have your assistant stabilize the body and all four extremities. Place a large rubber band around the circumference of the head just above the ears as a tourniquet. Stabilize the infant's head with one hand (Figure 2-2).

Figure 2-1 Palmar flex of infant's wrist, with thumb applying skin traction.

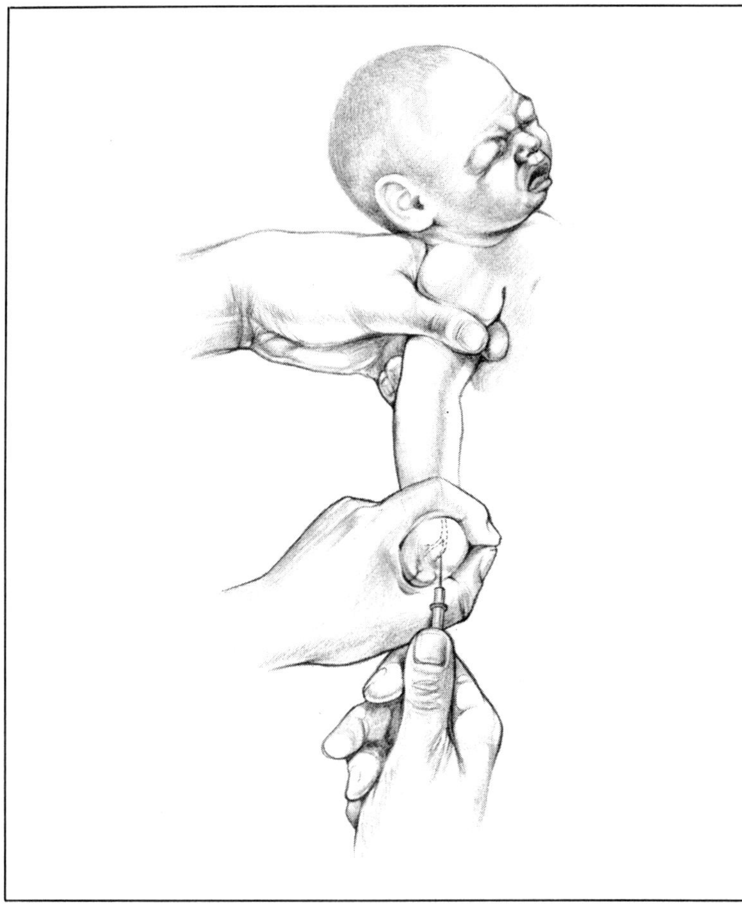

Figure 2-2 Positioning for scalp vein infiltration. Assistant gently immobilizes limbs while rubber band tourniquet is applied around circumference of head. Note that the infant's head is stabilized with the nondominant hand.

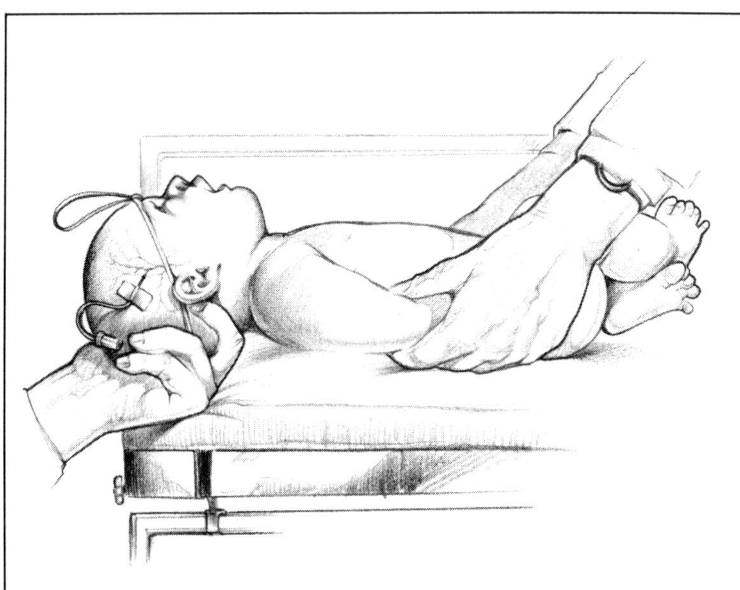

PROCEDURE

1. Locate a vein junction as you would in an adult and prepare the skin with an alcohol pad. Lidocaine HCl (Xylocaine) and other local anesthetics are of little use in the newborn; they only obscure the vein.

2. Prefill the catheter with sterile saline to maximize visualization of blood return when you enter the vein: Blood return is minimal in the low-pressure veins used for cannulation, and trying to tell when an infant's vein is cannulated by the feel of the catheter is difficult. If you use a butterfly, facilitate back flow by removing the tubing plug and leaving it open at a level lower than the point of insertion.

3. With the obturator in the cannula, pierce the skin about 1 cm (3/8 in.) distal to where you plan to pierce the vein for better anchoring of the catheter by the skin. Enter the vein in the direction of venous blood flow and remove the obturator. You don't need to insert the cannula more than 5–10 mm (3/16–3/8 in.) into the lumen of the vein.

4. Once blood return is visible, have your assistant release his tourniquet grasp. If you are using a butterfly, proceed to step 5. If you are using a catheter, slowly advance it 2–3 mm (1/16 in.) while flushing it with saline. As an alternative to flushing, rotate the catheter slightly as you advance it.

5. Test the position of the catheter tip by flushing a small amount of saline into the catheter with a syringe. A subcutaneous bleb at the vein entrance site indicates infiltration: Withdraw and restart the whole procedure at a different site. If no bleb appears, insert the catheter into IV tubing that has been preconnected via a rate-limiting device to a bottle of fluid and prefilled with solution.

6. If you are using a cannula and tubing, secure them as you would in an adult patient. Tape the cannula in position, wrapping 1/2-in. tape around the extremity at the insertion site or, if you are cannulating a scalp vein, crisscrossing strips of tape over the insertion site. Then tape a loop of IV tubing next to the cannula. If you are using a butterfly, place a piece of gauze between wings and skin to maintain the angle of the cannula as inserted, then apply tape over the wings to fix them to the skin. Cover the catheter where it enters the skin with a dressing of antibiotic ointment and gauze. If you cannulated an extremity, secure the arm or leg to the tongue-blade board with double-backed tape to prevent flexion of the joints near the insertion site.

Suggested Readings

Archibald ME: Intravenous technique, in Roberts PW (ed): *Useful Procedures in Medical Practice.* Philadelphia, Lea & Febiger, 1986, pp 547-565.

DeLorimier AA, Harrison MR: Special procedures: Intravenous cannulation, in Pascoe DJ, Grossman M (eds): *Quick Reference to Pediatric Emergencies,* ed 3. Philadelphia, JB Lippincott Co, 1984, pp 560-561.

Hughes WT, Buescher ES: *Pediatric Procedures*, ed 2. Philadelphia, WB Saunders Co, 1980, pp 87-115.

3

Emergency Intraosseous Infusion

Charles E. Driscoll, MD

First developed in the mid-1930s, intraosseous infusion has recently been rediscovered and is recommended for emergency administration of fluids in some cases. The technique is quick and easy to master. Even in darkness, paramedical personnel can perform it as an on-site emergency measure. Complications are minor.

Since bone marrow circulation communicates directly with general circulation, fluids administered into marrow are almost immediately absorbed. The circulation times of intraosseous and IV fluid injections are essentially the same.

With few exceptions, IV access—if possible—is still preferred. In situations when venous access is difficult or contraindicated, however, bone marrow infusion should be considered early in resuscitative efforts as an alternative to waiting for central surgical techniques or more sophisticated interventions.

Among its advantages, bone marrow infusion results in a secure access to the circulation that is difficult for an uncooperative patient to dislodge. The technique is preferred over IV infusion in severely burned patients because the small bone-marrow blood vessels act as a filter to prevent pulmonary emboli resulting from embolization of burned epithelial cells into the central circulation.

Intraosseous infusion has been used for administration of blood transfusions, saline, plasma, glucose, Ringer's lactate, thiopental sodium (Pentothal) 5%, dopamine HCl (Dopastat, Intropin), dobutamine HCl (Dobutrex), and various antibiotics. Nearly any drug administered by IV infusion can be administered by intraosseous infusion.

Indications

- When failure to achieve IV access may be life-threatening in any critically injured child or adult

- As an alternative to IV infusion in patients critically ill with burns, shock, or circulatory collapse

Contraindication

- Underlying infection, bony abnormality, or bone lesion

Materials

- Body or extremity restraints (for small children and uncooperative patients)
- Surgical skin cleanser scrub such as povidone-iodine (Betadine) or chlorhexidine gluconate (Hibiclens)
- Small basin and cotton balls for surgical scrub
- 1% lidocaine HCl (Xylocaine)
- 3-mL syringe with 25-gauge needle for administration of anesthesia
- Sterile rubber gloves
- Sterile towels (if available)
- IV infusion set with drip chamber and tubing
- Adhesive tape for securing intraosseous needle and IV tubing
- 10-mL syringe with 5 mL of sterile normal saline
- No. 11 scalpel blade
- Needles to enter bone marrow: Standard bone marrow needles, special Turkel trephine needles, 18- or 20-gauge short spinal needles, or standard 14-, 16-, or 18-gauge hypodermic needles

Note: Although the trephine bone needle is preferred, it is rarely available in emergencies, so the standard 16- or 18-gauge hypodermic needle is used more often. Since an open-channel needle may become obstructed with bone chips or marrow during introduction, you may have to introduce a second, smaller-gauge hypodermic needle through the lumen of the first needle to clear the obstruction.

PROCEDURE

1. If the patient is uncooperative or is a small child, apply appropriate restraints.

2. Clean the insertion site thoroughly with surgical scrub, and if convenient, drape the site with sterile towels. Wear a sterile rubber glove on the hand with which you palpate for landmarks.

Recommended insertion sites are the tibia and femur. On the tibia, locate the site in the midline on the flat tibial surface approximately 2 finger breadths—2–3 cm (¾–1 in.) below the tibial tuberosity (Figure 3-1). On the femur, locate the site in the inferior third about 3 cm (1 in.) above the external condyle in the anterior midline (Figure 3-2). Less desirable access sites are the iliac crest and the sternum.

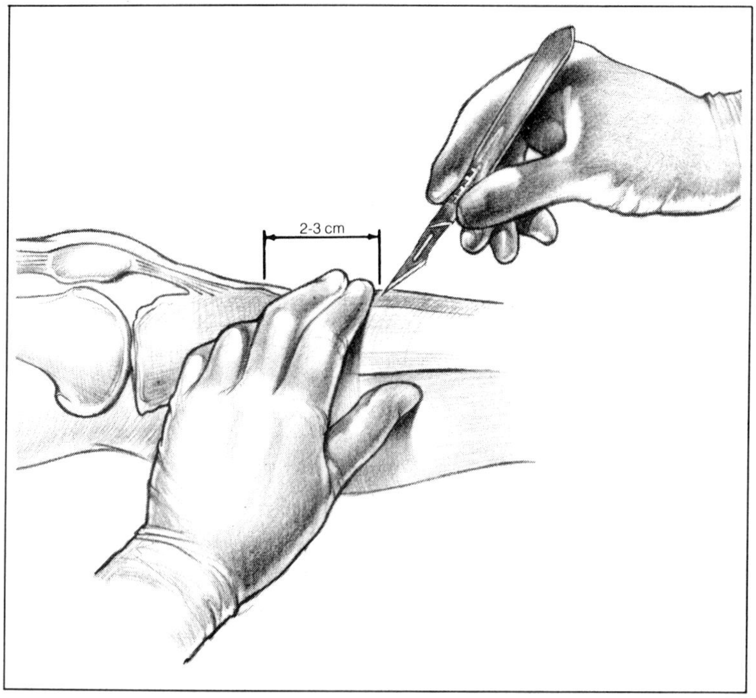

Figure 3-1 Insertion site on tibia. Find the point in the midline ¾–1 inch below the tibial tuberosity.

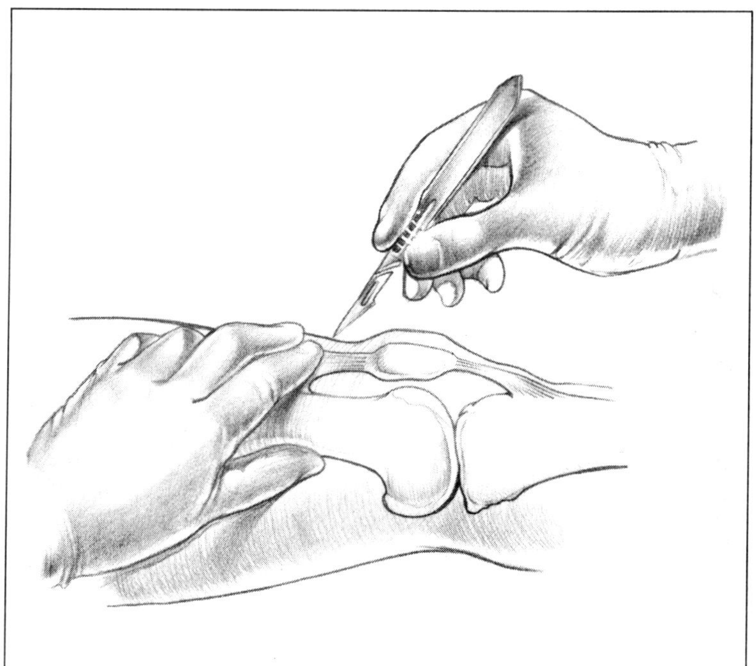

Figure 3-2 On the femur, locate the site in the inferior third, approximately 1 in. above the external condyle in the anterior midline.

3. Anesthetize the insertion site with 1% lidocaine, first raising a wheal in the dermis and then infiltrating the subcutaneous tissues down to and including the periosteum.
4. Make a small nick incision in the skin with a No. 11 blade to facilitate needle insertion.
5. Insert a 16- or 18-gauge hypodermic needle (or, if a trephine needle is available, the outer part of the needle with stylet in place) through the incision and down through the subcutaneous tissue until it meets with bone. In the tibia, direct the needle inferiorly, 45–60 degrees above the skin surface (Figure 3-3); in the femur, direct the needle superiorly at a similar angle (Figure 3-4).
6. Advance the needle into the marrow space as follows:

STANDARD HYPODERMIC NEEDLE Insert the needle well into the medullary cavity. Clean the lumen of the needle by inserting a 14-gauge needle through the larger needle.

TREPHINE BONE NEEDLE Remove the stylet, and introduce an inner trephine needle with its stylet through the outer needle. Turn the trephine needle to and fro in a drilling motion with firm downward pressure until sudden lack of resistance signals entry into the medullary cavity. Further advance the trephine needle until it is well within the medullary cavity.

Advance the outer needle through the hole made by the trephine needle. When the outer needle is firmly lodged in the medullary cavity, withdraw the trephine needle.
7. Attach the syringe containing 5 mL of sterile saline to the needle in the bone. Check to be sure marrow is easily aspirated and sterile saline is easily administered into the medullary cavity without significant subcutaneous infiltration.

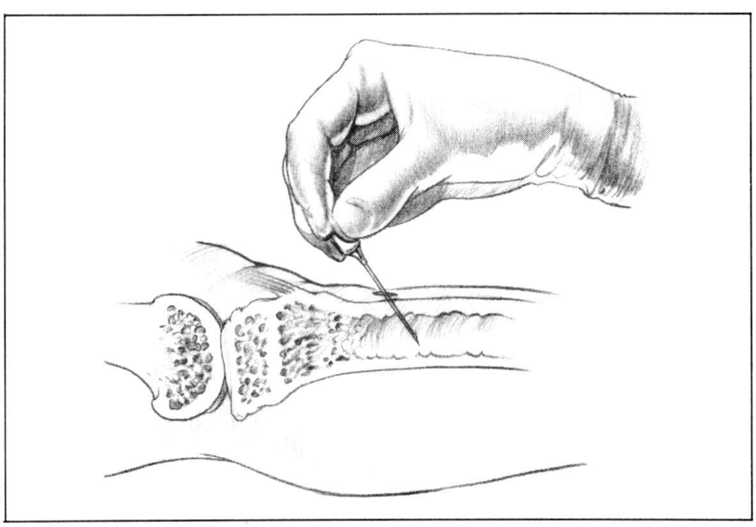

Figure 3-3 Through tibial incision, direct needle inferiorly, 45–60 degrees above the skin surface.

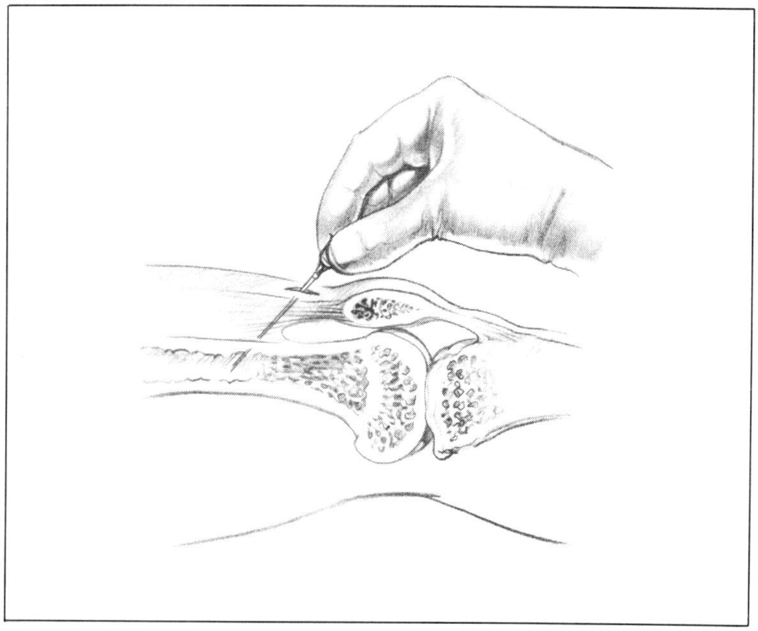

Figure 3-4 In the femur, direct needle superiorly, 45–60 degrees above the skin surface.

Other ways to assess needle placement before intramedullary infusion include noting a sudden give or lack of resistance as the needle passes through the bony cortex and noting that the needle stands erect without support and feels firmly locked into bone.

8. Detach the syringe, connect the IV line, and infuse sterile saline or other solution as desired. Use strips of adhesive tape to secure the needle and IV tubing to the skin.

Follow-up Care

- Use an intramedullary infusion site for as short a time as possible and for no more than 2–3 days at one site.
- When infusion is no longer necessary, withdraw the needle and cover the puncture site with a sterile dressing.
- Observe the puncture site for any indication of local inflammation.

Complications

Minor complications may include the following:

- Local abscess or cellulitis
- Subcutaneous leakage from around the needle
- Osteomyelitis
- Small needle-hole defect in the cortex, which may last for several months
- Sepsis, which can result from improper technique such as failure to observe an aseptic approach, prolonged use of one infusion site, or the infusion of hypertonic solutions

Suggested Readings

Berg RA: Emergency infusion of catecholamines into bone marrow. *Am J Dis Child* 1984;138:810-811.

Hughes WT, Buescher ES: *Pediatric Procedures*, ed 2. Philadelphia, WB Saunders Co, 1980, pp 117-119.

Turkel H: Emergency bone marrow infusions. *Am J Dis Child* 1985;139:438-439.

Turkel H: Emergency infusion through the bone. *Milit Med* 1984;149:349-350.

Turkel H: Intraosseous infusion. *Am J Dis Child* 1983;137:706.

4

Emergency Cannulation of the Femoral Vein

Advantages of the wire-guided catheter

Ronald B. Low, MD

The choice of catheter for central venous cannulation was formerly limited to the catheter-through-needle type. This device required a large-bore needle, and any inadvertent puncture of a structure adjacent to the vein could be serious. The newer wire-guided (Seldinger) catheter technique that is now recommended has important advantages:

- The exploring needle is small and thin-walled, minimizing chances of iatrogenic damage to adjacent structures.
- Most wire-guided catheterization kits now include an insertion wire with one end rounded into a J shape. Before insertion through the needle, this end is straightened, but it reverts to the J shape as the wire exits through the bevel of the needle. The rounded end is far less likely than a straight one to puncture the vein wall opposite the insertion site; it is also more likely to remain in the central circulation and out of small tributary veins as it is advanced toward the heart.
- The technique is adaptable; it can be used to insert a wide variety of intravascular devices.
- Large-bore lines can be inserted rapidly, allowing large volumes of fluid during a resuscitation.

Indications

In emergency situations:

- To provide a portal of entry for monitoring devices such as central venous pressure and Swan-Ganz catheters or for therapeutic devices such as pacemakers.
- To provide venous access when peripheral venous cannulation is inadequate—usually because peripheral veins cannot be cannulated or because an especially large venous cannula is needed to infuse IV fluids rapidly.

In nonemergency situations:
- To infuse particularly irritating cytotoxic agents or hypertonic feeding fluids.

Site Selection

Several sites are available for large-bore IV lines. Some clinicians prefer the subclavian vein because it is anatomically fixed, but the complication rate rises from the risk of pneumothorax and interthoracic bleeding. An alternative site is the internal jugular vein, which has a lower risk of pneumothorax, but this can be difficult to approach during a vigorous resuscitation. Advantages to using the femoral vein, particularly in emergency situations, are these:
- The chance of serious immediate complications is low with the femoral approach because it does not risk puncturing the lungs.
- While significant iatrogenic bleeding from the femoral vein or the adjacent femoral artery is possible, it seldom occurs and can readily be controlled by direct pressure over the vessel. In addition, hematoma development in this area is obvious, whereas bleeding from the subclavian or internal jugular vein may enter the chest and be invisible.
- While cannulating the femoral vein, you can easily remain out of the way of other medical personnel simultaneously treating the patient.
- This approach is particularly good if there are extensive upper body injuries that may have damaged blood vessels preventing adequate return or resuscitation fluids to the heart.

Risks

Although the femoral vein approach in general has lower risks than subclavian or internal jugular vein approaches, it is commonly done in an emergency situation and therefore has an increased rate of complications from this fact alone.
- The risk of bleeding exists from arterial puncture, coagulopathy, or a tear in the vein.
- Femoral lines have an increased rate of infection and should be removed as soon as possible to avoid risks of a line infection, particularly if put in during an emergency situation.
- If a femoral line is to be left in place, it is much harder to stabilize if the leg moves in the area of insertion.
- Particular care must be taken to avoid shearing of the guidewire or losing control of the guidewire, either of which would lead to a distal embolization.

Materials

For skin preparation

- Povidone-iodine solution (Betadine) or another antiseptic skin cleanser
- Sponges
- Drape
- Gloves
- Mask
- 5 mL 1% lidocaine HCl (Xylocaine HCl)
- 5-mL syringe with 25-gauge, ⅝-in. needle

For venipuncture

- Central vein catheterization kit with a wire-guided (Seldinger) catheter.[1] The kit should include the following components:
- An 18-gauge, 2½-in. thin-walled introducer needle
- A J wire (spring wire guide with straight tip on one end, J tip on opposite end, 0.89 mm diameter × 45 cm
- A J-wire straightener
- Dilator
- Indwelling catheter or sheath (usually 8.5 French for an adult)
- Syringes
- Needles
- Scalpel
- Suture material
- Sterile dressings
- Drapes
- Lidocaine HCl (Xylocaine HCl)

PROCEDURE

Technique

1. Check to make certain the lines for infusion are set up and flushed.
2. After donning mask and gloves, prepare and drape the area of insertion. Using a 5-mL syringe and ⅝-in. needle, inject lidocaine HCl at a point one finger width (1 cm) medial to the femoral pulse and usually about two finger widths (2–3 cm) below the inguinal crease.
3. Attach the thin-walled introducer needle to a 3-mL syringe, and insert it at the same point at 45 degrees to the skin surface, aiming it toward the umbilicus. Aspirate as you advance the needle; when you

[1]Note: Variations in kit design and equipment can dictate modifications in technique. The method described here can be altered to suit available equipment.

see dark blood in the syringe, you know you have entered the vein (Figure 4-1).

4. Straighten the J tip of the wire with the straightener. Disengage the syringe from the needle, leaving the needle in the vein. Insert the J wire through the needle, and advance it toward the heart. If you encounter resistance, rotate the wire and try again. Should resistance continue after a few tries, remove the needle then the wire (in that order) and start over. Do *not* pull the wire back through the needle; the J tip may shear off and cause an embolus. When you have advanced the wire several centimeters, stop. Enough wire should be in the vein to stabilize the catheter while enough should be left at the insertion site to allow you to thread on the dilator and catheter and to get a firm grasp on the end of the wire.

5. Withdraw the needle, leaving the wire in the vein (Figure 4-2). Do not at any time release your hold on the wire.

6. Make a small nick with a scalpel at the insertion site to facilitate insertion of the dilator.

7. Grasping the wire and the dilator firmly, thread the dilator over the wire, and advance it 20 cm (8 inches), or more if you desire, into the vein using a rotating motion. Hold the far end of the wire in place.

8. Withdraw the dilator, and place it inside the indwelling catheter or sheath. Grasp the wire and the indwelling catheter firmly. Thread the catheter and dilator over the wire back into the vein to the extent desired (Figure 4-3). Twirl the catheter or sheath slightly during insertion to facilitate entry.

9. Withdraw the wire and the dilator. If you don't see a free flow of blood from the catheter hub, attach a syringe and aspirate until good

Figure 4-1

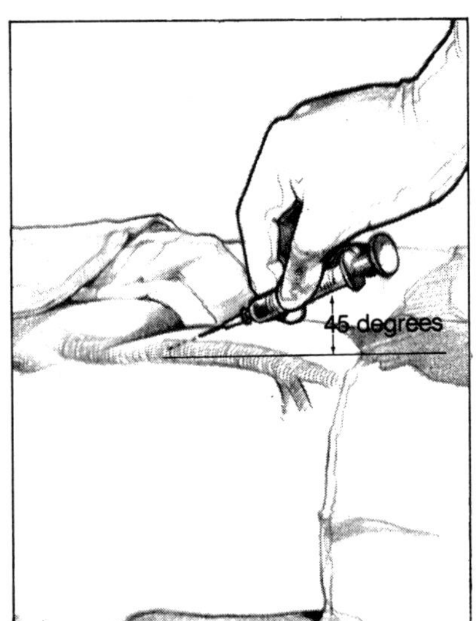

Figure 4-2

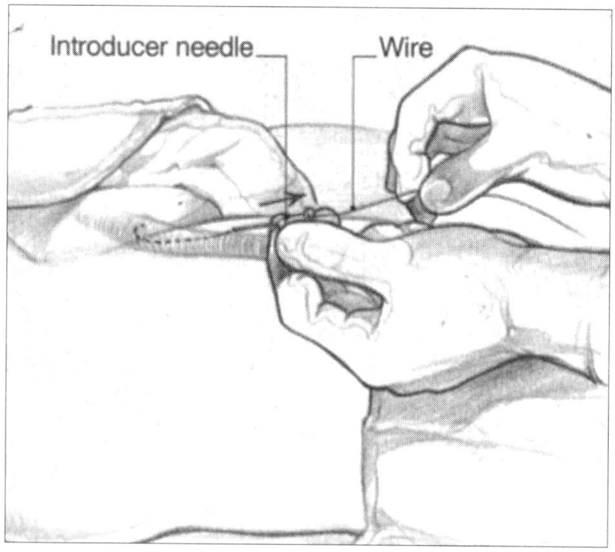

Figure 4-3

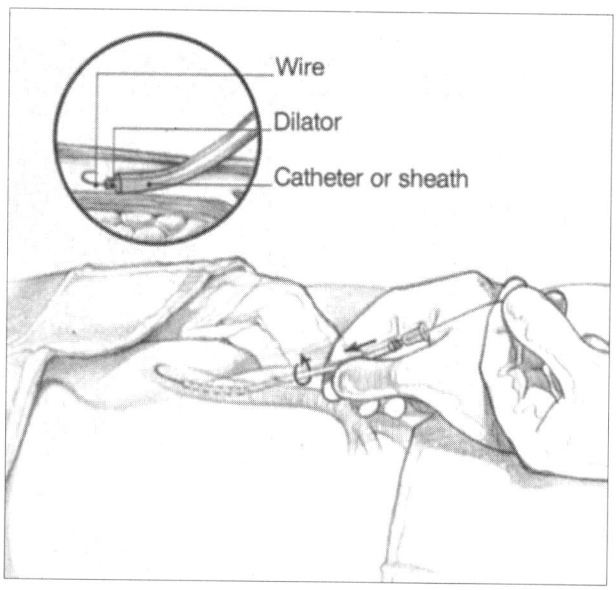

blood flow is established. Remember, excessive negative pressure can collapse the vein and prevent blood flow.

10. Once all the air is removed from the line, attach the catheter to the appropriate device or line.

11. Suture the catheter in place by placing a suture through the skin and through the opening or ring on the catheter hub. Remember, now is not the time to puncture the catheter with the suture.

12. Apply antibiotic ointment and a sterile dressing to the insertion site. Tape well.

Suggested Readings

American College of Surgeons: *Advanced Trauma Life Support Course*. Chicago, American College of Surgeons, 1988.

Gilston A: Letter: Cannulation of the femoral vessels. *Br J Anaesth* 1976;48:500-501.

Rosen M, Latto IP, Ng WS: *Handbook of Percutaneous Central Venous Catheterisation*. London, WB Saunders Co, 1981, pp 121-129.

5

Cardiopulmonary Resuscitation in Adults

Gayle Roggeveen Nelson, RN
Charles E. Driscoll, MD

These instructions are based on the assumption that you are the only person present who is qualified to deliver cardiopulmonary resuscitation (CPR) and that emergency medical facilities are not immediately available. If a qualified assistant is present, you can use this method with one person attending to ventilation and the other to chest compression (see Table 6-1, p. 34).

Note: In two-person CPR, the ratio of compressions to ventilations should be 5:1 rather than 15:1 as recommended in step 9 of the procedure.

PROCEDURE

1. Establish unresponsiveness by noting the absence of breathing, the absence of a carotid pulse for at least 5–10 seconds, and the resultant deathlike pallor.

   Note: If you find respiratory arrest without cardiac arrest, follow steps 2–5, and then ventilate once every five seconds.
2. Call for help immediately and have someone summon the nearest emergency medical service.

   Note: Do not delay beginning CPR to telephone for help. If no one else is immediately available, administer no more than one minute of CPR before leaving the victim to call for help. Rapid application of advanced life support procedures (specifically defibrillation) is critical to survival of out-of-hospital cardiac arrest.
3. Position the victim on a firm surface, moving him or her with care if you suspect a cervical spine injury.
4. Place one hand on the forehead, and with the other hand, grasp the bony prominence of the chin and lift to open the airway (Figure 5-1). The airway is likely to be blocked by the tongue when the uncon-

Figure 5-1 Position the victim on a firm surface. Place one hand on the forehead and with the other hand, grasp the bony prominence of the chin and lift to open airway.

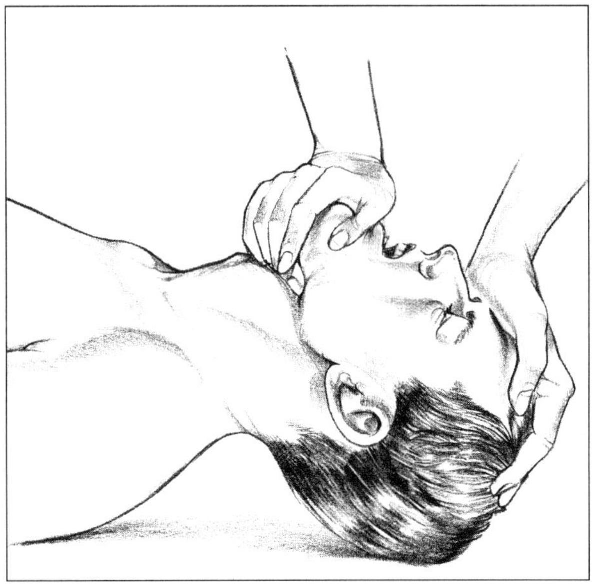

Figure 5-2 Check for absence of breathing by feeling for air movement. If you find no breath response, immediately begin mouth-to-mouth resuscitation.

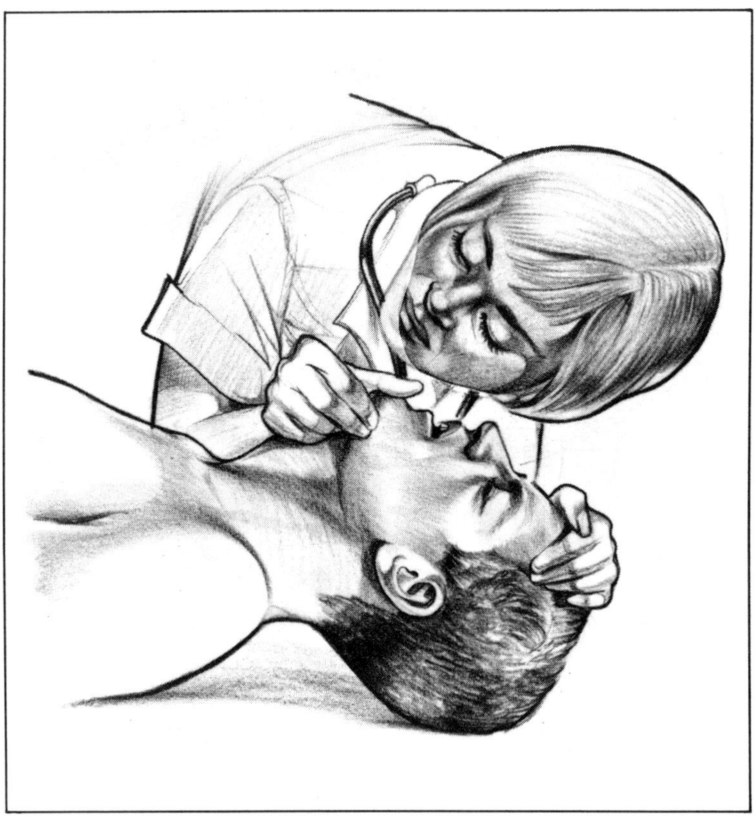

scious person is supine. Check again for breathlessness by watching chest movement and feeling for air movement (Figure 5-2).

Note: Avoid this maneuver if you suspect cervical spine injury. Open the airway by placing the fingers at the angles of the jaw and anteriorly displacing the mandible, keeping the neck in a neutral position.

5. If you find no breath response, immediately begin mouth-to-mouth resuscitation. Pinch the victim's nostrils closed with the thumb and forefinger as your hand rests on his forehead, and seal your mouth firmly over his (Figure 5-3). Blow air into his mouth, and watch for responsive chest movement. Listen for escaping air during exhalation as a further sign of lung responsiveness. Transmit two slow, full breaths allowing for lung deflation (1½ seconds each). If you do not see or feel results from your ventilatory efforts, reposition the head and neck and reventilate. If necessary begin obstructed airway procedures if a foreign body is present.

Note: Use mouth-to-nose ventilation when you cannot open the patient's mouth, when the mouth has been traumatized, or when edentia prevents you from keeping a tight mouth-to-mouth seal. Hold the mouth closed as you ventilate mouth-to-nose.

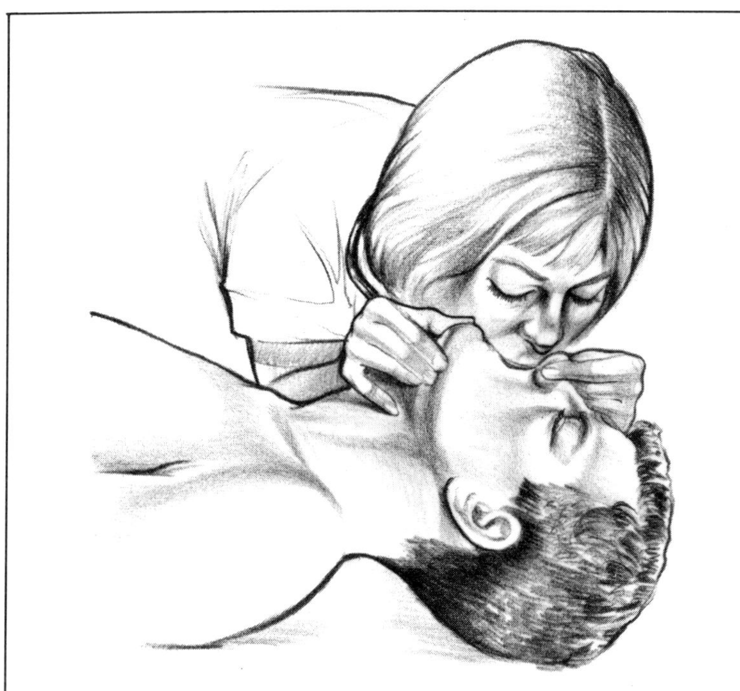

Figure 5-3 Pinch the victim's nostrils closed with thumb and forefinger and seal your mouth firmly over his. Transmit two slow, full breaths and allow for full lung deflation.

6. After initiating rescue breathing and carotid pulse check, begin external cardiac compression. Kneel or stand at the patient's side, locate the lower margin of the rib cage, and identify the xiphoid process.

7. Place the heel of one hand—the one closer to the victim's head—on the long axis of the sternum about two finger widths cephalad from the xiphisternal notch. Place your other hand on top of the first so that the fingers are parallel (Figure 5-4). Make sure only the heel of the bottom hand touches the chest.

8. Straighten your elbows and position your shoulders directly over your hands for more efficient application of force. Depress the sternum, and release the pressure completely without removing your hands. Aim for depressions of 4–5 cm (1½–2 in.) in an adult of average size. Repeat rhythmically and smoothly for a total of 15 compression-release cycles, trying to deliver the compressions at a rate of 80–100/min, so that the series of 15 takes from 8–12 seconds.

9. After the series of 15 compressions, pause to deliver two full ventilations in 4–7 seconds allowing the patient to partially exhale between breaths. Together, the 15 compressions and two ventilations should take from 12–19 seconds. Repeat the cycle of 15 compressions and two ventilations at least four times initially before stopping to check for spontaneous pulse and respirations. Thereafter pulse and respiration should be checked every 3–5 minutes.

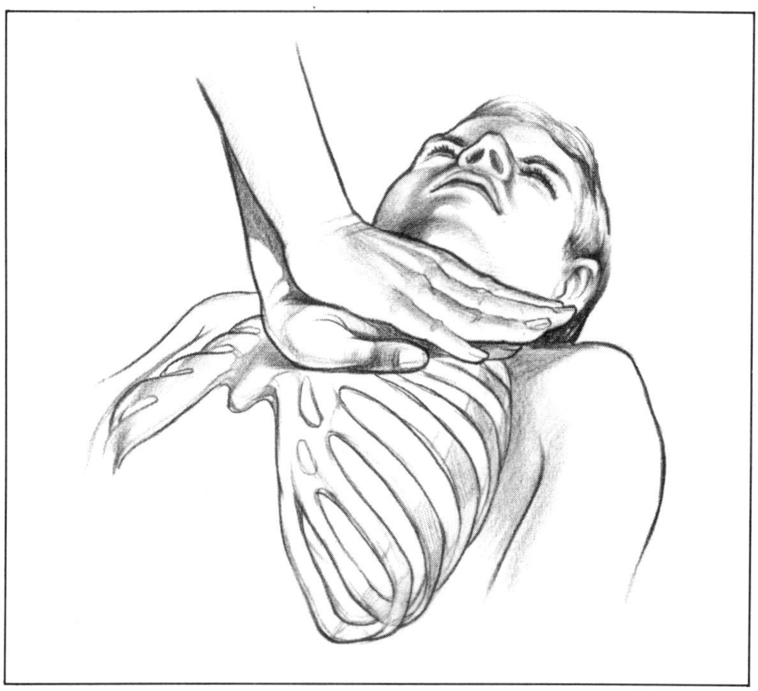

Figure 5-4 Place the heel of one hand on the long axis of the sternum approximately two finger widths cephalad from the xiphisternal notch. Place the other hand on top of the first so fingers are parallel.

Note: Do not interrupt CPR for more than a few seconds, except to institute endotracheal intubation or to transport the victim. In either case, allow no more than 30 seconds' interruption.

10. Continue CPR until emergency personnel and equipment for advanced life support take over or you pronounce the patient dead. Cardiovascular unresponsiveness is generally a more reliable basis for terminating CPR than the ominous signs of cerebral death. Continue CPR for longer periods in special cases, such as patients who are hypothermic; recovery has been achieved after long periods of unconsciousness in such patients.

Even with skillfully performed CPR, complications may occur, including rib fractures, pneumothorax, hemothorax, gastric distention, and lung contusions. Do not allow concern about possible complications to interfere with prompt administration of CPR.

Suggested Readings

Lampier TA: *Guidelines for Medical and Surgical Emergencies.* New York, Masson Publishing USA, 1983, pp 234-245.

Mills J, Ho MT, Trunkey DD: *Current Emergency Diagnosis and Treatment.* California, Lange Medical Publications, 1983, pp 1-22.

Safar P: *Cardiopulmonary Cerebral Resuscitation.* Philadelphia, WB Saunders Co, 1981.

Schwartz G, Safar P, Stone J, et al: The pathology of dying and reanimation, in *Principles and Practices of Emergency Medicine.* Philadelphia, WB Saunders Co, 1985.

Standards and Guidelines for Cardiopulmonary Resuscitation (CPR) and Emergency Cardiac Care (ECC). *JAMA* 1986;255:2915.

Wilkens E, Dineen J, Moncure A, et al: Cardiopulmonary resuscitation, in *MGH Textbook of Emergency Medicine.* Baltimore, Williams & Wilkins Co, 1983, pp 25-39.

6

Cardiopulmonary Resuscitation in Infants and Children

Gayle Roggeveen Nelson, RN

Basic cardiopulmonary resuscitation (CPR) techniques in infants and children younger than 8 years are similar to those for adults; those for children older than 8 years are identical (Table 6-1).

PROCEDURE

1. Determine the child's state of consciousness and ventilatory status. Note the absence of breathing, the absence of a carotid pulse (the brachial pulse in infants), and the resultant deathlike pallor.

Note: If you find respiratory arrest without cardiac arrest, follow steps 2–5, and then ventilate once every four seconds for a child or three seconds for an infant.

2. Call for help immediately and have someone summon the nearest emergency medical service.

Note: Do not delay calling for help. If no one else is immediately available, administer no more than one minute of CPR before leaving the victim to call for help. Rapid application of advanced life support procedures (specifically defibrillation) is critical to survival of out-of-hospital cardiac arrest.

3. Place the child on his or her back on a firm surface. If you suspect a cervical spine injury, move him or her with special care; and do not let the head roll, twist, or tilt backward or forward.

4. Open the airway.

- If there is any sign of neck injury, the safest way to open the airway is to move the lower jaw forward without tilting the head. Rest your elbows on the surface the child is lying on, and place two or

TABLE 6-1:

<table>
<tr><th colspan="5">CPR for Adults, Children, and Infants</th></tr>
<tr><th rowspan="2"></th><th rowspan="2">Objectives</th><th colspan="3">Actions</th></tr>
<tr><th>Adult (over 8 yr)</th><th>Child (1–8 yr)</th><th>Infant (under 1 yr)</th></tr>
<tr><td rowspan="5">A.
Airway</td><td rowspan="2">1. Assessment: Determine unresponsiveness.</td><td colspan="3">Tap or gently shake shoulder.</td></tr>
<tr><td colspan="2">Say, "Are you okay?"</td><td>Observe.</td></tr>
<tr><td>2. Get help.</td><td colspan="3">Call out "Help!"</td></tr>
<tr><td>3. Position the victim.</td><td colspan="3">Turn on back as a unit, supporting head and neck if necessary (4–10 sec).</td></tr>
<tr><td>4. Open the airway.</td><td colspan="3">Head-tilt/chin-lift (see Figure 5-1).</td></tr>
<tr><td rowspan="11">B.
Breathing</td><td>5. Assessment: Determine breathlessness.</td><td colspan="3">Maintain open airway. Place ear over mouth, observing chest. Look, listen, feel for breathing (3–5 sec).</td></tr>
<tr><td rowspan="3">6. Give 2 rescue breaths (see Figure 5-2).</td><td colspan="3">Maintain open airway.</td></tr>
<tr><td colspan="2">Seal mouth to mouth.</td><td>Mouth to nose/mouth.</td></tr>
<tr><td colspan="3">Give 2 rescue breaths, 1–1½ sec each. Observe chest rise. Allow lung deflation between breaths.</td></tr>
<tr><td rowspan="6">7. Option for obstructed airway.</td><td colspan="3">(a) Reposition victim's head. Try again to give rescue breaths.</td></tr>
<tr><td colspan="3">(b) Activate the EMS system (eg, dial 911).</td></tr>
<tr><td colspan="2" rowspan="2">(c) Give 6–10 subdiaphragmatic abdominal thrusts.</td><td>Give 4 back blows.</td></tr>
<tr><td>Give 4 chest thrusts.</td></tr>
<tr><td>(d) Tongue-jaw lift and finger sweep.</td><td colspan="2">Tongue-jaw lift, but finger sweep only if you see a foreign object.</td></tr>
<tr><td colspan="3">If unsuccessful, repeat steps (a), (c), and (d) until successful.</td></tr>
<tr><td rowspan="6">C.
Circulation</td><td>8. Assessment: Determine pulselessness.</td><td colspan="2">Feel for carotid pulse with one hand; maintain head-tilt with the other (5–10 sec).</td><td>Feel for brachial pulse; keep head-tilt.</td></tr>
<tr><td>9. Activate EMS system.</td><td colspan="3">If someone responded to call for help, send them to activate the EMS system.</td></tr>
<tr><td>Begin chest compressions:
10. Landmark check.</td><td colspan="2">Run middle finger along bottom edge of rib cage to notch at center (tip of sternum).</td><td>Imagine a line drawn between the nipples.</td></tr>
<tr><td rowspan="2">11. Hand position (see Figure 5-3).</td><td colspan="2">Place index finger next to finger on notch,.</td><td rowspan="2">Place 2–3 fingers on sternum, 1 finger's width below line. Depress ½–1 inch.</td></tr>
<tr><td>Two hands next to index finger. Depress 1½–2 inches.</td><td>Heel of one hand next to index finger. Depress 1–1½ inches.</td></tr>
<tr><td>12. Compression rate.</td><td colspan="2">80–100/min.</td><td>At least 100/min.</td></tr>
<tr><td rowspan="4">CPR cycles</td><td>13. Breath/compression ratio.</td><td>2 breaths to every 15 compressions.</td><td colspan="2">1 breath to every 5 compressions.</td></tr>
<tr><td>14. Number of cycles.</td><td>4 (52–73 sec).</td><td>10 (60–87 sec).</td><td>10 (45 sec or less).</td></tr>
<tr><td rowspan="2">15. Reassessment.</td><td colspan="2">Feel for carotid pulse (5 sec).</td><td>Feel for brachial pulse.</td></tr>
<tr><td>If no pulse, resume CPR, starting with 2 breaths.</td><td colspan="2">If no pulse, resume CPR, starting with 1 breath.</td></tr>
<tr><td rowspan="4">Option for entrance of 2nd rescuer</td><td>1st rescuer ends CPR.</td><td>End cycle with 2 rescue breaths.</td><td colspan="2">End cycle with 1 rescue breath.</td></tr>
<tr><td>2nd rescuer checks pulse.</td><td colspan="2">Feel for carotid pulse.</td><td>Feel for brachial pulse.</td></tr>
<tr><td>If no pulse, 2nd rescuer begins CPR.</td><td>Begin one-rescuer CPR, starting with 2 breaths.</td><td colspan="2">Begin one-rescuer CPR, starting with 1 breath.</td></tr>
<tr><td>1st rescuer monitors 2nd rescuer.</td><td colspan="3">Watch for chest rise and fall during rescue breathing, check pulse during chest compressions.</td></tr>
<tr><td>When pulse returns</td><td>If no breathing, give rescue breaths.</td><td>1 breath every 5 sec.</td><td>1 breath every 4 sec.</td><td>1 breath every 3 sec.</td></tr>
</table>

three fingers under each side of his jaw, just beneath the ears, and lift upward (Figure 6-1).

- If there is no sign of neck injury, place one hand on his forehead, and hook the fingers, not the thumb, of the other hand, under the bony prominence of the chin. Lift the chin gently while pressing down on the forehead, and tilt the head back, taking care not to close the mouth (Figure 6-2). The airway may be blocked by the tongue, so check again for breathlessness by watching chest movement and feeling for air movement.

Figure 6-1

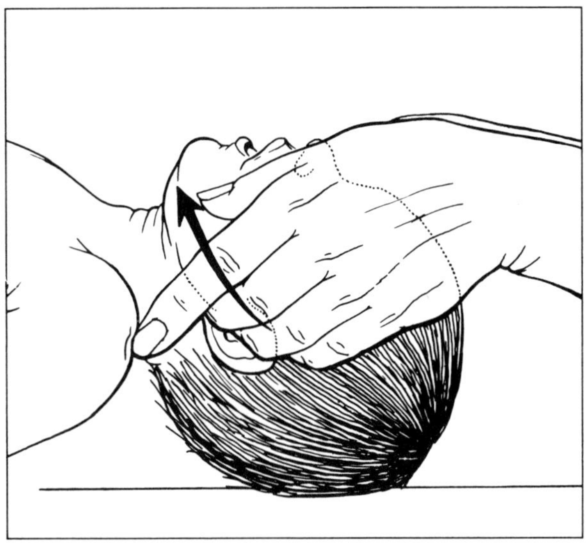

Figure 6-2

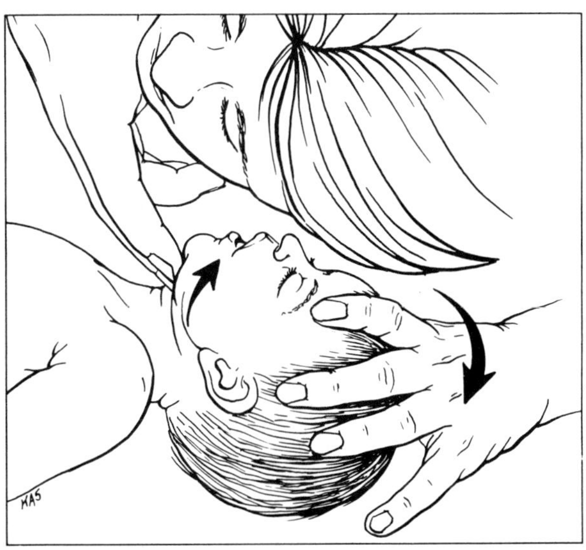

5. If the child is not breathing, immediately start mouth-to-mouth or mouth-to-nose resuscitation.

- For an infant, cover the mouth and nose with your mouth (Figure 6-3). Do not pinch the nostrils. Be sure your lips make a tight seal, and support the tip of his chin with your finger. Air will not reach the lungs without this support. Blow just enough air into the infant's mouth and nose to make his chest rise. Too much ventilatory pressure can cause gastric distension or pneumothorax. Breathe slowly to give enough air at the lowest possible pressure. Give two slow breaths between 1 and 1½ seconds per breath.
- For an older child, pinch his nostrils closed with the thumb and forefinger of your hand resting on his forehead. Take a breath, and seal your mouth firmly over his (Figure 6-4). Blow air into his mouth, and watch for responsive chest movement. Listen for escaping air during exhalation as a further sign of lung responsiveness. Blow two slow, full breaths allowing for lung deflation (1½ seconds each). If you do not see or feel results from your ventilatory efforts, reposition the head and neck and reventilate. If necessary begin obstructed airway procedures if a foreign body is present.

6. After initiating rescue breathing and checking the pulse, start external cardiac compression. Kneel at the patient's side, and locate the inferior margin of the rib cage.

- In an infant, imagine a line drawn between the nipples, and place 2–3 fingers on the sternum, one finger's width below the line (Figure 6-5). Depress ½–1 inch at least 100 times per minute.
- In a child younger than 8 years, locate the tip of the sternum by running your middle finger along the lower part of the rib cage to

Figure 6-3

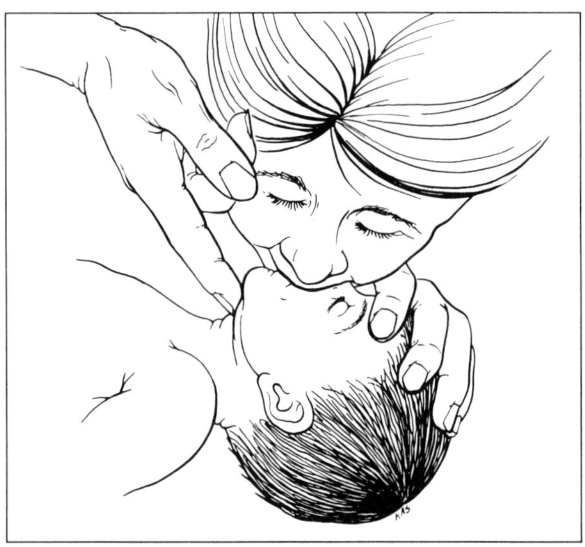

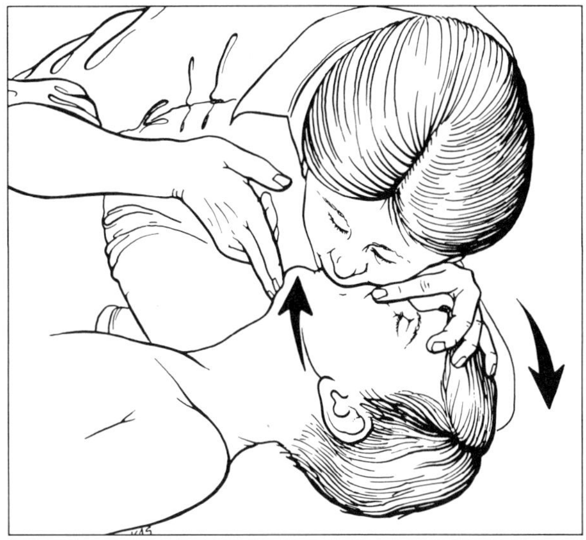

Figure 6-4

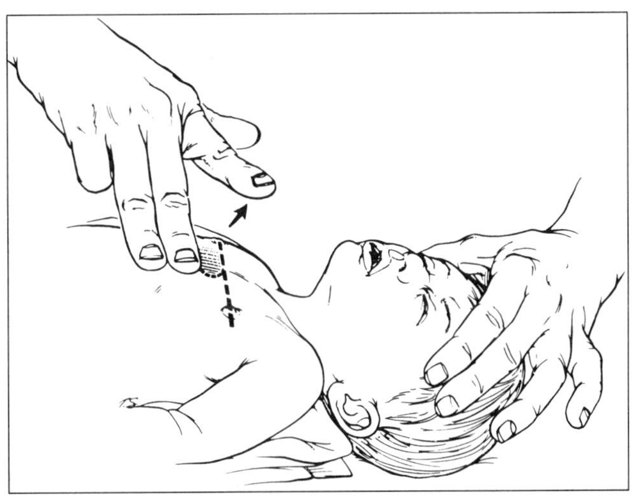

Figure 6-5 Locating the correct position for the fingers in chest compressions in the infant. (Reproduced with permission of the American Heart Association.)

the notch, and position the heel of the same hand next to the previous location of the index finger, and depress 1–1½ inches about 80–100 times per minute (Figure 6-6). You may maintain head position with your other hand on the child's forehead. This facilitates rapid movement between ventilation and compression.

- In older children, use the same technique as for adults (see "Cardiopulmonary Resuscitation in Adults," page 27). Place the heel of one hand—the one closer to the victim's head—on the long axis of the sternum about two finger widths cephalad from the xiphisternal notch. Place your other hand on top of the first so that the fingers are parallel, making sure only the heel of the bottom hand

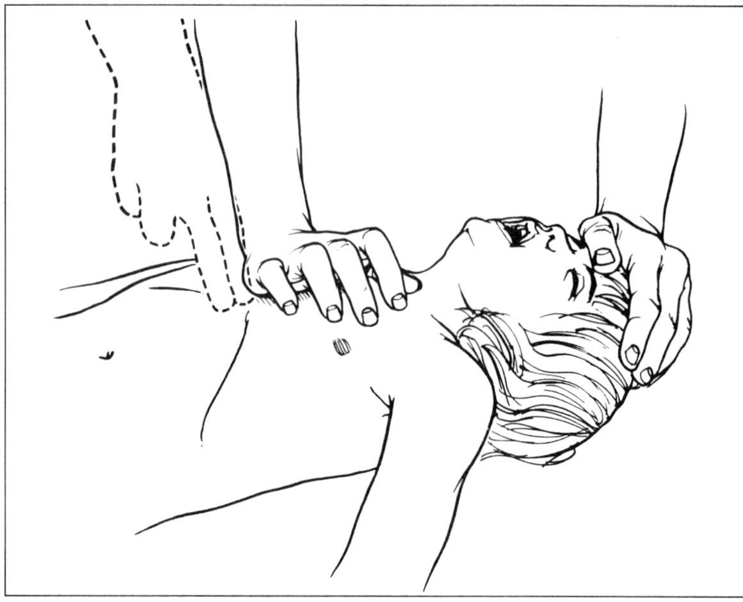

Figure 6-6 Locating the correct position for the hand in chest compressions in the child. (Reproduced with permission of the American Heart Association.)

touches the chest. Depress the sternum about 1½–2 inches, and release the pressure completely without removing your hands. Do this at a rate of 80–100 per minute.

7. Repeat the chest compressions rhythmically and smoothly.

- In infants and children younger than 8 years, perform five compression-release cycles, and stop to deliver a full breath. Repeat this cycle at least 10 times before stopping to check for spontaneous pulse and respirations. In infants, this would take 45 seconds; in children, 60–90 seconds.
- In children older than 8 years, perform 15 compression-release cycles, and stop to deliver two full ventilations allowing the patient to partially exhale between breaths. Together, the 15 compressions and two ventilations should take from 12–19 seconds. Repeat the cycle of 15 compressions and two ventilations at least four times initially before stopping to check for spontaneous pulse and respirations. Thereafter pulse and respiration should be checked every 3–5 minutes.

Note: Do not interrupt CPR for more than a few seconds, except to institute endotracheal intubation or to transport the victim. In either case, allow no more than 30 seconds' interruption.

10. Continue CPR until emergency personnel and equipment for advanced life support take over or you pronounce the patient dead.

Suggested Readings

Chameides L (ed): *Textbook of Pediatric Advanced Life Support.* Dallas, Texas, American Heart Association, 1988.

Heartsaver Manual. Dallas, Texas, American Heart Association, 1987.

Standards and Guidelines for Cardiopulmonary Resuscitation (CPR) and Emergency Cardiac Care (ECC). Part IV: Pediatric Basic Life Support. *JAMA* 1986;255:2954-2960.

Supplement to the Instructor's Manual for Advanced Cardiac Life Support. Dallas, Texas, American Heart Association, 1988.

7

Managing Airway Obstruction in Children

Gayle Roggeveen Nelson, RN

More than 90% of pediatric deaths from foreign body aspiration occur in children younger than 5 years, and 65% are in infants. Suspect the problem whenever infants and children experience acute respiratory distress associated with coughing, gagging, or stridor.

Controversy continues over the safest method to expel a foreign body from a child's airway, but the American Academy of Pediatrics currently recommends that abdominal thrusts are preferred in children older than 1 year while back blows can be used in infants.

PROCEDURE

FOR A CHILD OLDER THAN 1 YEAR

1. If another person is nearby, ask him or her to call for emergency medical help.
2. Place the child on his or her back, straddle his hips (for a larger child) or kneel at his feet (for a smaller one), and place the heel of one hand on the midline of his abdomen just above the umbilicus and below the rib cage.
3. With the other hand on top of the first, push rapidly inward and upward in 6–10 abdominal thrusts (the modified Heimlich maneuver) until the foreign body is expelled (Figure 7-1). Care must be taken to keep the thrusts in the midline and not to either side and to use gentler pressure in younger children.
4. In an older, larger child (usually older than 4 years) who is conscious, use the Heimlich maneuver with the child sitting or standing (Figure 7-2).
5. Wrap your arms around the child's waist with one hand made into a fist and the thumb side of the fist resting against his abdomen in the midline slightly above the navel and below the xiphoid process.

Figure 7-1

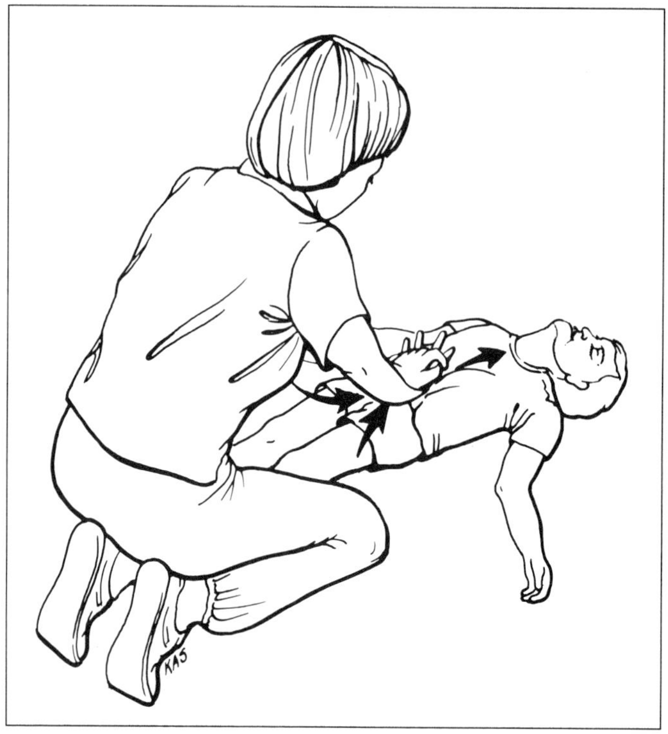

Figure 7-2

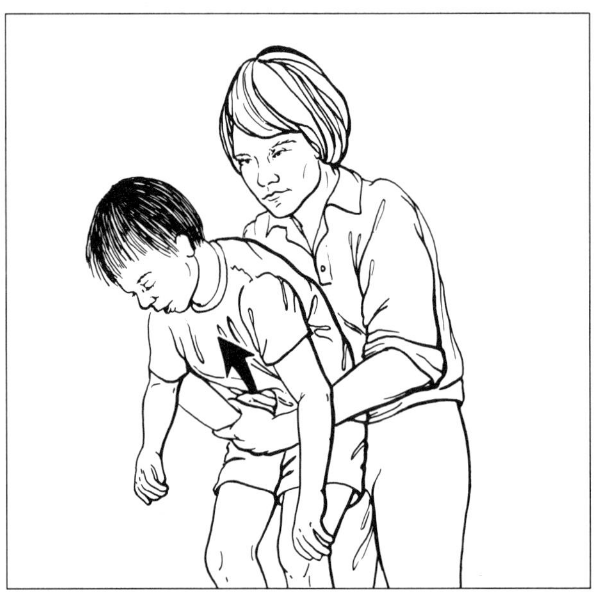

6. Grasp the fist with the other hand, and use quick upward thrusts, never touching the xiphoid process or lower margins of the rib cage to avoid injury to internal organs. Each thrust should be a separate, distinct movement.
7. If the airway is still obstructed, open the child's mouth by holding the tongue and lower teeth with your thumb and the lower jaw with your fingers. Pull the jaw up in a tongue-jaw lift (Figure 7-3). This should pull the tongue away from the back of the throat and may loosen the obstruction.
8. If you can see the object, try to remove it with a finger sweep.
Warning: Blind finger sweeps may push a foreign body farther into the airway and are to be avoided in infants and children.
9. If the child is not breathing on his own, start mouth-to-mouth resuscitation, and continue as necessary.

FOR AN INFANT YOUNGER THAN 1 YEAR

1. Place the infant on your forearm, face down with his head lower than his trunk. Stabilize the head and neck by resting your forearm against your thigh for support (Figure 7-4).
2. Using the heel of your hand, deliver four rapid blows to the infant's back high between the scapulas.
3. If the obstruction is not dislodged, compress the chest as follows:
- Turn the infant, and place on a firm surface or your thighs if more convenient, keeping his head lower than his trunk.

Figure 7-3

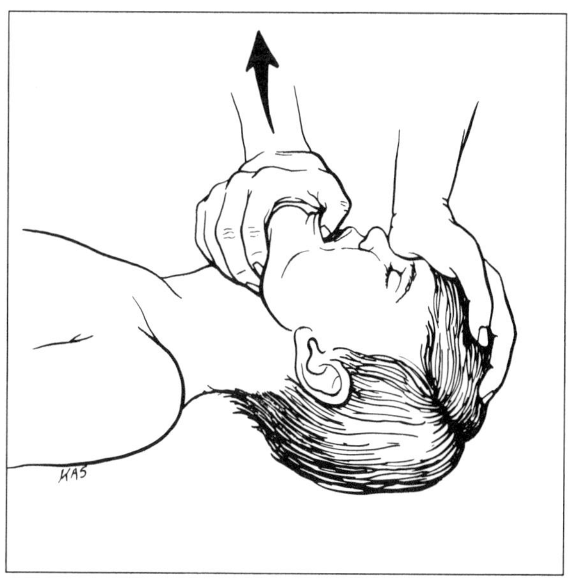

Figure 7-4

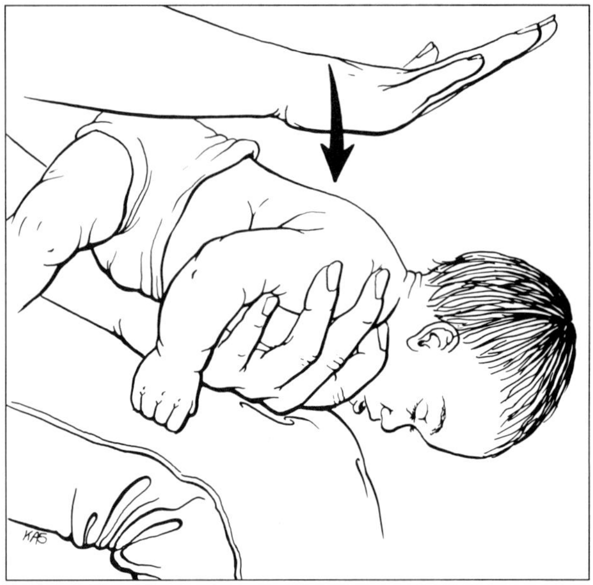

- Place your index finger on the infant's nipple line, and use the middle and ring fingers to deliver four rapid thrusts to the chest.

4. If the baby still is not breathing, look into his mouth, remove any foreign body that can be seen, and try to ventilate by mouth-to-mouth-nose resuscitation.

5. Continue ventilation efforts as necessary.

Suggested Readings

Chameides L (ed): *Textbook of Pediatric Advanced Life Support.* Dallas, Texas, American Heart Association, 1988.

Committee on Accident and Poison Prevention, American Academy of Pediatrics. Revised first aid for the choking child. *Pediatr* 1986;78:177-178.

Standards and Guidelines for Cardiopulmonary Resuscitation (CPR) and Emergency Cardiac Care (ECC). Part IV: Pediatric Basic Life Support. *JAMA* 1986;255:2954-2960.

Supplement to the Instructor's Manual for Advanced Cardiac Life Support. Dallas, Texas, American Heart Association, 1988.

8

Internal Jugular Vein Catheterization

Ralph Knudson, MD
Gayle Roggeveen Nelson, RN

The medical management of nearly all emergency conditions requires establishing reliable IV access to administer drugs and fluids. Cannulation of a large central vein provides the most versatility and stability; for this procedure, the American Heart Association recommends the internal jugular vein. Cannulation of the internal jugular vein does not require visualization of the vessel, so quick access to central circulation is possible even if peripheral veins are collapsed. But because the internal jugular vein is so close to the carotid and subclavian arteries, the lungs, and the lymphatic ducts and nerves, the risk of damage to these structures is high if the procedure is performed incorrectly. The rate of complications is also higher than for peripheral vein cannulation.

Indications

- To supply reliable access to the central venous system for administering drugs and fluids
- To insert emergency cardiac pacemaker and monitoring catheters (for example, Swan-Ganz)

Contraindications

- Acute infection at the site of venipuncture

Relative Contraindications

Inability to visualize landmarks for any of the following reasons:
- Trauma to the neck
- Hematoma

- Subcutaneous emphysema
- Scarring
- Gross obesity

Materials

- Needle at least 6 cm long with a 16-gauge catheter at least 15–20 cm long. If the catheter is inserted through the needle, a 14-gauge needle is required.
- Syringe to attach to the needle as the vein is being located
- IV solution and administration set to attach as soon as the IV line is placed
- Local anesthesia for alert patients (1% lidocaine HCl [Xylocaine HCl]) or normal saline, 5-mL syringe, 25-gauge 1-in. needle
- Suture to secure catheter after placement
- Povidone-iodine dressing (Betadine antiseptic gauze pads) and adhesive tape
- Sterile drapes, gloves, mask
- Surgical skin cleanser scrub (Betadine, Hibiclens)

Preparation

Place the patient in a 15–30 degree head-down position to distend the vein and decrease the chance of an air embolus to the cerebral circulation. Work on the right side of the neck because the pleura and dome of the right lung are lower than those of the left, the right atrium is more accessible, and the thoracic duct is not endangered.

The internal jugular vein emerges from the base of the skull, enters the carotid sheath posterior to the internal carotid artery, and lies posterior and lateral to the internal and common carotid artery. Near its termination, the internal jugular vein is lateral and somewhat anterior to the common carotid artery. Posterior, central, or anterior approaches to the jugular can be used. The method described here is the central approach, which is easiest to learn and use.

PROCEDURE

To position the catheter correctly, determine the depth of placement by measuring from the point of insertion to the manubrial-sternal junction; this places the catheter at the level of the superior vena cava. Measure 5 cm below that for insertion into the right atrium of the heart. If fluid resuscitation is your major goal, place the catheter in the vena cava above the right atrium.

1. Cleanse the area and prepare with sterile drape. Wear sterile gloves, face mask, and hair cover if possible.

2. If the patient is alert, infiltrate the area with local anesthetic.

3. Palpate the carotid artery, and turn the patient's head to the opposite side of insertion.

4. Insert the needle at the apex of the triangle found by palpating the clavicular (lateral) and sternal (medial) attachments of the sternocleidomastoid muscle (Figure 8-1). Direct the needle lateral to the carotid pulsation and at a 30-degree angle to the horizontal plane; aim toward the ipsilateral nipple.

5. Slowly advance the needle, maintaining slight negative pressure on the syringe until you obtain a blood return (Figure 8-2). Rapid backward movement of the plunger with the appearance of bright red blood obviously indicates arterial puncture. If this occurs, remove the needle, and apply pressure to the puncture site for at least 10 minutes.

Note: In the event of arterial puncture, do not attempt internal jugular vein cannulation again on either side. This precaution is necessary to avoid a bilateral hematoma that would compromise the patient's airway.

Figure 8-1 Insert needle at apex of the triangle found by palpating the lateral and medial attachments of the sternocleidomastoid muscle.

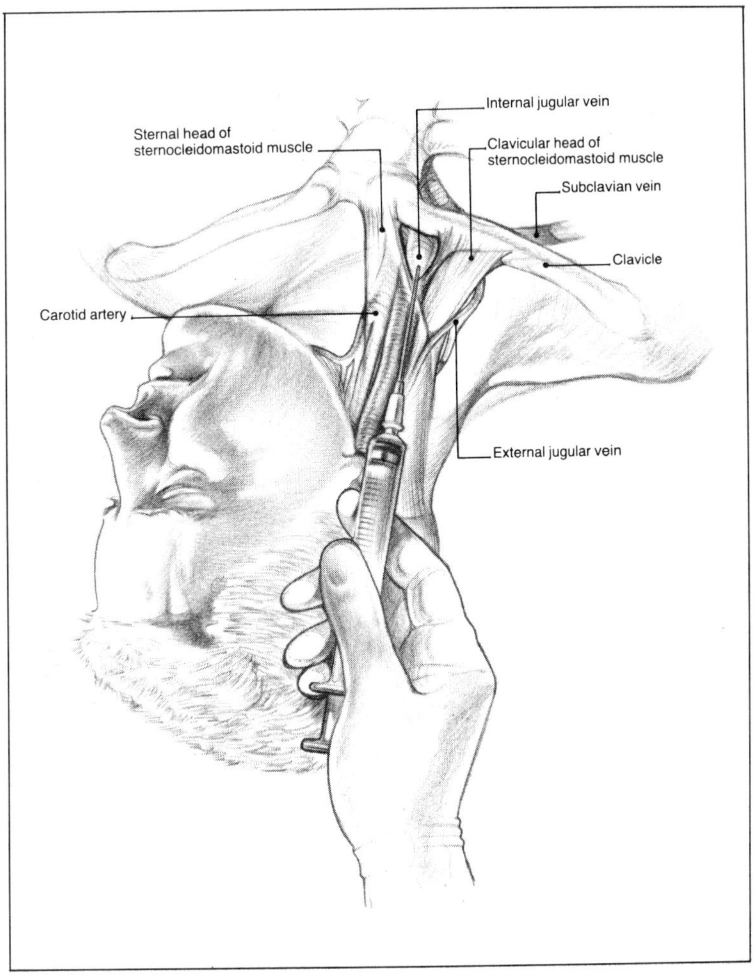

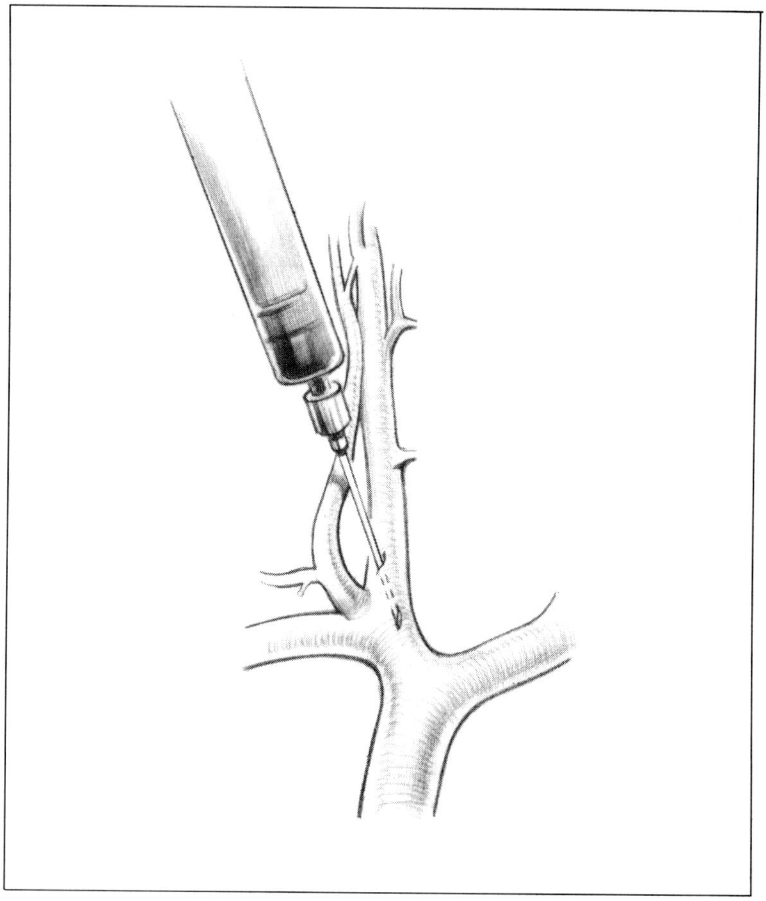

Figure 8-2 Slowly advance needle while maintaining slight negative pressure on syringe until you obtain blood return.

6. Remove the syringe from the hub of the needle, and with gloved finger quickly occlude the needle to prevent air embolization. If the patient is alert, you may have him hold his breath.
7. Insert the catheter through the needle until it reaches at least the superior vena cava (Figure 8-3).

Note: If the catheter does not thread easily, remove the entire needle and catheter as a unit to prevent the catheter's shearing and forming a fragment embolus.
8. Affix the catheter to the skin with suture, being careful not to occlude the lumen of the catheter, and attach IV tubing. You may apply a povidone-iodine dressing and tape the catheter IV-line assembly to the skin.

Complications

- Hematoma
- Air embolus
- Pneumothorax

Figure 8-3 Insert catheter through the needle at least to the depth of the superior vena cava.

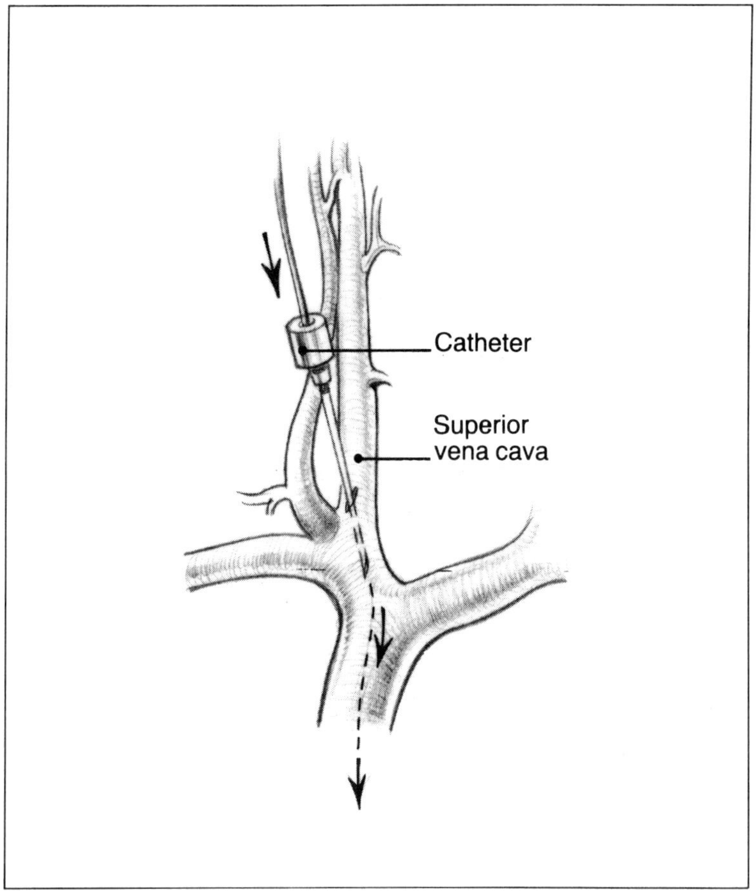

- Perforation of the right atrium
- Puncture of the lung

Follow-up Care

- A chest X-ray is recommended as soon as possible after completing the procedure to check for proper positioning of the catheter tip, absence of pneumothorax, and inadvertent puncture of the lung.

Suggested Readings

Textbook of Advanced Cardiac Life Support. Dallas, American Heart Association, 1983, pp 157-161.

Schwartz GR: *Principles and Practice of Emergency Medicine*, ed 2. Philadelphia, Saunders, 1986, vol 1, pp 430-431.

Standards and guidelines for cardiopulmonary resuscitation (CPR) and emergency cardiac care (ECC). *JAMA* 1986;255:2905-2989.

Wilkins EW: *MGH Textbook of Emergency Medicine*, ed 2. Baltimore, Williams & Wilkins, 1983, pp 926-927.

9

Emergency Defibrillation and Cardioversion

Gayle Roggeveen Nelson, RN

Electrical defibrillation, generally without drug therapy or endotracheal intubation, is the most effective method of terminating ventricular fibrillation (VF). Nevertheless, its success depends largely on how quickly it is initiated after onset of VF. The longer the heart is in VF, the greater the metabolic deterioration and the less likely survival.

In general, defibrillating a patient within a 6–8 minute window following onset of VF dramatically improves the survival rate. With immediate defibrillation—as in patients with implanted defibrillators—survival rates are 95% or better. Other factors influencing the success of defibrillation include reduction of transthoracic resistance, paddle size and position, and the amount of current delivered.

Transthoracic resistance is an important consideration because greater resistance means less current delivered. Several factors influence this resistance: delivered energy, electrode size and position, paddle-skin interface, number and timing of shocks, paddle pressure, phase of ventilation, and distance between paddles.

Some of these factors are under the operator's control; others are not. Energy-dependent resistance and paddle size are seldom under your control when using the defibrillator, but they are important to understand if you are responsible for purchasing the instrument. An electrode with a 13-cm diameter is the optimal size for adults. As for the paddle-skin interface, resistance is very high if bare metal electrodes are placed on the chest. Using electrode paste creates the lowest resistance, but some packaged defibrillator pads are also acceptable.

Previous countershocks lower transthoracic resistance. Firm pressure of about 25 pounds against the chest wall improves conduction, assures good skin contact, compresses the chest, and lessens the distance between the paddles. Remember, too, that resistance is at a minimum at full ventilatory expiration.

Paddle placement can be crucial. For adequate depolarization, the electrical current must pass through a critical mass of fibrillating myocardium (Figure 9-1). Standard paddle placement is anterolateral—one paddle to the right of the upper sternum under the right clavicle and the other left of the nipple in the midaxillary line over the apex of the heart (Figure 9-2). An alternative is anterior-posterior placement, with one paddle placed anteriorly over the precordium and the other placed behind the heart; this technique may be more difficult to use in an emergency because it necessitates turning the patient to position the posterior electrode.

VF is uncommon in children and rare in infants. Cardiac arrest in this age group is usually secondary to respiratory arrest, so pay particularly careful attention to correcting hypoxia and acidosis while supporting circulation by chest compression. If VF is present, use an energy level of 1 J/lb (2 J/kg), with electrode size guided by chest size.

Figure 9-1

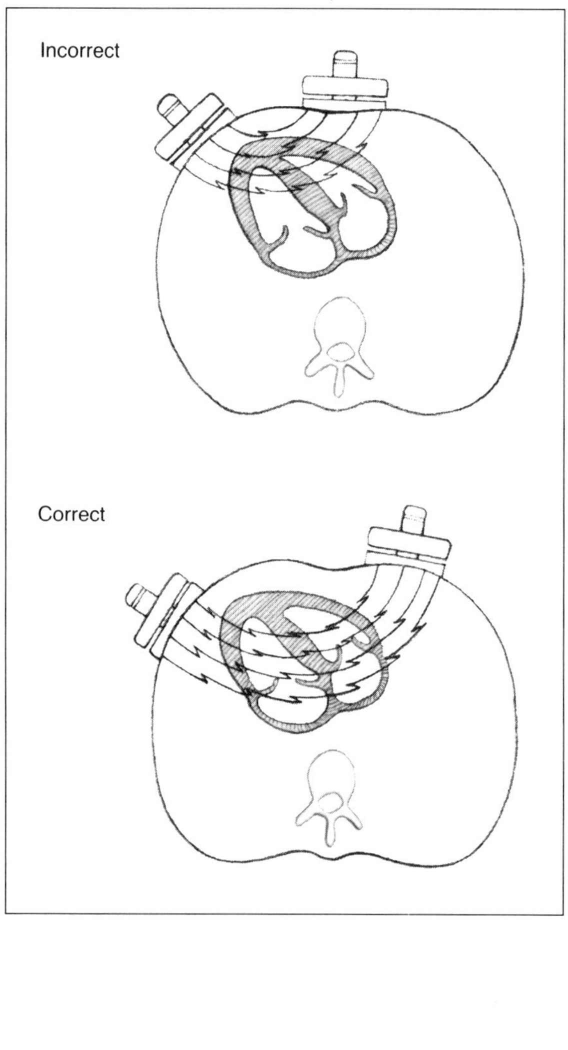

Figure 9-2

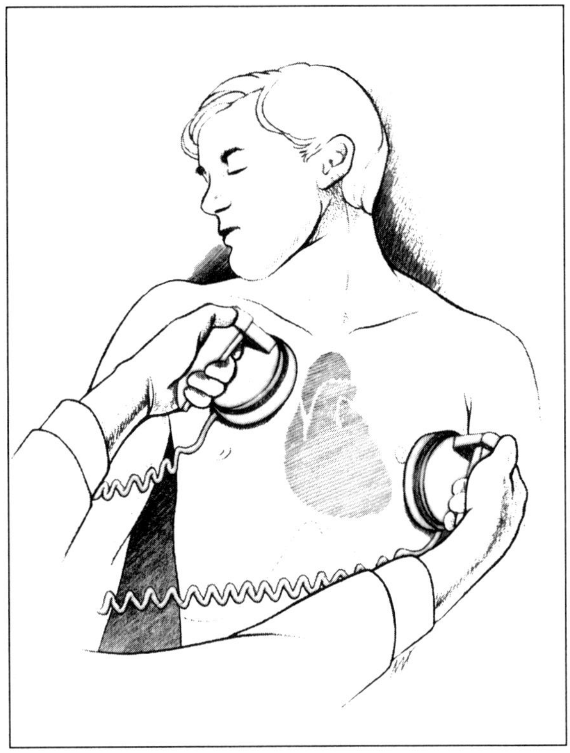

Indications

- Ventricular fibrillation
- Ventricular tachycardia without a pulse

Relative Contraindication

- Digitalized patient

Equipment

- Defibrillator (most are direct current; some are alternating current)
- Conductive medium

PROCEDURE

DEFIBRILLATION TECHNIQUE

1. Determine pulselessness, and verify VF on the monitor.
2. Turn on the defibrillator.

3. Apply conductive material to paddles as necessary.
4. Select the appropriate energy level, and charge the defibrillator.

Note: The American Heart Association recommends 200 J for the initial countershock in an adult. If that is unsuccessful, try the second at 200–300 J. If VF persists, deliver the third and subsequent shocks at up to 360 J. If the first or second shock is successful and the patient refibrillates, return to the energy level responsible for the successful conversion.

5. Place electrodes in the anterolateral position on the chest: one to the right of the upper sternum under the right clavicle, one left of the nipple in the midaxillary line over the apex of the heart (Figure 9-2).
6. For best conduction, apply about 25 pounds of firm pressure, being careful not to lean on the paddles and make them slip.
7. Clear the area, and announce loudly that you will defibrillate the patient on the count of three: "One" (check to be sure everyone is clear), "Two" (reverify the rhythm on the monitor), "Three" (check to make sure *you* are clear).
8. Deliver the countershock by simultaneously depressing the buttons on both paddles.
9. Check the patient's pulse and rhythm.

Note: Pulse is the most reliable indicator of patient status; if it is present, VF cannot be. If the monitor continues to show VF or asystole and you find a pulse, suspect that a loose electrode is causing the artifact.

URGENT SYNCHRONIZED CARDIOVERSION Electrical cardioversion is the treatment of choice for hemodynamically unstable tachydysrhythmias, ventricular or supraventricular. If the patient is pulseless, use the same technique as for VF. Generally, emergency synchronized cardioversion is used for rhythms that have not responded to drugs or vagal maneuvers. The synchronizing circuit makes it possible to deliver current during a "programmed" phase of the QRS complex on the ECG. The procedure is essentially the same as for defibrillation with these exceptions:

1. Since the patient is conscious, administer anesthesia or analgesia; diazepam (Valium) in a 5–10 mg IV bolus (injected slowly over one to two minutes) will suffice.
2. Activate the synchronizer circuit.
3. Adjust energy levels according to the dysrhythmia:

- Atrial fibrillations: 200 J initially, then 360 J
- Paroxysmal supraventricular tachycardia: 75–100 J
- Atrial flutter or ventricular tachycardia: 50 J initially, then 100, 200, up to 360 J if necessary.

Follow-up Care

- If VF occurs before or after emergency cardioversion, immediately turn off the synchronizer circuit, and defibrillate the patient.
- After defibrillation, continue monitoring and assessing cardiopulmonary status.

Suggested Readings

Ewy GA: Electrical therapy of cardiovascular emergencies. *Circulation* 1986;74(6 pt 2):IV 111-IV 116.

Stults KR, Brown DD, Schug VL, et al: Prehospital defibrillation performed by emergency medical technicians in rural communities. *N Engl J Med* 1984;310:219-223.

Textbook of Advanced Cardiac Life Support. Dallas, American Heart Association, 1987.

Weaver WD, Copass MK, Bufi D, et al: Improved neurologic recovery and survival after early defibrillation. *Circulation* 1984;69:943-948.

10

Exercise Treadmill Testing

Richard C. Dobyns, MD

Stress testing, once the almost exclusive province of cardiologists, has become a standard diagnostic procedure for many family practitioners. Major reasons for this are the continued high prevalence of coronary artery disease and the benefits of screening for early disease. For practitioners interested in formal training in exercise testing, several family practice residency programs now offer it, as the American Academy of Family Physicians usually does at its annual convention.

Potential morbidity and mortality of cardiac disease require a thorough assessment of all patients with multiple cardiac risk factors, complaints consistent with cardiac disease, or both. This often includes stress testing to help decide whether or not a patient should be referred.

Note: Costs of an exercise testing system vary by the degree of sophistication. In general, the treadmill costs from $2,000 to $5,000; the computer and software, from $3,000 to $15,000. Possible additional costs: cardiac resuscitation equipment, if not already available on-site, about $10,000; service contracts after the first-year warranty expires, an average of $1,800 per year. Most practices can recover the capital costs of exercise testing in 1–3 years.

Indications

- *Chest pain* Angina or equivalent symptoms are classic indications for exercise testing. Symptoms not typical for angina require testing when associated with coronary heart disease risk factors.
- *Known ischemic heart disease* Patients with known coronary artery disease require periodic reevaluation that includes exercise testing. Among them are

1. Patients with stable angina controlled by medications. Annual stress testing helps confirm the stability.

2. Patients who have had a myocardial infarction (MI). Timing of submaximal exercise testing varies, but generally all uncomplicated MI patients undergo testing 2–3 weeks after the event. A positive test result is associated with a 5–15% chance of reinfarction in the first year; a negative result, with a 2% risk. Maximal exercise testing 6–8 weeks after the event may provide additional prognostic information.

3. Patients with coronary bypass surgery or percutaneous transluminal coronary angioplasty. Periodic reevaluation of cardiac status is beneficial. Exercise testing can detect early signs of restenosis.

- *Exercise-related palpitations* Although Holter monitoring remains the standard of care, dysrhythmias provoked by exercise should be evaluated under comparable conditions. In addition, ventricular ectopy noted incidentally on resting ECG can be safely evaluated with submaximal exercise testing. Elimination of unifocal ectopy during exercise strongly suggests a benign process.
- *Silent ischemia* There are no firm indications on how to manage these patients, but the condition undoubtedly represents a good deal of cardiac disease in this country. Because the rate of false-positive results in exercise testing in men is approximately 30%, the testing should be limited to patients with a reasonable chance of developing coronary atheroma. To determine chances of a patient having silent ischemia, note these direct risk factors: male gender; hypercholesterolemia; age greater than 55; a family history of early cardiac disease; and a history of glucose intolerance, diabetes, hypertension, or smoking.

If you find more than four direct risk factors, use exercise testing to screen for silent ischemia. Remember, in half of all patients who go on to have coronary artery disease, the first symptom is MI or sudden cardiac death. This justifies at least screening for silent ischemia and prescribing appropriate health modifications.

- *Exercise prescription* In addition to diagnostic uses, exercise testing is indicated for assessment of functional capacity. Any patient older than 55 or younger patients with known cardiorespiratory ailments should be tested before undergoing a physical conditioning program, including entrance in cardiac rehabilitation programs.
- *Stimulation for behavior changes* Although exercise testing should not be done in patients who have no risk factors, it can be a powerful stimulus for behavior change in resistant patients.
- *Hypertension* Patients with suspected "white coat hypertension" can be unmasked under exercise testing. In true hypertensive patients, diastolic blood pressure will not change during exercise. In those with falsely elevated blood pressure, diastolic pressure initially falls at the beginning of the exercise, suggesting that these patients might benefit from exercise for blood pressure control but do not require antihypertensive medications.

Absolute Contraindications

- Unstable chest pain (acute MI or pericarditis)
- Unstable angina (progressive or crescendo)

- Rapid atrial dysrhythmias
- Second- or third-degree atrioventricular block
- Systemic illness (infection, hyperthyroidism, anemia)
- Inability to ambulate due to disease or deformity

Relative Contraindications

- Left ventricular outflow obstruction (aortic stenosis, idiopathic hypertrophic subaortic stenosis)
- Severe hypertension
- Severe ST-segment depression at rest
- Congestive heart failure

Exercise Protocols

- Bruce (modified and regular)
- Balke
- Ellestad
- Sheffield
- Astrand
- Naughton
- Kattus

These exercise protocols correlate total exercise time with total metabolic expenditure. For example, after nine minutes on the Bruce protocol the exercising patient has expended 10 metabolic energy equivalents ([METs]; 1 MET represents oxygen consumption at rest, or about 3.5 mL of oxygen per kilogram of body weight per minute).

The family practice department at the University of Iowa Hospitals routinely uses the regular Bruce protocol for a diagnostic test, changing treadmill speed and incline every three minutes to reach maximum heart rate within 10 minutes. Less conditioned patients, however, require more warm-up time, and for them the department employs the Balke and modified Bruce protocols, exercising the patients more gradually. The Naughton and Kattus protocols are generally used for patients who require a significantly reduced stress test, such as those who are post-MI or have significant cardiorespiratory compromise. Patients who are about to enter a phased cardiac rehabilitation program and need functional determinations often receive the Naughton or Kattus protocol. The protocol programmed into your exercise system depends on the manufacturer.

Materials and Personnel

TREADMILL The control console and any computer device are usually sold separately from the treadmill itself, which contains the motors that drive the tread and regulate the incline. Less expensive systems combine treadmill and controls in one unit. Railings are also available.

CONTROL AND COMPUTER CONSOLE Although additional features increase the cost, the preferred system is one that gives the clearest tracing of subtle waveform changes. This can be a system that computes an average of previous beats to eliminate any artifact, a valuable feature for less experienced physicians. Some users feel that other features such as ST slope and ST heart rate/slope computations augment the predictive value of stress testing.

RESUSCITATION EQUIPMENT Every exercise testing laboratory should have a complete crash cart with defibrillator and oxygen.

ASSISTANTS A registered nurse with some training in exercise testing or a registered cardiopulmonary technician should be available. He or she should be annually recertified in basic life support and preferably in advanced cardiac life support (ACLS) as well.

Note: Serious cardiac complications occur with exercise testing in fewer than one in 10,000 patients, but having a currently ACLS-certified physician in charge is recommended.

Patient Preparation

- Informed consent is mandatory.
- Have the patient wear loose-fitting clothing and comfortable walking shoes. Women should wear a comfortable bra.
- Ideally, exercise testing should be done on an empty stomach. Insist on no more than a very light meal two hours or longer before testing.
- Testing is better done early in the morning, when older patients are less likely to be fatigued. Recent studies have also shown an increased likelihood of ischemia during the late morning hours.
- Patients can generally continue their medications, but some cardiac drugs can affect the test interpretation. Among those that can cause false-positive results are digoxin (Lanoxin) and diuretics (due to decreased potassium). Among the drugs than can cause false-negative results are beta-blockers, diltiazem HCl (Cardizem), verapamil HCl (Calan, Isoptin), and vasodilators (although short-acting agents have little effect). To eliminate these effects, digoxin would have to be stopped 10 days before the exercise test; diuretics and beta-blockers; 3–5 days; verapamil and diltiazem, 2 days; and vasodilators, one day.

PROCEDURE

1. Place the 10 electrodes (Figure 10-1). Prepare the skin by shaving the areas and cleaning with alcohol. Abrade the skin with a commercial abrasive agent or gauze pad for good conductivity.

2. Explain the procedure, and warn the patient to alert you immediately if he tires quickly so you can safely stop the treadmill. Tell the patient that blood pressure will be taken at regular intervals and that the speed and incline of the treadmill will increase.

3. Before starting the test, take ECGs with the patient standing and supine using the proper electrode placement for a resting test. You may want to include an ECG with the patient hyperventilating, to detect ST-segment changes due solely to that condition, which will cause a false-positive result.

4. With the appropriate protocol in mind, start the treadmill, and have the patient straddle the moving tread. Tell him to gauge the speed by placing one foot on the tread.

5. Have the patient place both feet on the tread and start to walk. He should not grasp the railing with his hands, but rather rest his fore-

Figure 10-1

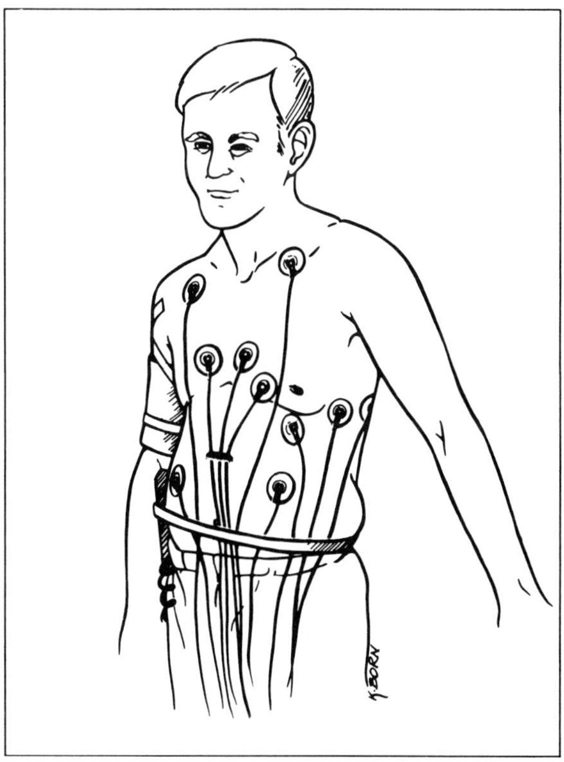

arms or wrists on it. Take blood pressure readings every minute or so, making sure the arm is hanging over the side of the railing (Figure 10-2).

6. Ask the patient to tell you if he experiences any symptoms that would warrant stopping the test, including chest pain, other angina-equivalent pain (in the neck or arm), palpitations, light-headedness, musculoskeletal pain, or fatigue.

Note: Fatigue is best measured by the Borg Scale of Perceived Exertion. It uses a scale of one to 20 and is available from cardiac rehabilitation laboratories or the American Heart Association.

7. If you are testing for diagnosis of coronary artery disease, exercise the patient to 85% of his estimated heart rate. Many patients are able to go beyond this rate, so the 85% is not an absolute limit. If the patient's limit is significantly lower than 85%, the test can be interpreted as submaximal.

8. Terminate the test for any of these reasons:

- Couplets or ventricular tachycardia
- Supraventricular tachycardia or new atrial fibrillation
- Onset of second- or third-degree heart block
- Progressive angina
- ST-segment depression greater than 6 mm
- Progressively dropping blood pressure
- Fatigue, dyspnea, or musculoskeletal pain beyond the patient's tolerance

Figure 10-2

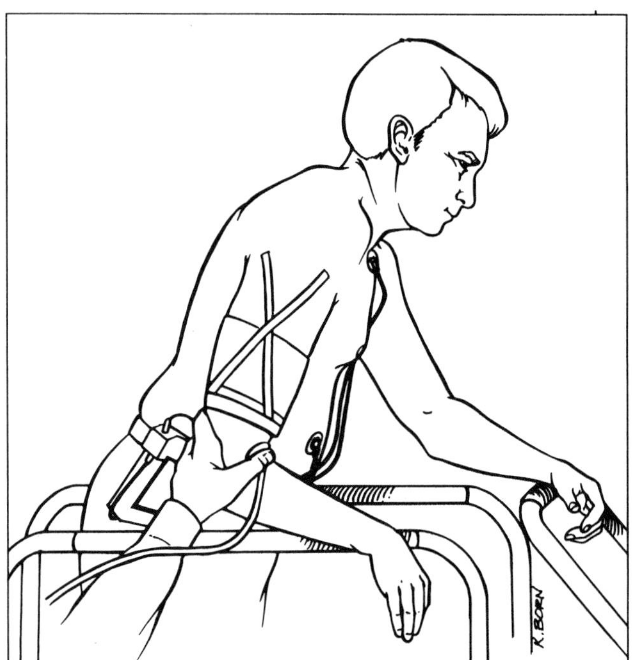

- A clammy or vasoconstricted appearance in the patient
- The patient's reaching or exceeding the maximum predicted heart rate

9. Recovery takes 10 minutes after exercise stops. Let the patient slow down gradually while you take a final standing blood pressure, then have him sit in a reclining chair with his legs elevated to increase venous return. This increases the heart work load and heightens the sensitivity of the test. Have oxygen at hand in case it is needed.

10. Monitor heart tracings continuously for 10 minutes, or longer if complications arise. If you note worrisome ECG changes, be sure the patient returns to resting levels before you discontinue monitoring.

Follow-up Care

- Have the patient avoid showering for several hours after stress testing to avoid temperature fluctuations that might induce syncope.
- If the patient chooses to shower, recommend lukewarm water.
- Advise no further exercise for the day; the testing is a substantial workout.
- Remind the patient to call you if cardiac-related symptoms occur after the test.

Suggested Readings

American College of Sports Medicine: *Guidelines for Exercise Testing and Prescription*. Philadelphia, Lea & Febiger, 1986.

Buring RE: Choosing an in-office treadmill system. *Diagnosis* 1988;10(8):49-57.

Ellestad MH: *Stress Testing: Principles and Practice,* ed 3. Philadelphia, FA Davis Co, 1985.

Gubin SS, Judge RD: Graded exercise testing. *AFP* 1987;35(4):123-129.

II

PULMONARY PROCEDURES

11

Thoracentesis for Fluid Removal

Leslie E. Weber, MD

When a patient has a pulmonary effusion of unknown origin, it is essential to classify it: A complicated (or infectious) effusion must be drained, and an uncomplicated effusion will resolve spontaneously. Fluid should be drawn for protein, specific gravity, lactate dehydrogenase, glucose, and amylase determinations; a WBC count with differential; and a Gram's stain and culture to determine the presence and type of bacteria.

Thoracentesis is simple to perform, and it can be done unaided. It should not be done in patients with severe coagulopathy and is best postponed or deferred in those who have a small effusion that is not growing, in those who are physically agitated and cannot hold still, and in those who are already responding to drug therapy.

Materials

- Sterile gloves
- Antiseptic skin preparation such as povidone/iodine (Betadine)
- Sponges
- Sterile drape or towels
- Local anesthetic such as 1% lidocaine HCl (Xylocaine HCl)
- 5-mL Luer-Lok syringe
- 25-gauge, ⅝-in. needle
- 22-gauge, 2-in. needle

For thoracentesis

- 50 mL Luer-Lok syringe
- 22-gauge, 2-in. needle
- 18-gauge, 2-in. needle
- 15-gauge, 2-in. needle
- Two curved clamps
- Three specimen tubes with stoppers
- Three-way stopcock with rubber tubing attached to stopcock side-arm
- Specimen bowl
- Pressure pads
- Sterile sponge dressings
- Adhesive strips
- Vacuum bottle (optional)

PROCEDURE

1. Get an upright chest X-ray no more than a day before the procedure is scheduled to determine the extent and location of the effusion.

Caution: Although thoracentesis is not especially difficult, it does require a high degree of cooperation on the part of the patient: You can accidentally puncture a lung if the patient is agitated. Delay the procedure in anyone who is coughing or hiccuping.

2. Have the patient sit leaning forward. One convenient arrangement is to have him or her sitting on the edge of the bed and leaning on a pillow placed on a bedside stand (Figure 11-1). He should be resting as comfortably as possible with arms elevated.

3. Impress upon the patient the importance of remaining as still as possible to avoid puncturing the lung, and tell him to expect some discomfort when you enter the pleura. Warn him against coughing, and ask him to tell you if he feels a cough coming on.

4. Select the thoracentesis site at a point well below the level of the fluid as indicated on the chest film. In the posterior approach, the site is often the seventh or eighth interspace on the posterior axillary line. A slightly higher site may be used, but to be sure of intercepting the pleura, do not use a site lower than the ninth interspace.

5. With the patient properly positioned, put on the sterile gloves, and prepare the skin with antiseptic solution, covering an area about 20 cm in diameter around the selected site.

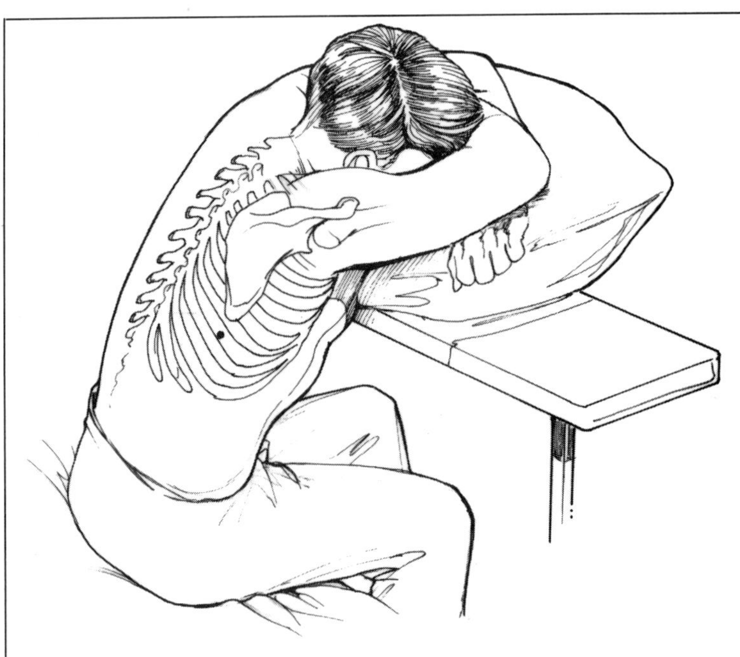

Figure 11-1 Patient in correct position for thoracentesis. He or she should be as comfortable as possible, with arms raised on a pillow.

6. You can use a drape with a hole 10 cm in diameter cut in it, taping the upper margins to the patient's skin. This has a tendency to fall off, and a preferable alternative is simply to attach a sterile towel across the patient's back below the site of needle entry.

7. Anesthetize the skin with 1% lidocaine HCl (Xylocaine HCl), using a 5-mL Luer-Lok syringe and a 25-gauge, ⅝-in. needle to raise a wheal. Then inject about 1–3 mL down through the muscles of the chest wall. Direct the needle just above the upper margin of the rib below the selected interspace; if the needle enters too close to the inferior rib margin, it might compromise the adjacent vascular structures (Figure 11-2). You will want to aspirate periodically as the needle goes in to confirm that you are not encountering blood vessels.

8. Switch to the 22-gauge, 2-in. needle, and anesthetize the deeper structures with 3–5 mL of lidocaine. When you reach the pleura, the patient almost always feels pain, which will alert you to the needle-tip position. You will not necessarily feel the often-mentioned popping sensation as you puncture the pleura.

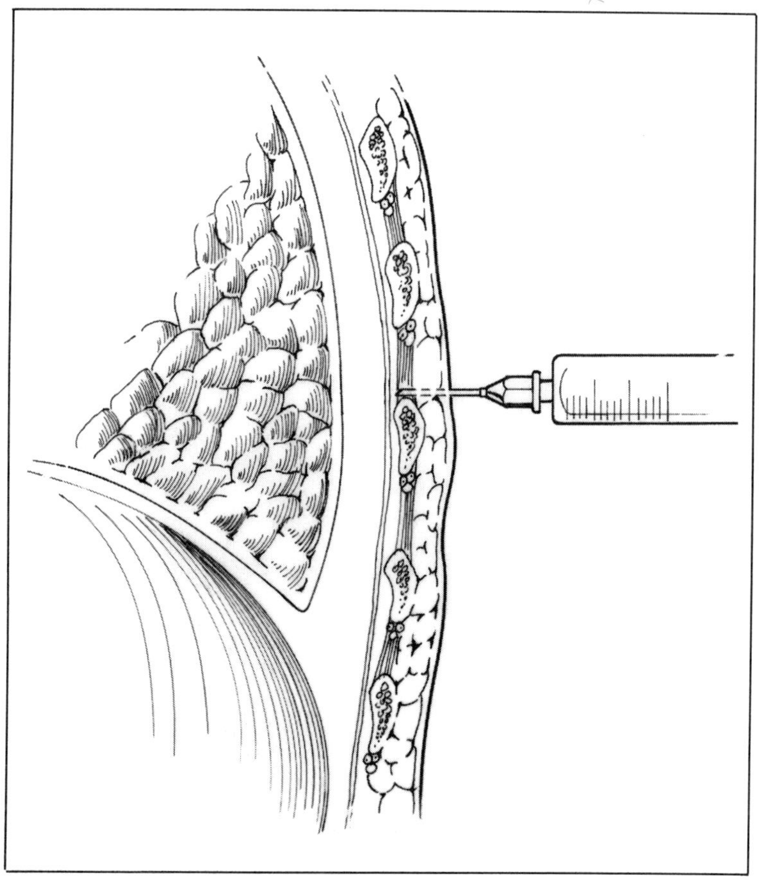

Figure 11-2 To inject anesthetic, select a point of insertion directly above the upper margin of the rib that lies directly below the interspace you wish to enter. Aspirate periodically as you advance the needle to confirm that you are not entering blood vessels.

9. Try carefully to aspirate by using negative syringe pressure. If the aspirate is not pleural fluid, reposition the needle and reaspirate. When you get pleural fluid return, mark the needle depth with a curved clamp, and withdraw the needle (Figure 11-3).
10. Attach the appropriate thoracentesis needle to the 50-mL syringe (22- or 18-gauge for sampling; 15-gauge for removing large quantities of fluid); mark the proper depth by clamping the needle at the same depth as on the anesthetizing needle (Figure 11-4); and insert the needle.
11. To sample pleural fluid, withdraw enough fluid to fill the specimen tubes.
12. To remove a large amount of fluid, aspirate 50 mL and then turn the stopcock to let the syringe empty through the rubber tubing into the specimen bowl. Repeat as necessary.

A vacuum bottle is occasionally useful if you are sure you will be aspirating a large amount of fluid: Connect the bottle to the 15-gauge needle with rubber tubing, first having clamped off the tubing. With the needle in the pleural space, open the tubing clamp, allowing the

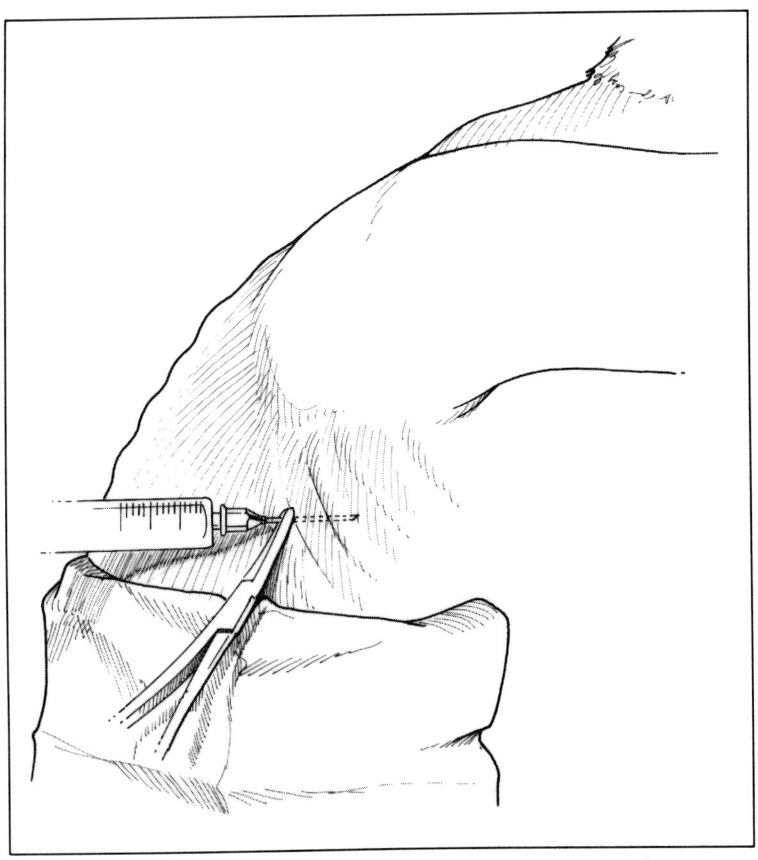

Figure 11-3 When you think you have entered the pleural space, attempt to aspirate fluid. Reposition the needle if the aspirate is not pleural fluid. Upon pleural fluid return, mark the depth of the needle with a curved clamp and withdraw.

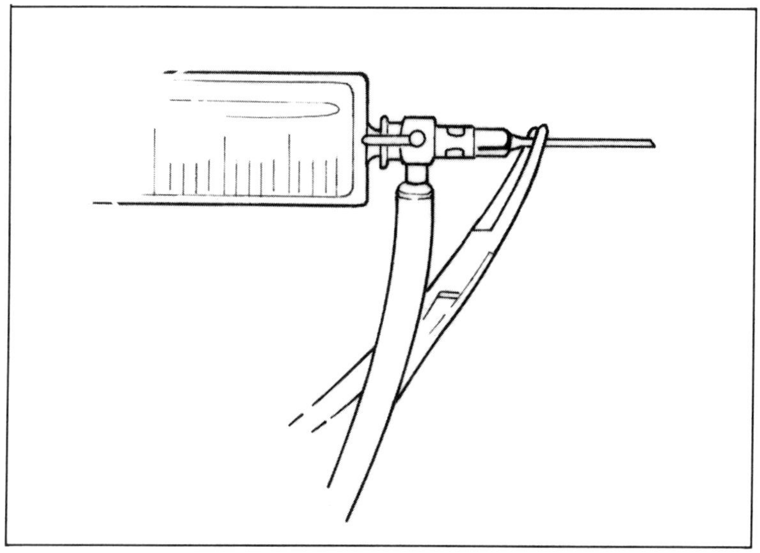

Figure 11-4 Mark the thoracentesis needle with a clamp in the same position as the clamp on the anesthetizing needle.

vacuum to aspirate the fluid. This method benefits the patient by speeding up the aspiration.

13. When enough fluid has been aspirated, withdraw the needle, and apply finger pressure over the puncture site to keep air from entering. Hold the pressure for a few moments to close the site; then apply a pressure pad with adhesive strips. When the procedure is complete and the patient is resting, instruct the nursing staff to observe him closely and check vital signs often for the next hour or so. Patients who have had large amounts of fluid removed may develop pulmonary edema. Watch for shortness of breath, which can indicate developing pneumothorax. If this should occur, only a small amount of air is usually lost, even when the lung is inadvertently punctured.

Bleeding may very occasionally occur. You can avoid this complication by selecting the puncture site carefully and directing the needle over the superior margin of the rib.

Suggested Readings

Orland MJ, Saltman RJ (eds): *Manual of Medical Therapeutics,* ed 25. Boston, Little Brown & Co, 1986, pp 173-174.

Pories WJ, Thomas FT (eds): *Office Surgery for the Family Physician.* Boston, Butterworth Publishers, 1985, pp 149-152.

Roberts PW (ed): *Useful Procedures in Medical Practice.* Philadelphia, Lea & Febiger, 1986, pp 449-455.

Wright CV, Mitts DL: Pleural effusions and empyema thoracis, in Rakel RE (ed): *Conn's Current Therapy.* Philadelphia, WB Saunders Co, 1986, pp 127-128.

12

Endotracheal Intubation

Timothy Nagel, MD
Charles E. Driscoll, MD

Endotracheal intubation is the definitive procedure for airway management during cardiopulmonary resuscitation (CPR). With proper equipment and training, you can rapidly establish a patent and protected airway, providing for active and effective regulation of ventilation.

Indications

- To ensure airway patency
- To prevent aspiration
- To facilitate suctioning and pulmonary hygiene
- To permit active regulation of ventilation
- To administer drugs

Relative Contraindications

- Suspected or actual cervical spine injury
- Mechanical upper airway obstruction
- Laryngeal or tracheal trauma
- Inability to open patient's mouth
- Excessive difficulty in previous attempts
- Lack of skill

Materials

- Endotracheal tube of proper size (approximately 6.5–7.0 mm for women; 7.5–8.0 mm for men) with inflatable cuff
- Laryngoscope with removable curved (McIntosh) or straight (Miller, Guedel) blade
- 10-mL syringe
- Hemostat

- Stylet to stiffen endotracheal tube (optional)
- Bite block or oral airway
- Magill forceps
- Several precut strips of adhesive tape
- Tank or wall source of 100% oxygen
- Bag-valve-mask or pocket mask

PROCEDURE

Note: An intubation attempt should take no longer than 15–20 seconds. Hold your breath when you begin. If the procedure is not completed when you become uncomfortable, remove equipment and ventilate the patient for a few minutes with 100% oxygen, using a tank or wall source and a bag-valve-mask or a pocket mask. Then make another attempt.

1. With the patient supine, place a hand behind the neck and gently pull up to extend it so that the head is tilted slightly backward; avoid hyperextending the neck and take special care to protect the neck if you suspect a cervical spine injury. Place a folded towel or small pillow under the head to keep the mouth, pharynx, and larynx aligned and the neck extended at the atlanto-occipital joint, and alignment commonly called the sniffing position (Figure 12-1).
2. Stand at the patient's head with the laryngoscope in your left hand and use your right hand to open the patient's mouth as wide as possible. Gently insert the blade into the mouth along the right side, and let the blade push the tongue gently to the left. Do not allow the tongue to drop back onto the open side of the blade.

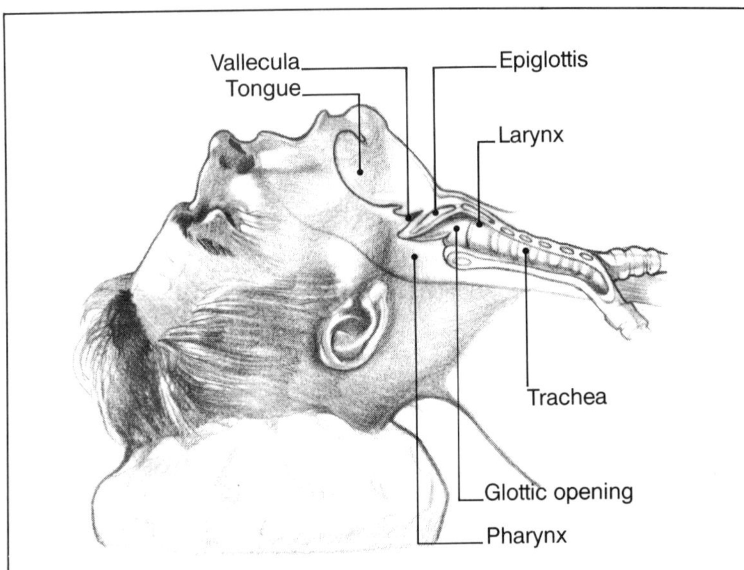

Figure 12-1 A pillow or folded towel placed under the neck keeps the mouth, the pharynx, and the larynx aligned.

3. When the blade is at the midline, exert gentle traction upward at a 45-degree angle to the floor of the mouth, and slowly advance the blade without levering against the teeth. If using a straight-blade laryngoscope, place the tip of the blade over the epiglottis to lift it and expose the vocal cords (Figure 12-2). If using a curved-blade laryngoscope, insert the tip between the base of the tongue and the epiglottis to lift them both and visualize the cords (Figure 12-3). If a foreign body obstructs the airway, remove it with the Magill forceps.
4. With the arytenoid cartilages and vocal cords in view, use your dominant hand to insert the endotracheal tube from the right-hand corner of the mouth, through the vocal cords into the trachea (Figure 12-4). Be sure you see the vocal cords clearly as you move the tube along (Figure 12-5). Pass the cuff about 2.5 cm (1 in.) beyond them.

You may want to place a stylet inside the tube before insertion to stiffen the curve. The most likely indications for using a stylet include emesis or blood in the airway, an unusually pliant endotracheal tube, and a narrow or constricted passageway through the vocal cords. When using a stylet, make sure that the end of the stylet rests at least 1 cm (⅜ in.) back from the end of the endotracheal tube. Remove the stylet after the tube is passed beyond the vocal cords.

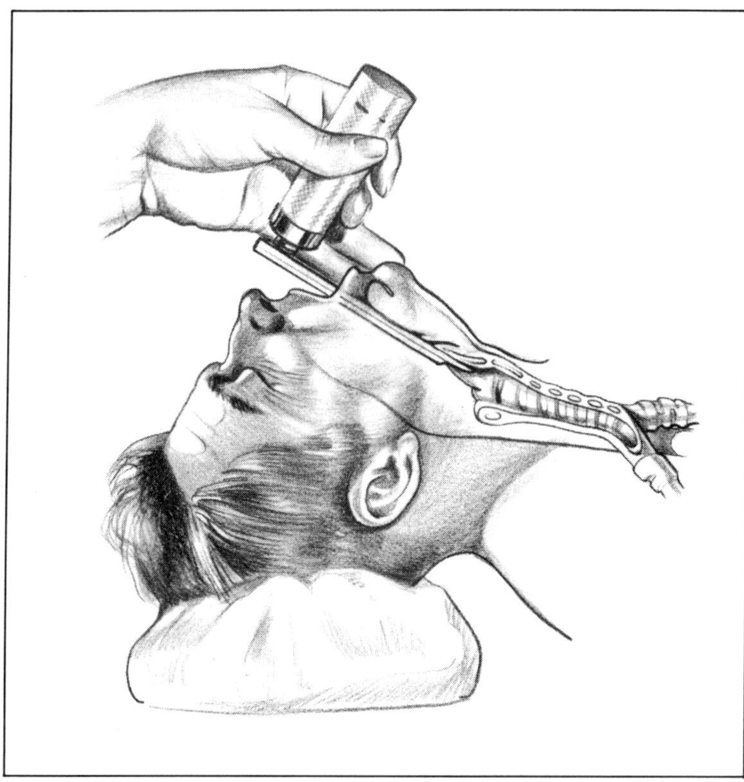

Figure 12-2 When the blade is at the midline, apply gentle traction upward at a 45-degree angle to the floor of the mouth. Slowly advance the blade over the epiglottis to expose the vocal cords.

Figure 12-3 Using a curved-blade laryngoscope. Insert the tip between the base of the tongue and the epiglottis to lift them both and expose the vocal cords.

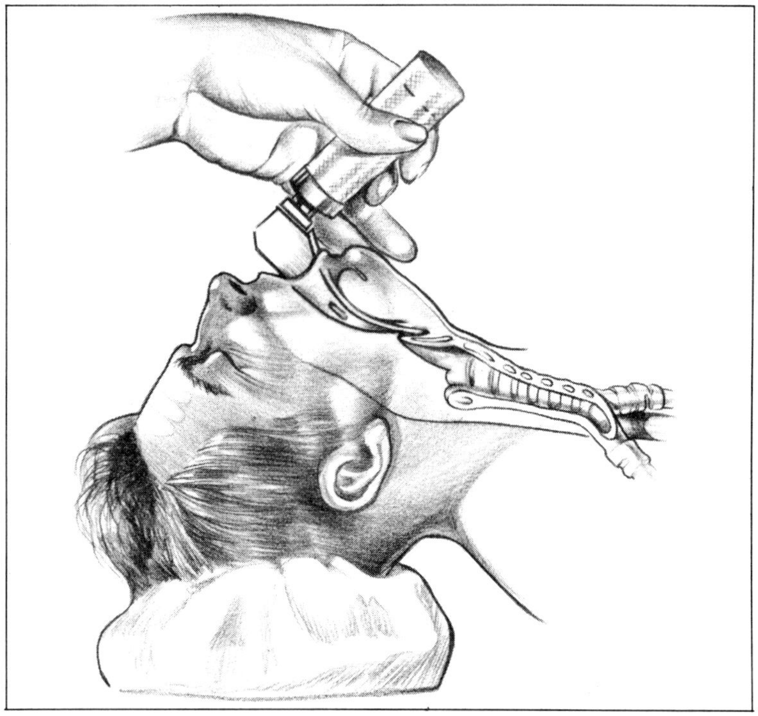

Figure 12-4 Use right hand to insert the endotracheal tube from the right-hand corner of the patient's mouth.

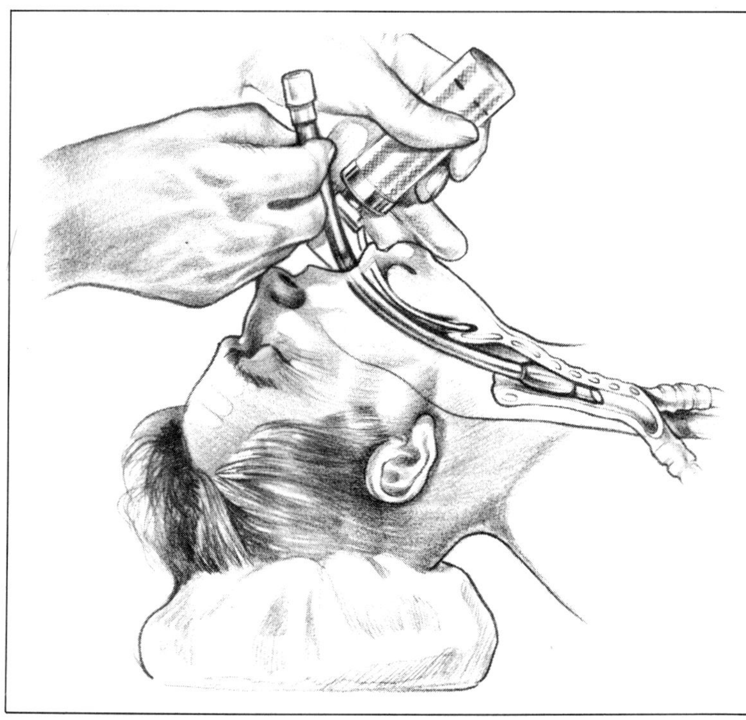

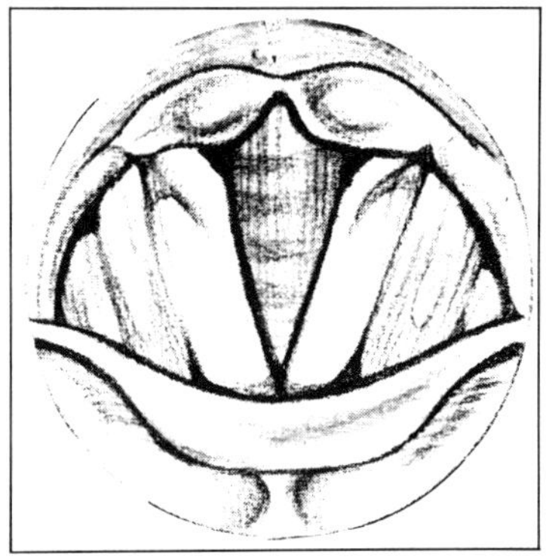

Figure 12-5 Be sure you can see the vocal cords clearly as you advance the tube.

5. Use the 10-mL syringe to inflate the cuff with 5–8 mL of air, and clamp off the inflation line with a hemostat.
6. Make sure the endotracheal tube is placed properly. As a quick assessment, look for symmetric chest rise with ventilation, and auscultate to confirm that breath sounds are equal bilaterally. If breath sounds are absent bilaterally, the cuff is most likely in the esophagus: Deflate it immediately, remove the tube, and ventilate the patient with 100% oxygen for at least three minutes using a tank or wall source and a bag-valve-mask or pocket mask before the next attempt. If you hear breath sounds on one side only (usually the right), the tube has probably entered a main bronchus: Deflate the cuff and very slowly pull the tube back while ventilating, until breath sounds are equally audible on both sides of the chest. Then reinflate the cuff.
7. Use one hand to secure the tube by applying adhesive tape; do not remove your other hand until the tube is taped securely. Insert a bite block or oral airway to prevent the patient from biting the endotracheal tube and obstructing airflow.
8. With a standard 15-mm adapter on the end of the endotracheal tube, you can attach the tube to a bag-valve device or to a mechanical respirator and continue ventilation with 100% oxygen from a tank or wall source.

Complications

Some complications are common, but they can be avoided or ameliorated by use of the proper equipment and technique:

- Cardiopulmonary arrest secondary to hypoxia from prolonged or improper tube placement
- Interruption of CPR
- Aspiration of blood/vomitus during procedure
- Endobronchial intubation
- Vocal cord spasm
- Teeth fractures

Suggested Readings

Textbook of Advanced Cardiac Life Support. Dallas, American Heart Association, 1983.

Raehl CL: Endotracheal drug therapy in cardiopulmonary resuscitation. *Clin Pharm* 1986;5:572-579.

Rosen P, Baker FJ, Braen R, et al (eds): *Emergency Medicine: Concepts and Clinical Practice.* St. Louis, CV Mosby Co, 1983.

13

Emergency Cricothyroidotomy

Lawrence W. Steinkraus, MD
Gayle Roggeveen Nelson, RN

The cricothyroid is an excellent site for securing an emergency surgical airway. It is usually easy to identify in the adult; the trachea is most superficial at the cricothyroid; and serious bleeding can be minimized since major vessels are located elsewhere. By contrast, emergency tracheostomy is difficult, usually results in profuse bleeding, and may take too long to perform.[1]

Indications

- Inability to intubate the trachea when an emergency airway is needed.[2]
- Edema of the hypopharynx, epiglottis, or glottis; fracture of the larynx; or profound oropharyngeal bleeding may obstruct the upper airway and necessitate surgical opening for ventilation.
- Suspicion of injury to the cervical spine, with or without concomitant head and facial injuries, makes other modes of intubation hazardous.

Materials

- No. 10 and No. 11 scalpel blades and handle
- 7-mm endotracheal or 5–7 mm tracheostomy tube

---

[1]In children younger than 12 years, needle cricothyroidotomy, also referred to as the jet insufflation method, is a good alternative to the surgical method. Use a catheter-over-needle cannula of at least 12–14 gauge and a syringe. Insert the needle through the cricothyroid membrane, aiming caudally. When you can easily aspirate air into the syringe, advance the catheter into the trachea. This technique is similar to cannulating a vein.

Connect the catheter to an oxygen source with either a Y-connector or tubing in which a side hole has been cut. For intermittent ventilation, cover the open end of the Y-connector or the hole in the tubing periodically. This technique should not be used for more than an hour because exhalation is inadequate and excess carbon dioxide may accumulate.

[2]For a discussion of the procedure where intubation is possible, see "Endotracheal intubation," page 67.

- 4 × 4-in. gauze sponges
- Local anesthetic with syringe and needle
- Povidone-iodine solution (Betadine)
- Adhesive tape and/or twill tape
- Sterile gloves
- Suction machine and catheters
- Hemostats

PROCEDURE IN ADULTS

1. Place the patient supine with neck neutral. Slight hyperextension may facilitate locating the thyroid notch, but be sure to rule out cervical spine injury if you place the neck in anything but the neutral position. Monitor the patient, have suction available, and have an assistant for sponging and instrument handling whenever possible. Palpate the thyroid notch, cricothyroid space, and sternal notch (Figure 13-1). Clean the area with povidone-iodine, and if the patient is conscious, inject local anesthetic.
2. Stabilize the thyroid cartilage, and with the belly of the knife blade, make a horizontal skin incision that extends across the cricothyroid membrane (Figure 13-2). Incise quickly and deeply to expose the membrane.
3. With the blade point, stab through the membrane into the trachea. If the patient is making a respiratory effort, you will hear air escape when you enter the trachea.
4. You may open the wound with a curved hemostat or by inserting the knife handle and rotating it 90 degrees. The opening must be large enough to accommodate a 7-mm endotracheal tube or a 5–7 mm tracheostomy tube. The standard endotracheal tube is preferred, since it usually is readily available, is easy to use, and can be cut to size (Figure 13-3).
5. With either tube, inflate the cuff and secure it by ties to prevent dislodging or accidental extubation.

Note: Check ventilation immediately after placing the tube to confirm tracheal cannulation. If the incision is not deep enough to penetrate the trachea, you may unknowingly place the tube in a subcutaneous track created by pressure used to insert the tube. If this happens, you will hear no breath sounds during ventilation, and subcutaneous emphysema may be evident at the cannulation site. If you use an endotracheal tube, be sure it is not placed too deeply into the right mainstem bronchus.

6. Once you secure the airway and note resumed ventilation, provide 100% oxygen by either bag-valve-tube or ventilator. Monitor the patient's arterial blood gases to guide ventilation therapy.

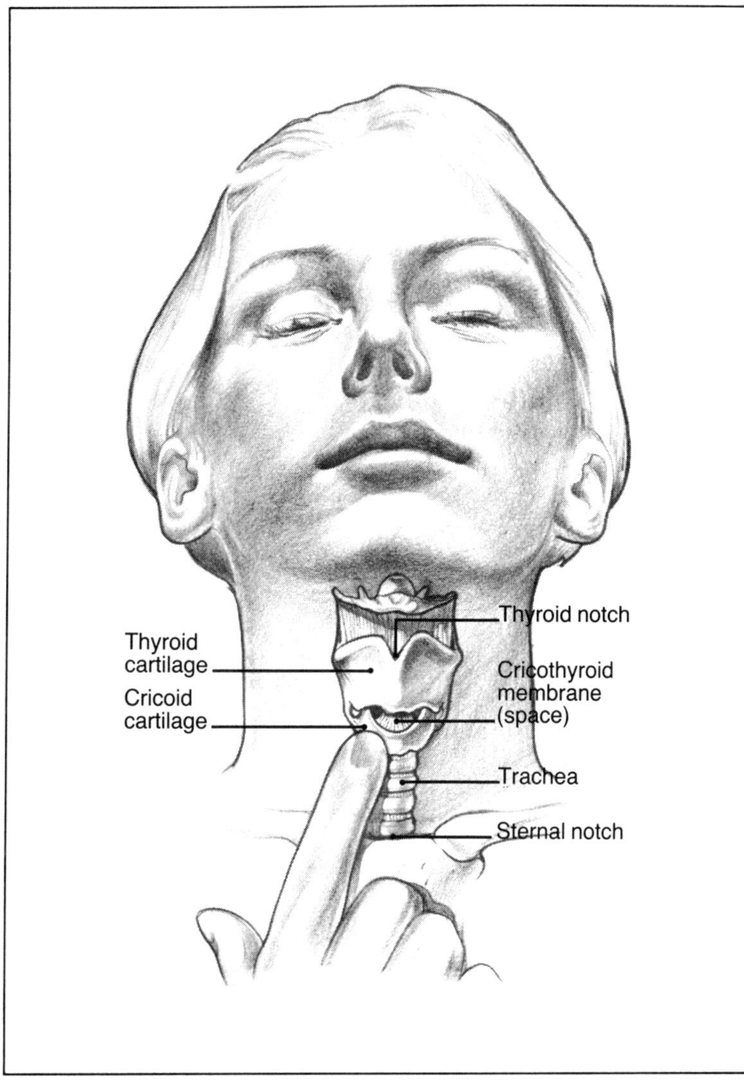

Figure 13-1 Palpate the thyroid notch, cricothyroid space, and sternal notch.

Complications

Possible complications with surgical cricothyroidotomy include the following:

- Asphyxia
- Aspiration
- Hemorrhage
- Hematoma formation
- Stenosis and laceration of the trachea or the esophagus

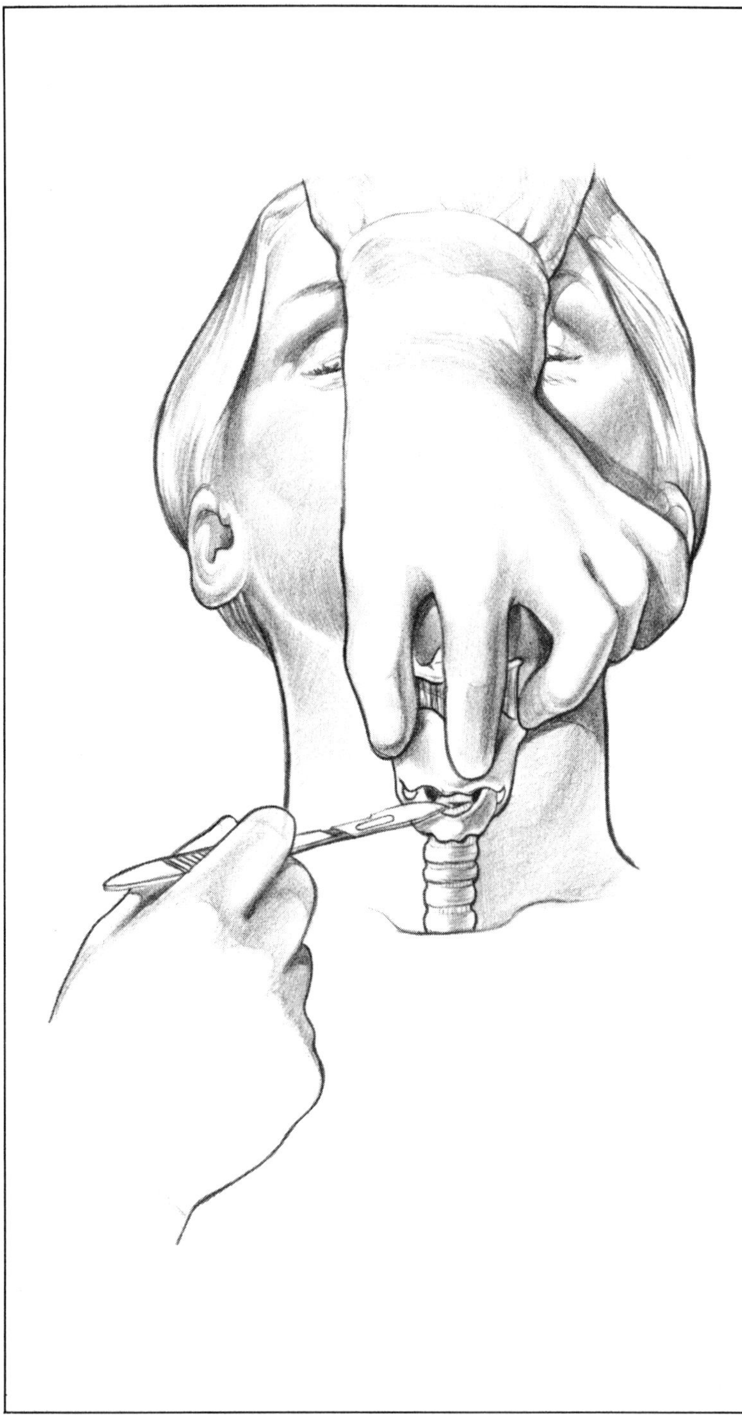

Figure 13-2 With the belly of the knife blade, make a horizontal incision across the cricothyroid membrane. With the blade point, stab through the membrane into the trachea.

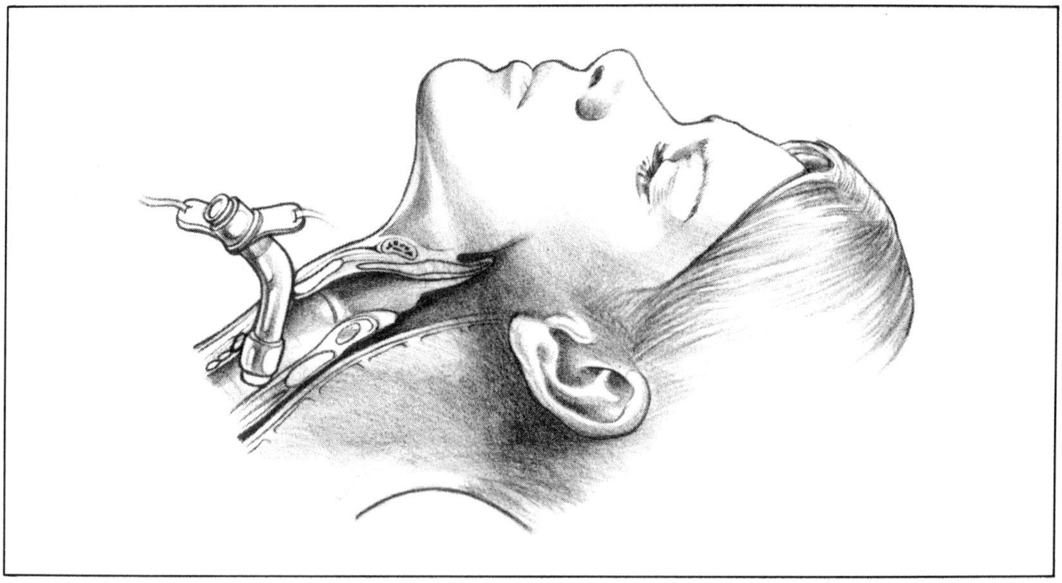

Figure 13-3 After enlarging the opening, insert a 7-mm endotracheal tube. Once ventilation is noted, provide 100% oxygen by either bag-valve-tube or ventilator.

Emergency cricothyroidotomy is, however, a life-saving procedure intended to secure an airway in a profoundly compromised individual. The alternative to performing the procedure may be death of the patient.

Suggested Readings

American College of Surgeons, Committee on Trauma: *Advanced Trauma Life Support Student Manual*. Chicago, American College of Surgeons, 1984.

Advanced Cardiac Life Support Instructor Manual. Dallas, American Heart Association, 1983.

Schwartz GR, Safar P, Stone JH, et al (eds): *Principles and Practices of Emergency Medicine*, ed 2. Philadelphia, WB Saunders Co, 1986.

Wilkins EW: *MGH Textbook of Emergency Medicine*, ed 2. Baltimore, Williams & Wilkins Co, 1983.

14

Spirometry

George C. Xakellis, MD

Spirometry today is a simple, inexpensive way to evaluate a patient's pulmonary status in your office. The most frequently used parameters are FEV_1 (forced expiratory volume in one second) to measure air flow and FVC (forced vital capacity) to measure lung volume. From these two measures you can usually classify the patient's pulmonary abnormality, response to therapy, and prognosis.

Indications

- To screen patients at risk for lung disease
- To diagnose pulmonary disease in symptomatic patients
- To classify pulmonary abnormalities as either obstructive or restrictive
- To monitor effectiveness of therapy for pulmonary function
- To follow progression of a patient's pulmonary disease
- To determine a patient's prognosis

Relative Contraindications

- Active pulmonary infections
- Unstable cardiovascular disease
- History of hypersensitivity or other untoward reactions to inhaled bronchodilators

Materials

- Dry bellows or diaphragm spirometer
- Manual or computerized recording system
- Noseclip
- Breathing tube
- Disposable mouthpiece
- Selective $beta_2$-adrenergic inhalational agent
- Recording materials (pens and chart paper for manual systems, compatible hardware for computerized systems)
- Reference nomogram of predicted values for FEV_1 and FVC

PROCEDURE

For dry spirometer, diaphragm type, and manual recording:

1. Place the spirometer on a flat surface. Align the recording pen and chart paper, connect the breathing tube to the spirometer, and attach a disposable mouthpiece to the breathing tube.

2. Have the patient remove a coat or jacket, loosen tight clothing such as a collar, bra, or corset, and remove oral appliances. He or she may stand or sit for the test. Demonstrate the proper method of inhaling and forcefully exhaling. Place the noseclip on the patient, occluding both nostrils.

3. Instruct the patient to

- Inhale deeply
- Place his mouth around the mouthpiece, forming an airtight seal
- Exhale as forcefully and completely as possible (coaching often improves performance)
- Remove the mouthpiece and hold it away from his face while the spirometer empties.

4. Do three successive tests, and use the best performance for calculating results.

5. Give two metered doses of the beta$_2$-adrenergic inhalational agent, and repeat the test in about 20 minutes.

Interpreting Results

- The most important variables measured by this test are FEV$_1$ and FVC. Compare these values with the predicted normal values for the patient's age, sex, and height (Figures 14-1 and 14-2). Calcu-

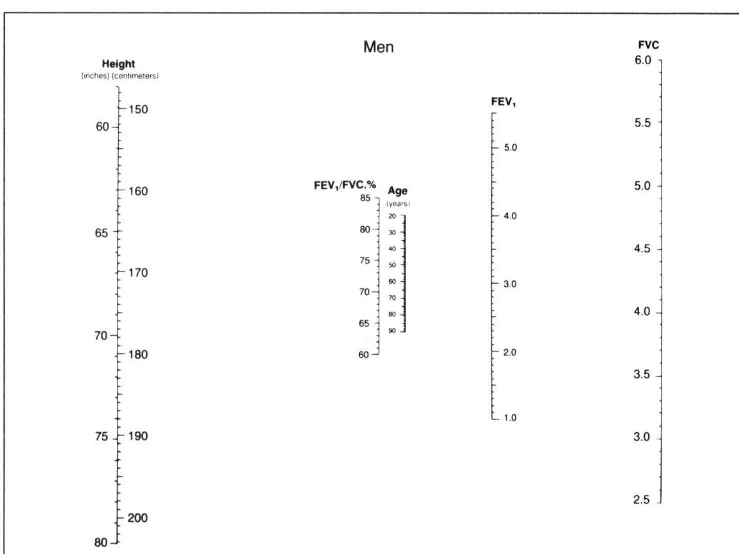

Figure 14-1 Adapted with permission from Morris JF: Spirometry in the evaluation of pulmonary function. *West J Med* 1976; 125:114.

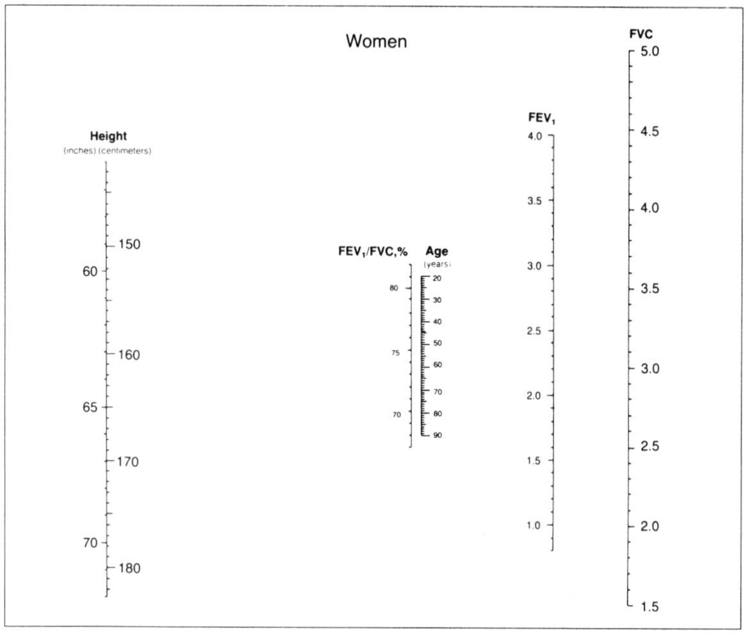

Figure 14-2 Adapted with permission from Morris JF: Spirometry in the evaluation of pulmonary function. *West J Med* 1976; 125:115.

late the FEV_1/FVC ratio, and compare it with the predicted normal values. If any measurements are abnormal, you must decide whether the patient has restrictive, obstructive, or mixed pulmonary disease.

- In restrictive disease, the patient has decreased FVC. Because a drop in FVC also decreases the maximal potential value of the FEV_1, this parameter may also be reduced, but the ratio of FEV_1/FVC remains normal at greater than 75%.
- In obstructive disease, the patient's expired airflow is reduced, which shows up as a decreased FEV_1. In mild obstructive disease, FVC is preserved, but the ratio of the FEV_1/FVC is reduced to abnormal levels of less than 75%. In severe obstructive airway disease or a mixture of obstructive and restrictive disease, all three parameters are abnormally low.
- Assess response to bronchodilators. If you find improvement, the patient is likely to benefit from bronchodilator therapy. But even if you see no evidence of improvement, a course of bronchodilators with or without corticosteroids may help the patient's pulmonary function.
- You can use the ratio of FEV_1/FVC to develop a prognosis. If the patient has an FEV_1 of less than 1.15 L, his five-year survival is reduced by one third. If the FEV_1 is less than 750 mL, the five-year survival is reduced by two thirds. An FEV_1/FVC ratio of less than 60% also means a less favorable prognosis (Table 14-1).

TABLE 14-1

Age-specific, Crude, and Age-adjusted Mortality Rates (%)*

	FEV$_1$/FVC (%)		
Age interval	**<60**	**60–74**	**>75**
20–29	0	0	0
30–39	20.0	0	0
40–49	16.7	8.0	9.1
50–59	30.8	10.0	7.1
60–69	13.3	11.8	8.3
Crude rate	19.5	7.6	4.3
Age-adjusted rate	18.1	6.3	5.3

*For 3 categories of FEV$_1$/FVC (%) in 1967, regardless of chronic bronchitis

Adapted with permission from Petty TL, Pierson DF, Dick NP, et al: Follow-up evaluation of a prevalence study for chronic bronchitis and chronic airway obstruction. *Am Rev Respir Dis* 1976;114:881-890.

Follow-up Care

Use serial testing to determine whether a patient's pulmonary function is stable or deteriorating.

Suggested Readings

Burrows B, Earle RH: Course and prognosis of chronic obstructive lung disease: A prospective study of 200 patients. *N Engl J Med* 1969;280:397-404.

Good JT Jr, Petty TL: Office spirometry. *Am Fam Physician* 1980;21(4):111-114.

Morris JF: Spirometry in the evaluation of pulmonary function. *West J Med* 1976;125:110-118.

Petty TL, Pierson DJ, Dick NP, et al: Follow-up evaluation of a prevalence study for chronic bronchitis and chronic airway obstruction. *Am Rev Respir Dis* 1976;114:881-890.

Statement of spirometry: A report of the section on respiratory pathophysiology. *Chest* 1983;83(3):547-550.

15

Chest Tube Insertion

Charles E. Driscoll, MD

Traumatic chest injuries are among the most complex to diagnose and treat. Intrathoracic structures may be injured by penetrating trauma or by significant blunt forces to the chest wall, with little evidence of external injury. As many as 25% of motor vehicle accident (MVA) deaths result from chest injury, and it may be a contributing factor in 25–50% of the remainder. In urban areas, violent crime also accounts for a significant percentage of chest trauma cases.

To reduce the morbidity and mortality of chest injury, carefully evaluate injured patients for signs of respiratory insufficiency. The patient usually appears agitated and restless, and he or she may be in shock and respiratory distress with the potential for respiratory and cardiac arrest.

Be alert for cyanosis, paradoxical movement of the chest, crepitus of the chest wall, altered sounds of percussion of the chest wall, altered breath sounds, deviation of the trachea, and distended neck veins. Internal bleeding (hemothorax) sometimes masks these physical signs, increasing the difficulty of diagnosis.

Observing these signs and acting urgently will significantly reduce mortality. It is wise to have a strong suspicion of underlying intrathoracic injury in any major injury such as MVA, severe crush injury, or gunshot wound. A patient who is deteriorating rapidly is a likely candidate for chest tube insertion even before a chest X-ray is carried out. Two procedures are usually recommended for the emergency treatment of compromised respiratory function: needle decompression of tension pneumothorax and insertion of a chest tube.

Indications

Compromised respiratory function due to

- Intrapleural air (tension pneumothorax or pneumothorax)
- Intrapleural fluid collection (pleural effusion or hemothorax)

- A combination of the first two
- Any severe chest injury and signs of rapid deterioration, even before a chest X-ray has been done.

Contraindication

- Equivocal diagnosis in a non-life-threatening situation

Materials

- Antiseptic skin preparation such as povidone-iodine (Betadine) or surgical scrub
- Sterile 4 × 4-in. pads for cleansing skin and as dressings
- Sterile gloves
- Sterile drape or sterile towels
- 10 mL of local anesthetic such as 1% lidocaine HCl (Xylocaine HCl)
- 100-mL Luer-Lok syringe with 21-gauge, 2-in. needle

For needle thoracentesis

- 14-gauge over-the-needle catheter 3–6 cm long
- 50-mL Luer-Lok syringe

For chest tube insertion

- Scalpel handle and No. 11 stab blade
- Two large curved Kelly clamps
- Suture scissors
- Mayo scissors
- Needle holder
- A No. 28–40 French chest tube, size determined by the size of the intercostal space (No. 32 is average)
- An underwater seal device (a three-bottle system or commercial model such as Pleur-evac or Thoradrain). If no underwater seal is available, a Penrose drain temporarily attached to the chest tube acts as a clamp, allowing air to exit but not enter the chest.
- Petroleum jelly to apply to sterile 4 × 4-in. gauze pads, or petrolatum gauze
- Suction apparatus
- No. 00 silk suture with cutting skin needle
- Tubing to connect chest tube and vacuum source to underwater seal device

PROCEDURE

NEEDLE THORACENTESIS

1. Determine the presence of tension pneumothorax by noting the signs of respiratory distress, tracheal deviation, distended neck veins, unilateral absence of breath sounds, and hypertympanic percussion note over the affected chest cavity. Tension pneumothorax is a clinical diagnosis and is treated emergently with needle decompression.

2. If time permits, prepare the skin in the midclavicular line on the side of the pneumothorax.

3. Identify the second intercostal space in the midclavicular line, lateral to the sternal angle.

4. If the patient is conscious and time permits, anesthetize the skin with 1–2 mL of 1% lidocaine; if the patient is unconscious and his condition is deteriorating, do the procedure without anesthesia.

5. Attach the 14-gauge over-the-needle catheter to the 50-mL Luer-Lok syringe.

6. Position the patient semiupright if tolerated and if cervical spine injury has been ruled out. This will help move the heart and great vessels away from the puncture site.

7. Insert the needle through the skin directly into the chest cavity, over the top of the lower rib bordering the second intercostal space (Figure 15-1). You may feel a pop as the parietal pleura is punctured.

8. Aspirate as much air as possible with the 50-mL syringe to relieve acute symptoms. In severe tension pneumothorax, allow the air to rush out of the catheter hub without extraction.

9. Once the patient is stabilized, prepare for chest tube insertion. Leave the plastic over-the-needle catheter in place while withdrawing the syringe and needle. A bandage or small dressing may be placed over the plastic cannula left open to atmospheric pressure.

Figure 15-1

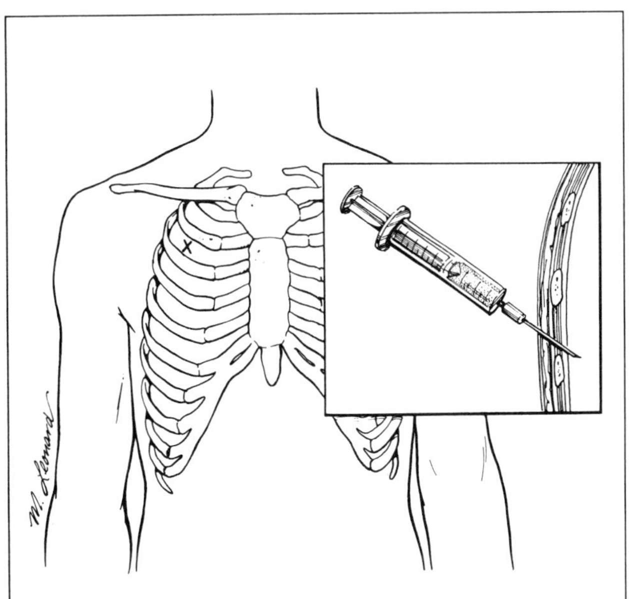

CHEST TUBE INSERTION

1. The most commonly recommended insertion site is in the fifth intercostal space just anterior to the midaxillary line of the affected lung (Figure 15-2).

2. Using sterile gloves, prepare the skin with antiseptic, and do the rest of the procedure in aseptic fashion. Drape the chest with sterile towels or drape. Regularly monitor vital signs during the procedure; these patients are generally unstable.

3. Anesthetize the skin directly over the surface of the sixth rib, injecting anesthetic into the skin, subcutaneous tissue, and periosteum of the sixth rib and moving the needle track above the superior border of the sixth rib. Also infiltrate the area of the fifth intercostal space. Then make a 1½-in. transverse incision through the anesthetized skin overlying the sixth rib and through the subcutaneous tissues to the point that just overlies the bony surface of the sixth rib.

4. Blunt dissect the subcutaneous tissues with a gloved finger or a large curved Kelly clamp. Aim and tunnel the clamp toward the superior border of the sixth rib and the intercostal space just above the rib (Figure 15-3a). Some practitioners prefer a longer tunnel, entering at the level of the seventh rib and tunneling subcutaneously to the fifth intercostal space before entering the chest cavity. The latter technique may reduce the likelihood of pneumothorax after the chest tube is removed.

Caution: To avoid the intercostal neurovascular bundle just inferior to each rib, stay close to the superior edge of the rib in making the subcutaneous tunnel and placing the tube.

Figure 15-2

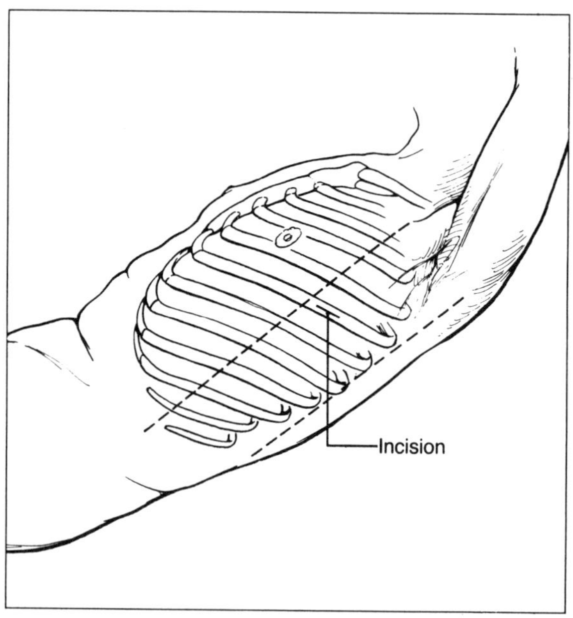

Figure 15-3

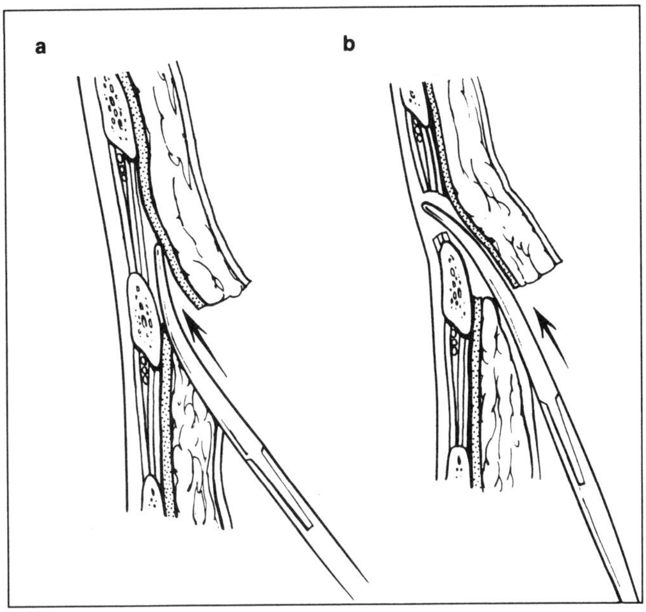

5. Enter the pleural cavity with the closed Kelly clamp, orienting the direction of insertion superiorly and turning the clamp with a screwlike movement (Figure 15-3b). Control insertion depth by placing your middle finger on the chest wall to stop too deep a puncture. Expect a sudden drop in resistance and a pop when entering the pleural cavity.

6. You may insert a gloved finger through the incision, the intercostal space, and parietal pleura to check for adhesions or unanticipated findings such as the diaphragm.

7. If necessary before placing the tube, enlarge the opening by inserting the closed Kelly clamp, and opening and spreading it in different planes.

8. Use the second Kelly clamp to close the proximal end of the chest tube. Grasp the distal tip of the chest tube with the first Kelly clamp, and advance it through the incision, the subcutaneous tissue, and the parietal pleura so the tip lies within the pleural cavity (Figure 15-4).

Note: Some chest tubes come with an intraluminal trocar inserter. These are not recommended because of a higher chance of inadvertent intrathoracic injury.

9. Withdraw the clamp, and advance the tube within the pleural cavity to the desired depth. Be sure all the holes in the tube are inside the chest. Look for fogging of the exit tube with respirations, or listen for air movement through the tube.

10. Connect the chest tube to the drainage system via plastic tubing, and set the device to get approximately 220 cm of H_2O suction

Figure 15-4

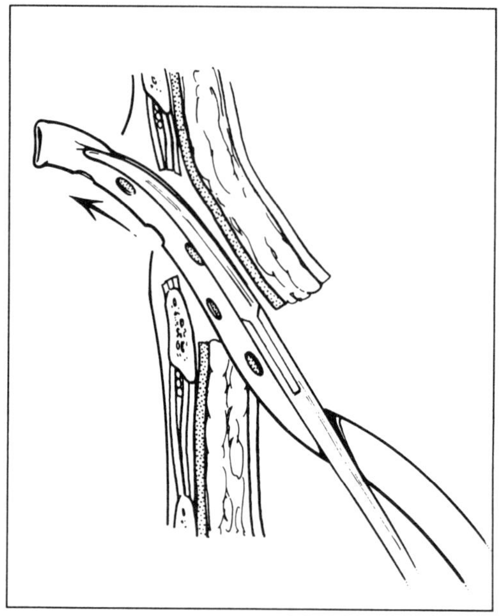

pressure. Air bubbles in the water of the chest draining unit during both inspiration and expiration confirm proper hookup (Figure 15-5).

11. Secure the chest tube to the chest wall with skin suture, using a suture on either side of the incision and wrapping the long ends of each suture around the tube several times in crisscross fashion (Figure 15-6). Apply an occlusive dressing with petrolatum gauze or petroleum jelly applied to sterile 4 × 4-in. gauze pads, and secure with tape in an H pattern (Figure 15-7).

12. Obtain a chest X-ray to document proper positioning of the tube and reinflation of the lung.

Figure 15-5

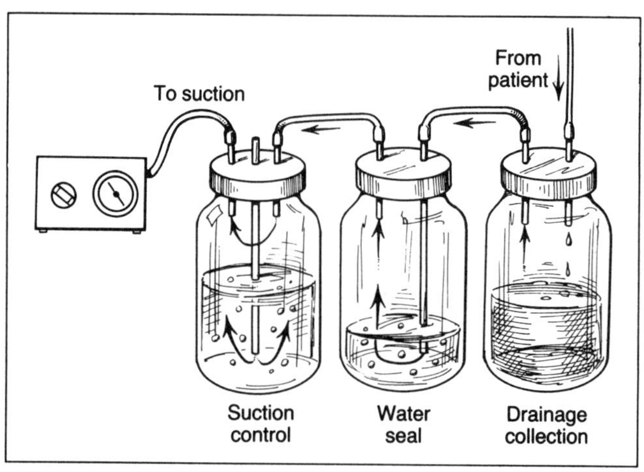

Figure 15-6

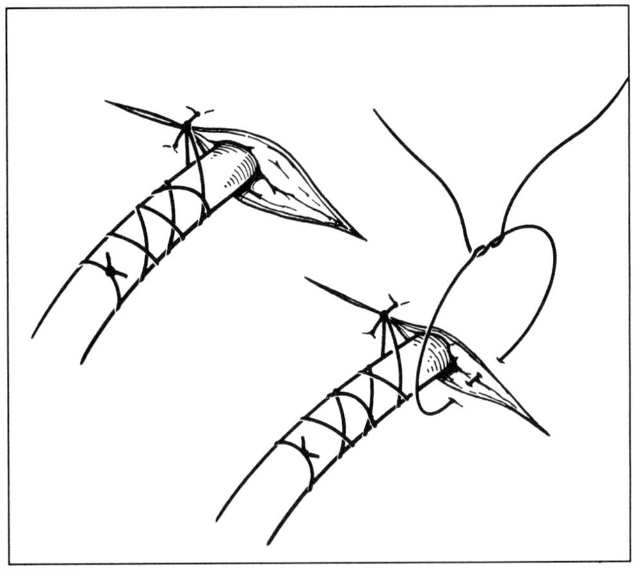

13. When the procedure is complete, the patient and drainage unit should be observed regularly. The drainage unit should bubble consistently in both phases of respiration. When the fluid drainage trap fills, the tube leading to the chest should be clamped and the unit emptied or replaced and reconnected. When therapy is complete, the tube should be carefully removed to avoid recurring pneumothorax.

Figure 15-7

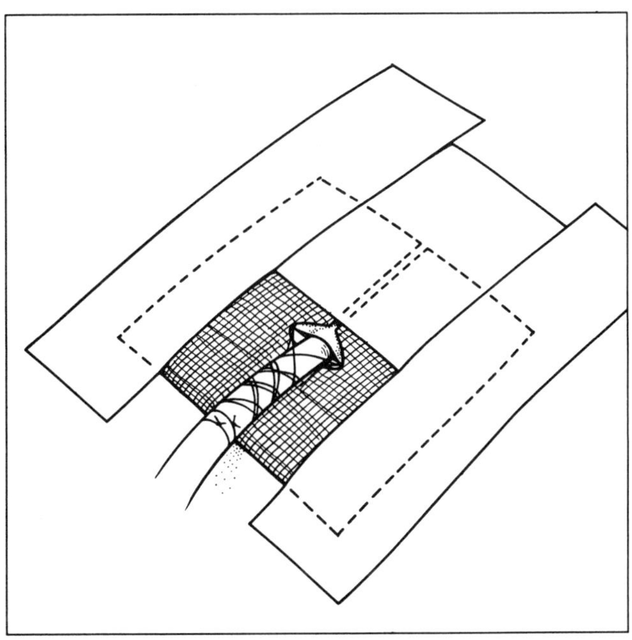

Chest Tube Removal

1. Premedicate the patient with an analgesic to lessen discomfort on withdrawal.
2. Remove all dressings, including the petrolatum occlusive dressing.
3. Prepare the skin near the chest tube with antiseptic solution.
4. Cut the anchoring suture, leaving the chest tube in place.
5. Be sure the patient is alert and cooperative before removing the tube. He must follow directions carefully.
6. Using folded sterile petrolatum gauze in double or triple thickness, place the gauze on the skin over the chest tube. Cover the superior aspect of the entry site.
7. Instruct the patient to take a maximum inspiration and not to exhale until told. During inspiration, quickly twist and remove the tube with one hand, and use the other hand to cover the wound with the petrolatum gauze pad. The patient may then exhale and breathe normally. Press down firmly with a slight circular motion to reapproximate the skin edges, and cover completely with the petrolatum occlusive dressing.
8. Cover the dressing with several thicknesses of sterile 4 × 4-in. gauze pads, and tape securely in place.
9. Using sterile scissors, cut off the distal 1-in. of the chest tube tip, and place it in a sterile culture tube for culture and susceptibility studies.
10. Obtain a chest X-ray study after the tube is removed.

Complications

NEEDLE DECOMPRESSION

- Local cellulitis
- Local hematoma
- Pleural infection
- Internal mammary artery laceration
- Pneumothorax

Note: Since this is usually a rapidly performed emergency procedure, it is easy to lose aseptic technique; prophylactic coverage with antibiotics may be indicated in these situations. Complications are infrequent.

CHEST TUBE INSERTION Any of the preceding, plus:

- Damage to an intercostal nerve, artery, or vein
- Damage to the internal mammary vessels if the puncture is too close to the sternum
- Intercostal myalgia

- Laceration or puncture of intrathoracic organs (heart, lungs, great vessels)
- Persistent pneumothorax with a large leak
- Subcutaneous emphysema
- Recurrent pneumothorax upon removal of the chest tube
- Penetration of diaphragm, liver, or spleen by too low an insertion.

Caution: The drainage system and underwater seal device should always be kept below the level of the chest to keep fluids from flowing back into the intraperitoneal space and predisposing the patient to empyema. Also, be sure that the chest tube does not clog with clots or material from the chest and that the tubing does not kink or disconnect. Most of the complications in this procedure are related to improper selection of a puncture site and failure to protect the drainage system.

Suggested Readings

Advanced Trauma Life Support Course Student Manual. Chicago, American College of Surgeons Committee on Trauma, 1984, pp 73-91.

Fishman NH: *Thoracic Drainage: A Manual of Procedures*. Chicago, Year Book Medical Pubs Inc, 1983, pp 32-37.

Kohn MS: Management of Chest Injuries. *Topics in Emergency Medicine* 1979;1:79-94.

Nussbaum MS: *The Mont Reid Handbook: University of Cincinnati Surgical Manual*. Chicago, Year Book Medical Pubs Inc, 1987, pp 526-532.

16

Tactile Orotracheal Intubation

John Littler, MD
Charles E. Driscoll, MD

Tactile orotracheal intubation is an important technique for airway control in an unconscious or paralyzed patient. It requires only a few seconds to perform and is easily mastered, particularly if you already know the more difficult technique of direct laryngoscopy.

Because airway control is the first and often most important step in the management of critically ill patients, several techniques are available to the physician for different situations. Standard options include the two nonsurgical techniques of endotracheal intubation by direct laryngoscopy and nasotracheal intubation, either blind or with direct laryngoscopy and the use of Magill forceps. The surgical options include cricothyroidotomy and tracheostomy. Percutaneous transtracheal ventilation is an invasive but nonsurgical option.

The greatest usefulness of tactile intubation is in an unconscious patient with significant facial trauma and potential or actual cervical spine injury—a setting that traditionally has called for a surgical airway. Orotracheal and nasotracheal intubation with direct laryngoscopy carry some risk because you must assume cervical spine injury. Facial trauma also suggests the possibility of basilar skull fracture; in such a case, blind nasotracheal intubation might result in inserting the tube into the cranial vault. Tactile orotracheal intubation, however, can be done in this setting without difficulty.

In addition, if the patient is not breathing spontaneously, blind nasotracheal intubation is extremely difficult. Percutaneous transtracheal ventilation can provide temporary ventilation but does not protect the airway from aspirating blood or secretions from the oropharynx. Tactile intubation is a good alternative and can be done with the appropriate cervical spine stabilization mechanisms in place, even before cervical spine X-ray, if necessary.

Tactile orotracheal intubation is also useful in patients who have short or obese necks that make laryngoscopy difficult and when secretions, blood, or other materials interfere with adequate visualization of such landmarks as the vocal cords.

Indications

- This technique can be performed safely only in unconscious or paralyzed patients.
- Standard indications for endotracheal intubation apply: a patient unable to protect his own airway, a need for prolonged ventilatory support and for an alternative route for administering medication, and a need to assure patency of the airway.
- In an unconscious patient with potential or actual cervical spine injury and significant facial trauma, this might be considered the nonsurgical procedure of choice.
- In any unconscious patient requiring airway control, this procedure can be either the last alternative before attempting a surgical airway or the first choice when an airway is needed very quickly or with a minimum of equipment.

Contraindications

- A conscious, unparalyzed patient because of the risk of biting injuries to the person doing the intubation.
- Significant anterior neck trauma suggesting the possibility of laryngeal fracture. This is a contraindication for all methods of endotracheal intubation; performing a tracheostomy is the procedure of choice.

Materials

Essential
- Endotracheal tube of appropriate size, as for direct laryngoscopy (a 7.5-mm tube for most adults)
- 10-mL syringe to inflate the tube cuff

Useful but not essential
- Stylet for the endotracheal tube
- Gloves
- Oral airway to use as a bite block

Additional (for maintaining the airway)
- Stethoscope to check tube placement
- Suction
- Tape for securing the tube

PROCEDURE

1. Select an endotracheal tube and insert a well-lubricated stylet, if available, bending the stylet into a gentle curve and inserting it about 1–2 cm proximal to the distal tip of the tube. Oxygenate the patient.

2. Stand or kneel near the patient's right shoulder, facing his head. Place the oral airway sideways in the left corner of his mouth to serve as a bite block if desired.
3. Insert the index and long fingers of your left hand into the patient's mouth, following the midline of the tongue back into the oropharynx until your long finger strikes the epiglottis. Let your hand slip into the right corner of the patient's mouth; this gives more room to manipulate the tube and helps you reach the epiglottis if you have short fingers.
4. Lift the epiglottis anteriorly, primarily with the long finger.
5. Insert the endotracheal tube, following the surface of the tongue, on the palmar side of your left hand. Use the radial side of your long finger and volar surface of your index finger to guide the tube (Figure 16-1). As it passes posterior to the epiglottis, shift the long finger to the posterior surface of the tube.
6. As the tube passes down the airway, apply pressure on the posterior aspect of the tube with index and long fingers to lift it anteriorly above the cords. When the tube is in the midline of the airway and above the cords, it usually passes easily through the glottic opening.
7. As you advance the tip of the tube into the larynx, it will distort the surface of the neck above the sternal notch. Withdraw the stylet at this point to minimize trauma to the anterior portion of the trachea, and insert the tube to about the 22-cm mark at the incisors.
8. Inflate the cuff, assess placement, and secure the tube in place. Auscultate the epigastric region, and palpate the sternal notch during inflation to help confirm placement (Figure 16-2).

Figure 16-1

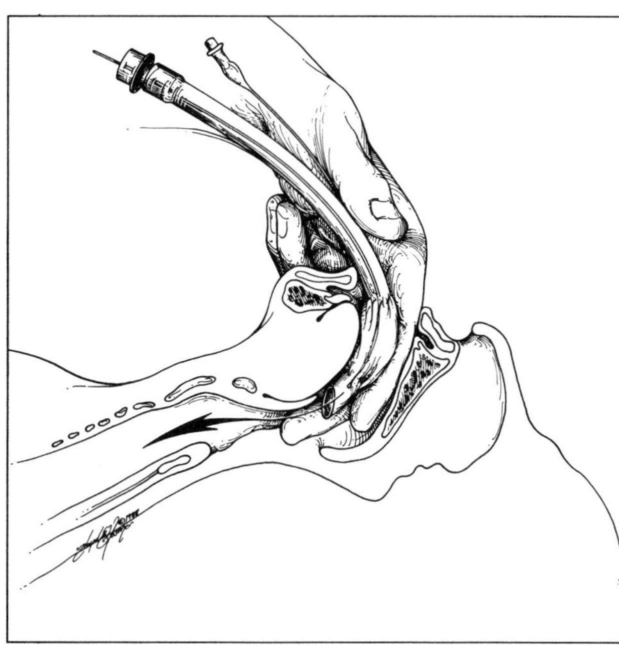

Figure 16-2

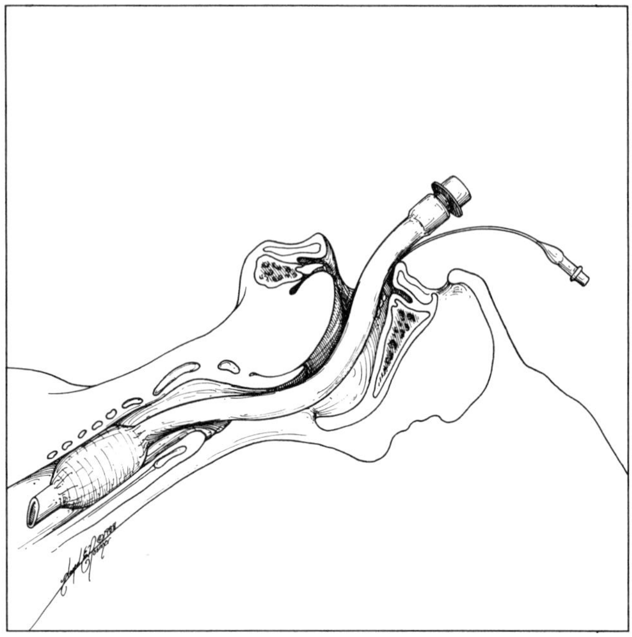

Note: Since this is a blind technique, assess results carefully, auscultating lung fields in the midaxillary lines and anteriorly at both apices.

Complications

- A biting injury to the practitioner, which is unique to this procedure. You can avoid this by using the technique only on unconscious or paralyzed patients or by using a bite block.
- Esophageal or piriform recess intubation because this is a blind technique. Pay careful attention to proper tube placement.
- Other possible complications shared with other methods of endotracheal intubation: airway trauma, hypoxia from prolonged attempts, and intubation of the right main-stem bronchus.

Suggested Readings

Rosen P, Baker FJ II, Barkin RM (eds): *Emergency Medicine: Concepts and Clinical Practice*. St. Louis, CV Mosby Company, 1988, pp 41-68.

Siddall WJ: Tactile orotracheal intubation. *Anaesthesia* 1966;21:221-222.

Stewart RD: Tactile orotracheal intubation. *Ann Emerg Med* 1984;13:175-178.

17

Arterial Puncture for Blood Gas Specimens

George C. Xakellis, MD

Indications

- To determine arterial PO_2, PCO_2, or pH
- To evaluate the oxygenation, ventilation, or acid-base status of patients with serious conditions that affect gas exchange or result in acid-base disturbance, such as respiratory failure
- To detect a change in clinical status in a patient who has a chronic condition that affects gas exchange or acid-base balance, such as chronic obstructive pulmonary disease
- To determine the need for home oxygen therapy, an assessment that can also be made by ear oximetry

Relative Contraindications

- Bleeding disorders
- Anticoagulant therapy
- Poor perfusion from the ulnar artery when the radial artery is the puncture site
- A possibility that thrombolytic therapy might be used

Materials

- 3-5-mL glass syringe
- 25-gauge needle
- 1 mL heparin (1,000 U/mL)
- Sterile gloves
- Antiseptic skin preparation such as povidone/iodine (Betadine)
- 1% lidocaine HCl (Xylocaine HCl) without epinephrine (optional)
- 3-mL syringe with 25-gauge needle for lidocaine
- Sterile 4 × 4-in. gauze pads
- Rubber stopper to cap syringe
- Bag of crushed ice

Patient Preparation

- Locate the puncture site. Recommended sites, in descending order of preference, are the radial, brachial, and femoral arteries.
- Do an Allen test to assess the adequacy of collateral circulation (Figures 17-1 and 17-2). Have the patient clench his or her fist to blanch the hand. Simultaneously compress both the radial and ulnar pulses, then have the patient release his fist. The palm of the hand should look pale. Release pressure on the ulnar artery. If perfusion from the ulnar artery alone is adequate, the hand will reperfuse in five seconds or less; if it takes longer than seven seconds, consider another site.
- Prepare the glass syringe with the 25-gauge needle attached by drawing up 1 mL of heparin. Rinse the barrel with heparin. Hold the syringe vertical, needle pointing up, and slowly eject air and heparin from the syringe. Enough heparin will remain to fill the dead space in the syringe. Be sure no air remains in the syringe.

Figure 17-1

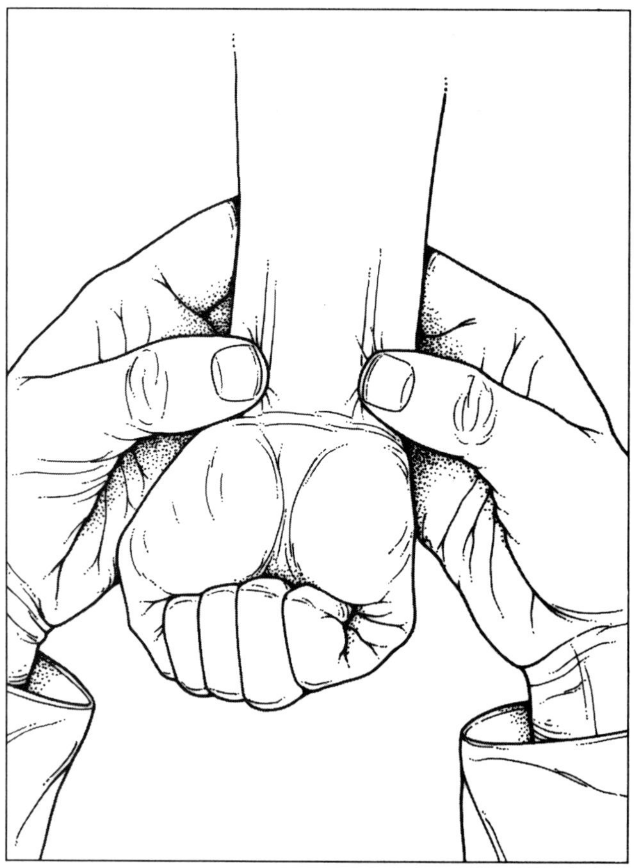

Figure 17-2

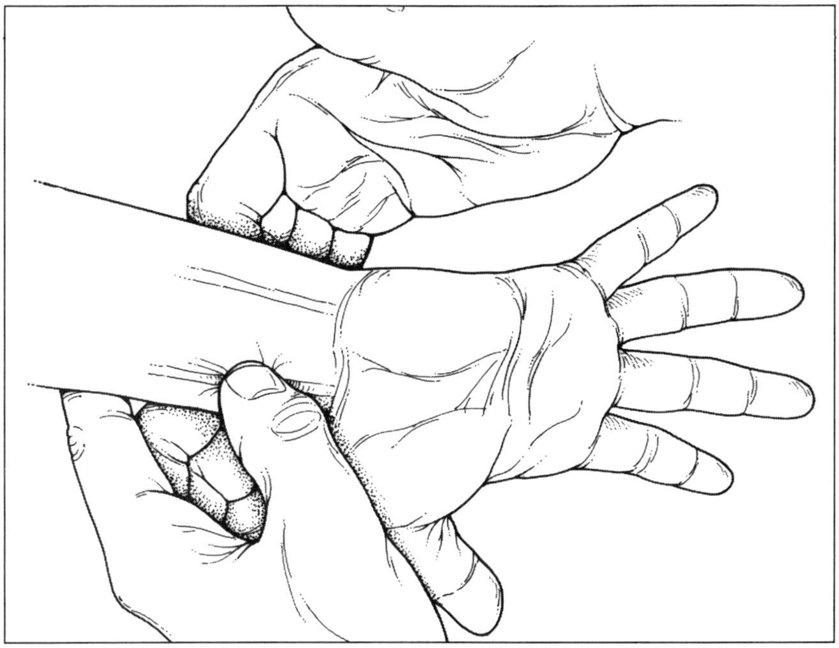

PROCEDURE

1. Have an assistant extend and hold the patient's wrist. Palpate the position of the radial pulse, which should be ½–1-in. proximal to the wrist crease.
2. Wearing sterile gloves, cleanse the site with povidone/iodine. Raise a skin wheal with a small amount of lidocaine (optional).
3. Palpate the patient's radial pulse with your left hand. While you are holding the heparinized syringe with your right hand (reverse hands in these directions if you are left-handed), puncture the skin at approximately a 60-degree angle, directing the needle toward the radial pulsation (Figure 17-3).
4. Slowly advance the needle until you obtain arterial puncture, noted by blood entering the syringe under arterial pressure.
5. Obtain 3 mL of blood.

Note: Do not aspirate. Depend on arterial pressure to produce the specimen.

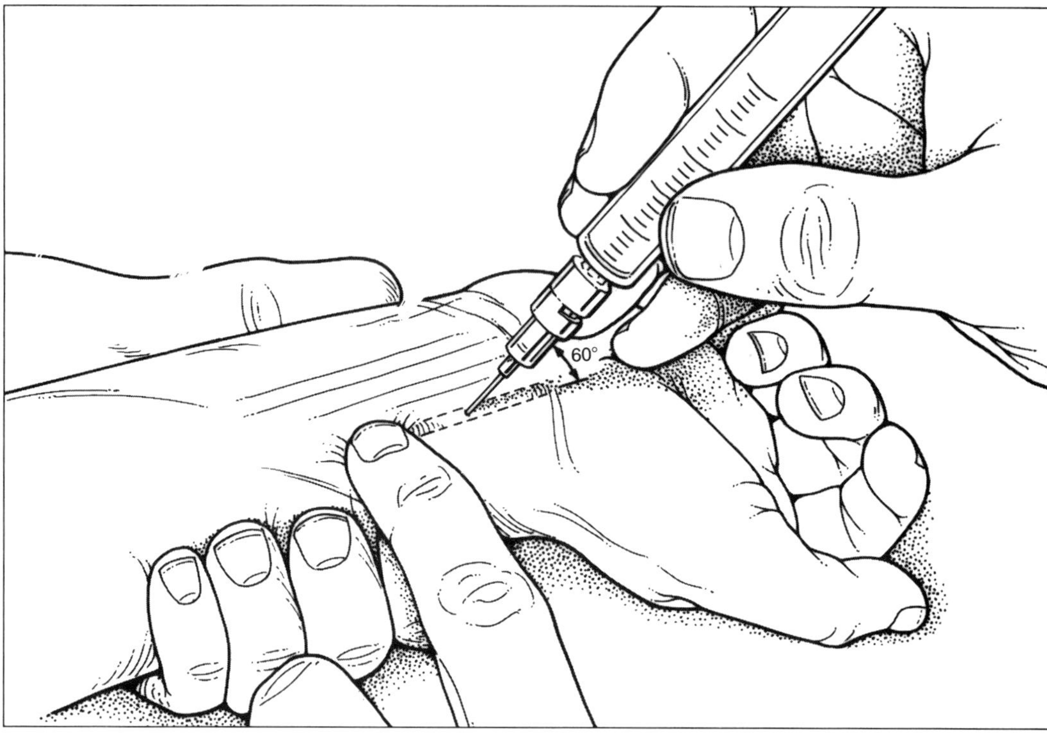

Figure 17-3

6. Withdraw the needle, and have your assistant immediately apply pressure to the site for 5–10 minutes using sterile 4 × 4-in. gauze pads. Be sure the assistant is wearing gloves.

7. Hold the syringe upright, and expel any air bubbles. Remove the needle from the syringe using precautions in accordance with your hospital's infection control policy. Cap the syringe with a rubber stopper, place the syringe on ice, and transport it immediately to the blood gas laboratory for analysis.

Complications

- Most common is hematoma at the puncture site.
- Bleeding, arterial thrombosis and occlusion, or infection may occur.
- The blood gas specimen may give inaccurate results if any air was left in the syringe, if too much heparin was in the syringe (heparin has an acid pH), or if there was too much delay between drawing and analyzing the specimen (leukocytes may metabolize the oxygen in the specimen and lower the PO_2).

Suggested Readings

Textbook of Advanced Cardiac Life Support. Dallas, Texas, American Heart Association, 1988.

Raffin TA: Indications for arterial blood gas analysis. *Ann Intern Med* 1986;105:390-398.

III

GASTROINTESTINAL PROCEDURES

18

Emergency Gastric Intubation

Richard W. Niska, MD

There are two diagnostic and three therapeutic reasons for performing gastric intubation on an emergency basis.

Indications

Diagnostic

- For blood in the stomach, to help diagnose a gastric or esophageal bleed.
- In suspected poisoning or overdosing with medication, to identify the ingested substance.

Therapeutic

- For symptomatic relief from vomiting in a patient to be hospitalized and for prevention of aspirating of vomitus into the lungs in a patient whose condition or position makes this likely, especially when the patient has a suspected neck fracture and must be immobilized.
- In lavage, to remove gastric contents, especially ingested poisons or excessive medications, or to instill iced saline to constrict bleeding vessels in gastric hemorrhage. Iced fluid lavage has also been reported as effective in the treatment of heatstroke, as it rapidly reduces the body's temperature.
- In decompression, to prevent gastric rupture during cardiopulmonary resuscitation (CPR) due to air pressure in the stomach or to improve the effectiveness of ventilation during CPR through the reduction of gastric distention and pressure on the lungs.

One other common indication, though seldom an emergency, is insertion of a soft, small lumen tube or intercatheter for feeding.

Contraindications

Base the decision to proceed with intubation on the patient's condition and the risk/benefit ratio involved.

- In patients with severe otolaryngologic or cranial trauma, the tube can be passed inadvertently into the cranial vault. Avoid this by visualizing the tube in the oropharynx, looking through the mouth.
- In esophageal varices or known prior esophageal trauma such as a corrosive burn, the inserted tube may further traumatize the esophagus and cause bleeding or perforation.

Materials

- For decompression: Levin tube (single lumen, with holes in the gastric end), size 10-16 French
- For aspiration of gastric contents: Sump tube (double lumen), size 18 French (Figure 18-1)
- For aspiration of large pills, capsules, or other semisolid materials: Ewald tube, size 26-36 French; use scissors to cut holes in this tube for maximum aspirating capacity if needed. For the conscious patient: diazepam (Valium) injectable
- General: 50-mL syringe with catheter tip; drinking water in a glass with a straw; lubricating jelly; adhesive tape; tincture of benzoin (optional)

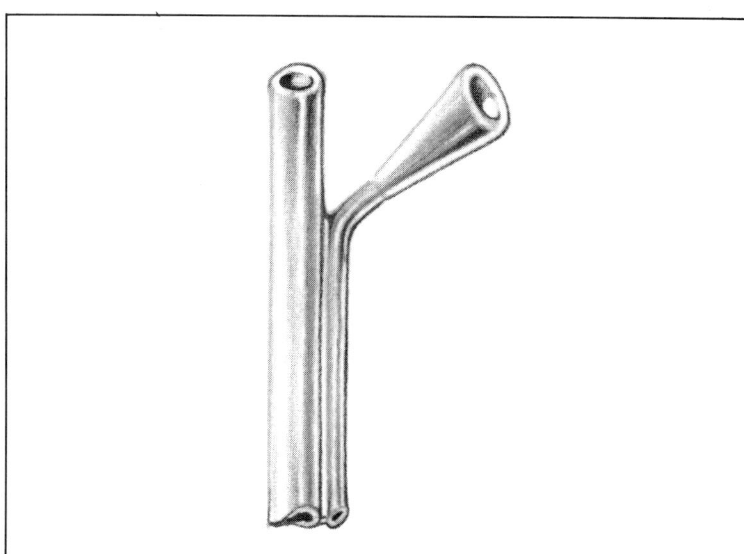

Figure 18-1 Sump tube (double lumen).

PROCEDURE

NASAL APPROACH This approach is most often used in conscious patients for decompression of the stomach or aspiration of stomach contents other than large pills or capsules.

1. Examine the nose for septal deviation and select the naris on the side away from deviation to afford more room for passage of the tube.
2. Have the patient sitting, with neck flexed. This places the esophagus, rather than the trachea, in a direct line from the oropharynx.
3. Lubricate the tube with lubricating jelly.
4. Advance the tube carefully along the floor of the nasal airway until it encounters the posterior nasopharynx.
5. Use firm, steady pressure against the nasopharynx to make the tip of the tube slide gradually downward along the pharyngeal wall (Figure 18-2).
6. At this point, have the patient swallow as you advance the tube fairly rapidly. Water sipped through a straw or administered through the tube may facilitate swallowing.

Note: The patient may regurgitate the tube into his or her mouth. If so, pull the tube back into the nasopharynx, recheck neck

Figure 18-2 Firm, steady pressure against the nasopharynx passes the tube downward along the pharyngeal wall.

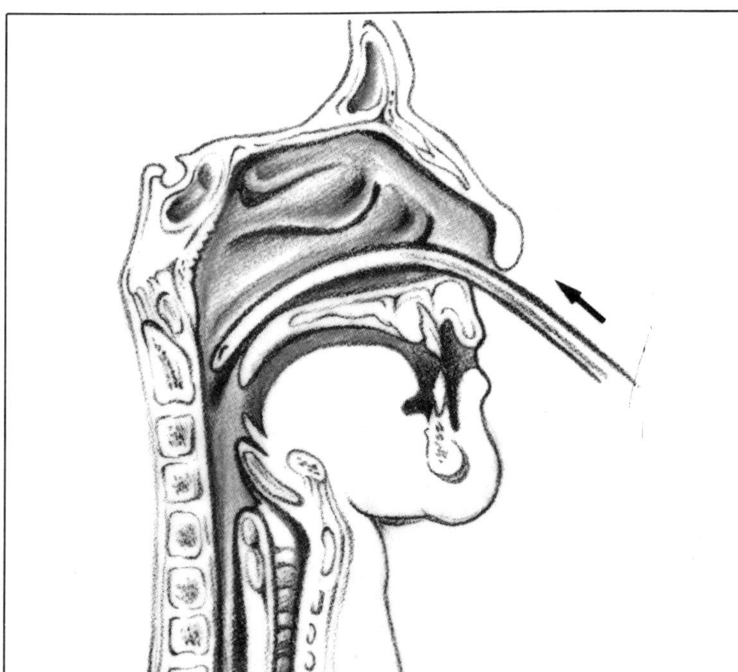

flexion, and try again. To avoid passing the tube into the trachea, advance it between the patient's respirations, when the epiglottis is closed.

7. Once the tube is in the esophagus, advance it until the tip is in the stomach. Inject air into the tube with a 50-mL syringe while auscultating over the epigastrium (Figure 18-3), the characteristic bubbling sound of air passing into the stomach will confirm that the tube is in the proper position.

ORAL APPROACH This method can be used in unconscious patients when nasal insertion is difficult or in conscious patients when very large-bore tubes must be passed for pill or capsule removal.

1. If the patient is conscious, sedate him with 5–15 mg diazepam IV, administered slowly, determining the dosage by his size and response. Watch for the respiratory depression and cardiac arrest that may occur as a result of injecting diazepam. Be prepared to control the airway or to institute CPR as needed.

2. Place the bite block that comes with the Ewald tube kit in the patient's mouth between the teeth (Figure 18-4).

3. Position the patient's head so that the neck is flexed.

4. Advance the lubricated tube into the oropharynx through the lumen of the bite block. Using the same technique as for nasogastric (NG) intubation, advance the tube into the stomach.

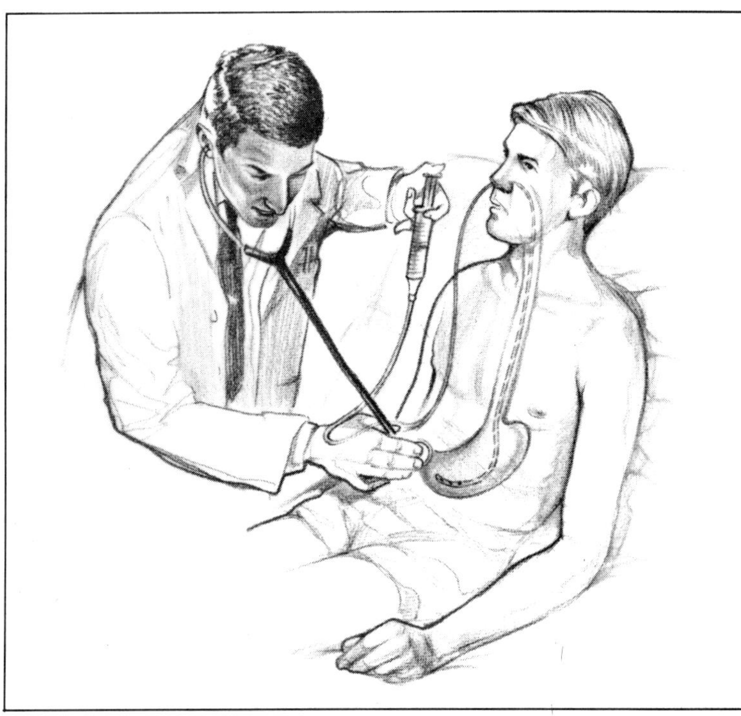

Figure 18-3 Air injected into a tube that has reached the stomach will make a bubbling sound over the epigastrium.

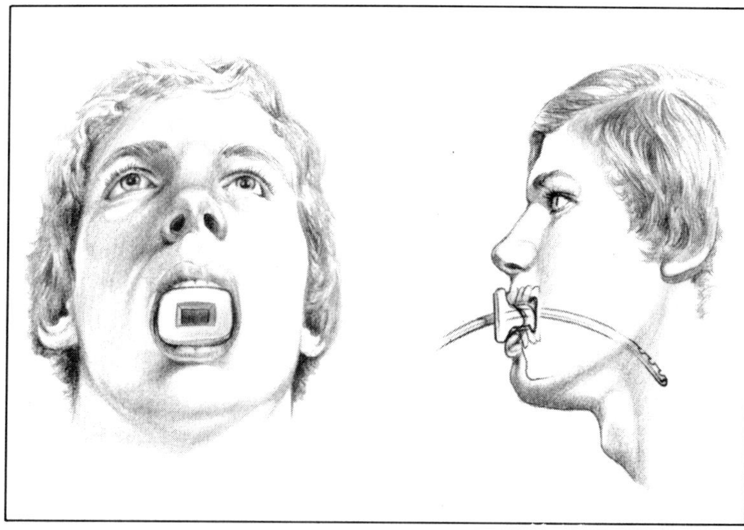

Figure 18-4 Bite block in place. Advance tube into the oropharynx through the lumen.

Taping

Fasten the NG tube to the patient's nose or cheek with tape. One method is to wrap a long piece of tape around the tube once, leaving two wings of tape that can be used to fasten the tube to the nose (Figure 18-5). Another method is to cut a wide piece of tape down the

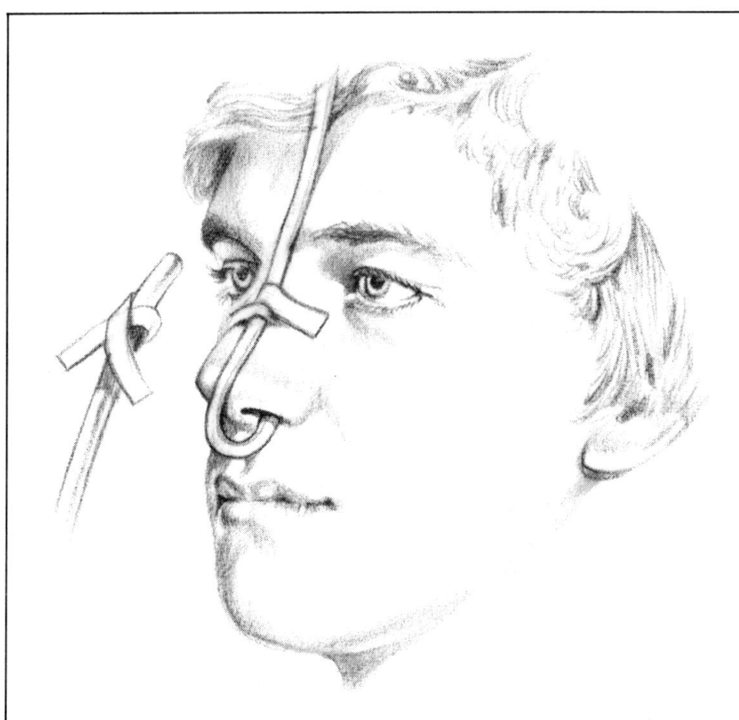

Figure 18-5 Insert is an example of one taping method. Wrap a length of tape once around the tube, with two wings of tape left hanging to fasten to nose.

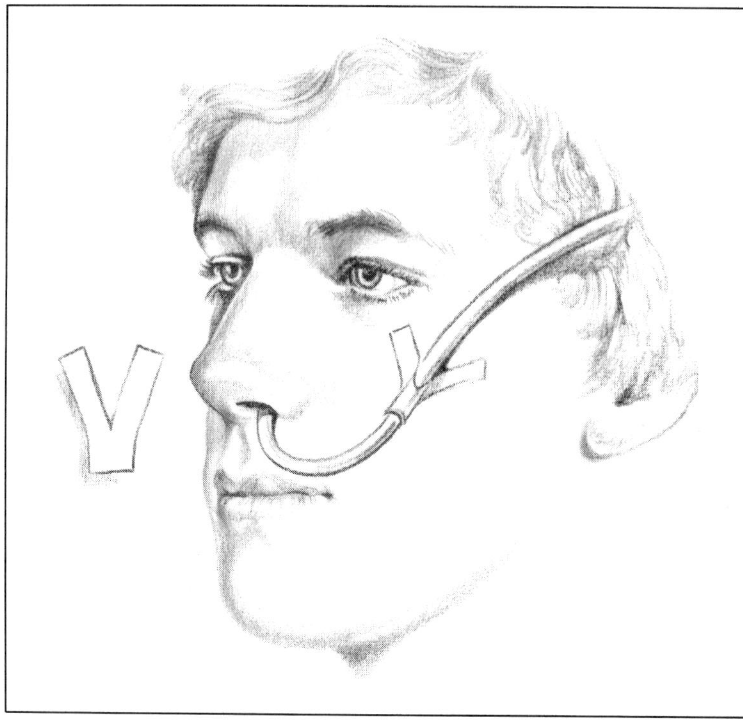

Figure 18-6 An alternative taping method. Split a wide piece of tape through the center, halfway down its length. Wrap the unslit half around the tube, and affix the flaps to the patient's cheek.

middle for half its length (Figure 18-6), wrap the uncut end around the tube, and use the split ends for taping to the patient's nose or cheek.

For security, add an extra piece of tape over each wing of tape to keep it down. If you have problems with the tape adhering, apply tincture of benzoin to the skin, and press the tape on when the benzoin has dried enough to be tacky.

Attachment

Connect the external end of the gastric tube to wall suction, syringe, or siphon apparatus as indicated. Whenever possible, use intermittent suction. This allows the tube to fall away from the gastric lining when suction is removed and prevents aspiration of gastric lining into the tube, thereby also helping prevent occlusion.

Complications

Although NG tube insertion is a safe, routine procedure, certain complications can arise, even when no specific contraindication exists.

ASPIRATION The tube may stimulate vomiting and secondary aspiration. In an obtunded patient without a gag reflex, the airway should be secured with an endotracheal tube, before passage of the NG tube. In a conscious patient, upright positioning will facilitate clearing of vomitus from the airway.

HEMATEMESIS AND PERFORATION Even in a patient with healthy esophageal and gastric mucosa, passage of an NG tube may traumatize these surfaces. In addition, suction applied to the tube may draw areas of gastric mucosa into the lumen, causing lacerations. A gentle technical approach is the key to minimizing these complications.

TRACHEAL INTUBATION The tube may pass anteriorly towards the trachea, in the hypopharynx, resulting in an inadvertent tracheal intubation. Recognizing the problem involves the obvious signs of cough and laryngospasm, as well as more subtle signs such as cyclic clouding of the lumen with respirations.

KINKING AND LODGING The tube may double back on itself in the pharynx or stomach and become lodged in the esophagus or nasopharynx on retrograde traction. Prevention of injury requires refraining from applying excessive force in removing a lodged tube. Esophagoscopy may be necessary to remove the tube safely. Nasopharyngeal kinks may be managed by oral visualization, grasping the tube with a Magill forceps, and bringing the kinked section out through the mouth.

DYSRHYTHMIAS Vagally mediated bradydysrhythmias, as well as adrenergically mediated ventricular ectopy, may occur as a result of NG intubation.

Suggested Readings

Askenasi R, Abramowicz M, Jeanmart J, et al: Esophageal perforation: An unusual complication of gastric lavage. *Ann Emerg Med* 1984;13:146.

Calvanese JC: Midesophageal kinking and lodgement of a 34-F gastric lavage tube. *Ann Emerg Med* 1985;14:1123-1126.

Syverud SA, Barker WJ, Amsterdam JT, et al: Iced gastric lavage for treatment of heatstroke: Efficacy in a canine model. *Ann Emerg Med* 1985;14:424-432.

19

Flexible Fiberoptic Sigmoidoscopy

Charles E. Driscoll, MD

Primary care physicians are using flexible fiberoptic sigmoidoscopy increasingly as the usual sites of colorectal cancer—the most common internal malignancy—shift. Not long ago, some 50% of bowel cancers were detectable by digital rectal examination. Today, only 10% are detectable this way because common sites of colon cancer have moved from the left toward the right side of the colon over the past two decades. Rigid sigmoidoscopy can theoretically detect up to 50% of colon cancers—those in the distal 25 cm. Yet rigid sigmoidoscopy generally reaches only 15–17 cm, decreasing the theoretical yield.

As colorectal cancer develops at more proximal levels, we must rely more on other detection methods such as occult blood testing, radiologic study using the air-contrast barium enema, and flexible fiberoptic sigmoidoscopy. The latter can extend the examination field to 77 cm and permit detection of 75% of large-bowel cancers.

Note: The technique can be learned easily but does require one-on-one training. Properly done, the procedure has an extremely low complication rate. Improperly done in a patient with a friable bowel, however, flexible sigmoidoscopy may be more likely to dispose toward perforation. Flexible sigmoidoscopes come in lengths of 35, 60, 65, 70, and 77 cm and range in price from $3,150 to $4,300, including light source and biopsy forceps. The longer (60–77 cm) scopes are preferred despite claims of the technique being easier with 35-cm models. Manipulating the scope during the first 35 cm of insertion is the most difficult part of the procedure; extending your view to 60–77 cm should produce no added difficulty or complications and generally increases the yield. Very few 35-mm scopes are now being sold.

Indications

The American Cancer Society recommends that every asymptomatic person have sigmoidoscopy at age 50, again one year later, and then every 3–5 years, assuming negative results from the first two examinations. In addition, flexible or rigid sigmoidoscopy is indicated in patients with any of the following conditions:

- Dark, tarry stools or bright red blood passed per rectum
- GI pain or cramping
- Change in bowel habits such as frequency, reduced stool caliber, constipation, or diarrhea
- Unexplained weight loss or anemia
- Positive fecal occult blood test
- A colorectal lesion discovered on X-ray
- Suspected foreign body

Routine periodic sigmoidoscopic examination is also recommended for patients with either a:

- Personal history of colorectal lesions such as cancer, polyps, or inflammatory bowel disease
- Family history of polyps or colorectal cancer

Contraindications

- Acute fulminating bowel disease

Note: While full insertion is contraindicated, the scope may be inserted safely as far as 15 cm.

- Acute diverticulitis with fever
- Suspected perforation of the bowel
- Paralytic ileus
- Peritonitis
- Severe cardiovascular disease or recent myocardial infarction
- Ischemic bowel disease
- Large aortic or iliac aneurysms
- Multiple abdominal surgeries and radiation therapy
- Suspected complete intestinal obstruction
- Toxic megacolon
- Prosthetic heart valves—unless the patient has received prophylactic antibiotics one hour before examination.

Note: Depending on the depth and ease of insertion, rigid sigmoidoscopy is sometimes permissible despite these conditions; digital examination is almost never contraindicated.

Materials

- Adjustable examining table; ideally proctologic
- Water-soluble lubricant
- Gloves

- Occult blood-test materials
- Anoscope
- Flexible fiberoptic sigmoidoscope with light source
- Suction machine
- Air and water sources; best when incorporated in the light source
- Biopsy forceps and brush
- Camera attachment or teaching head (optional)

Preparation

Inadequate bowel preparation is the most common cause of unsuccessful visualization of the colon. To ensure adequate preparation

- Have the patient take two sodium phosphate-type enemas (Fleet): one at two hours before the procedure, the other at one hour before, repeating enemas until evacuated fluid is clear.
- For patients who are inactive or have chronic constipation, order a clear liquid diet for 24 hours before the procedure, a bisacodyl suppository (Dulcolax, Fleet Bisacodyl, Theralax, etc.) at 3 PM the day before the procedure. In addition, 10 oz of citrate of magnesia may be given in the late afternoon of the day before.

PROCEDURE

1. Patient cooperation is mandatory. Have the patient on the examining table in a left lateral decubitis, Sims', or knee-chest position, or supine with the right leg flexed, whichever you prefer and the patient finds comfortable. In any but the knee-chest position, the patient's buttocks should be at the edge of the table nearer you.
2. With the patient positioned, insert a well-lubricated gloved finger into the rectum for digital examination, which helps relax the anal sphincter. Check for adequate bowel preparation and determine the exact direction of the rectum. Test any material on your glove for occult blood.
3. Perform anoscopy to visualize the distal 8 cm, an area difficult to inspect with a flexible sigmoidoscope.
4. Generously lubricate the anal opening and adjacent buttocks; also lubricate the distal 5–10 cm of the sigmoidoscope, taking care to avoid the lens.
5. Hold the control head of the sigmoidoscope in your left hand so the controls for suction, air, water, and tip deflection are at your fingertips. Use your right hand to advance and withdraw the shaft of the sigmoidoscope (Figure 19-1).
6. With the shaft in straight extension, insert the scope under direct visualization, always keeping the lumen in view. Insufflate minimal amounts of air to distend the bowel and allow visualization. Warn the patient not to strain against the instrument, and instruct him or her to report any significant discomfort during the procedure. (Pain is not

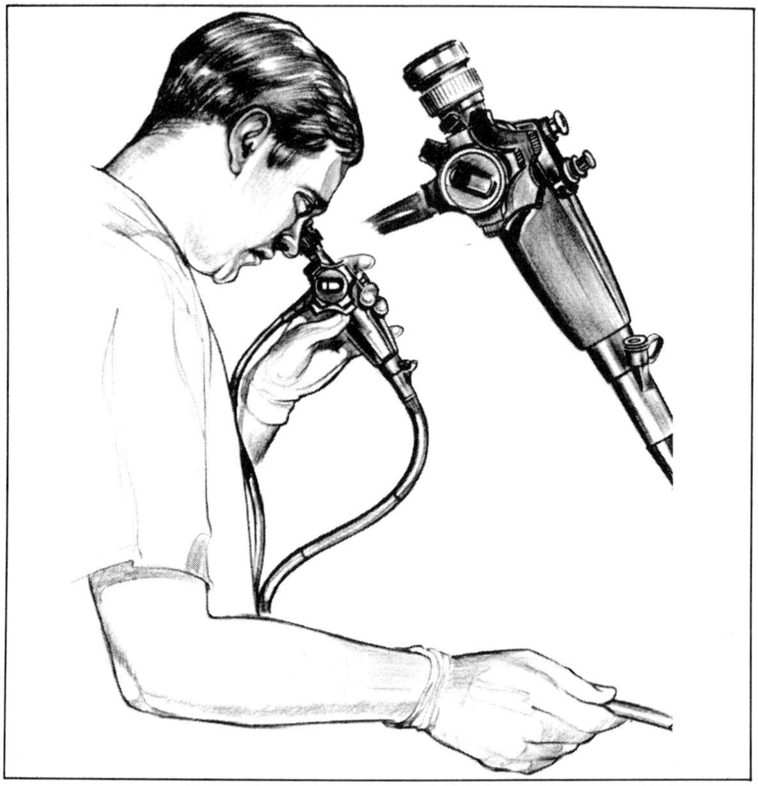

Figure 19-1 Insert is detail of scope head. Use the left hand to manipulate controls of sigmoidoscope, and the right hand to advance and withdraw the scope shaft.

customary with flexible sigmoidoscopy and may indicate too much pressure against the colon wall or too much stretching of the bowel on its peritoneal attachments. Aspirate air if the patient complains of cramping. If the patient at any point has extreme discomfort or intolerance, discontinue the insertion procedure.)

7. Stop just inside the rectum. Move the tip of the scope up and down until you completely visualize the posterior wall. If the lens becomes clouded or obscured by mucus or stool, squirt water over the lens to clear it, or use suction to clear thin mucus. In most scopes, the tip can be flexed 180 degrees, so you can look back to see the anal verge and entry of the scope through the anus. Reorient the scope and continue advancing it under direct visualization until you reach the recto-sigmoid junction (about 20–25 cm), where you must be prepared to negotiate a sharp angle.

As you continue the procedure, use "dithering" and "torquing" movements to advance the scope. Dithering is a smooth and gentle insertion of the instrument shaft 5–6 cm alternating with slow partial withdrawal—a jiggling motion that pleats the colon along the shaft and permits easier advancement. Torquing combines a clockwise or counterclockwise twist of the shaft with forward or backward motion.

This technique helps shorten turns of the colon and permits easier passage between the sigmoid and descending colon.

8. Negotiate the rectosigmoid fold by dithering and torquing or by hooking the fold with the tip of the scope and gently pulling. This straightens the rectosigmoid angle somewhat and facilitates entry into the sigmoid colon (Figures 19-2, 19-3, and 19-4). Study colon walls for arcuate shadows and bubbles of flatus to help you find and follow the lumen. Withdraw the scope slightly, and redirect it whenever you encounter any of the following:

- Resistance to movement of the scope. Make sure you can see the colonic mucosa sliding easily by the tip.
- "Redout"—a reddening that obscures your field of view. This indicates that you are pushing the tip of the scope against the bowel wall.
- Blanching of the colonic mucosa in your field of view. This indicates that you're putting the wall of the colon under too much pressure, which may lead to perforation. Also check for blind pouches indicative of diverticulosis; they may be large, and you can enter them inadvertently with the scope if you confuse them with the lumen. This can lead to excessive pressure, distension, and possibly perforation. Pouches usually have a slightly ovoid portal of entry and may contain stool.

9. There are landmarks and characteristics to help you as you advance the scope. You'll note the reticular pattern of blood vessels beneath the mucosa in the rectosigmoid area. Look for tubular folds in the sigmoid colon. Expect the descending colon to be pale pink because of its lack of prominent vascularity. While the rectosigmoid colon appears round to oval, the descending colon often appears slightly triangular.

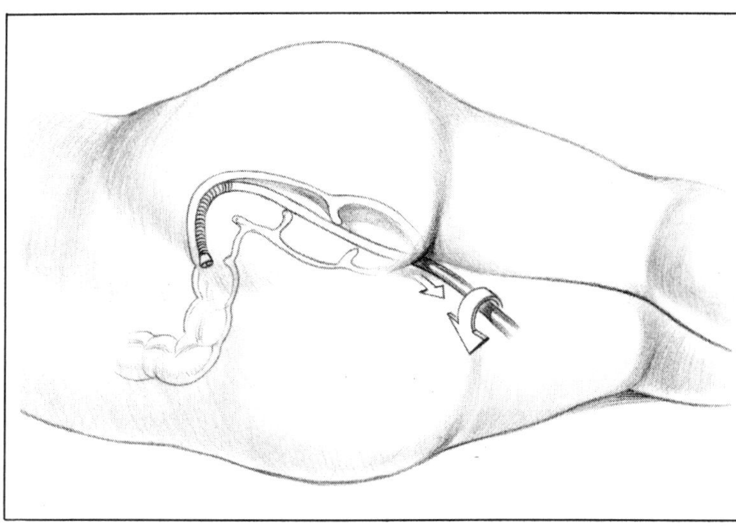

Figure 19-2 Arrows indicate direction of scope motion to advance. Note slight withdrawal with simultaneous downward rotation.

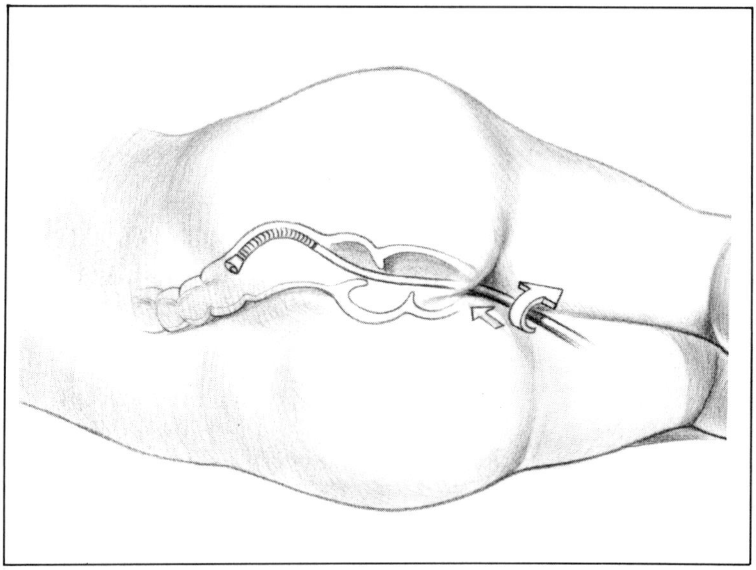

Figure 19-3 Immediately change direction by gently advancing scope while reversing rotation direction.

10. Torque the scope clockwise to help advance it into the sigmoid colon. Advance the scope through the sigmoid colon, which averages 35 cm in length, to the junction of the descending colon. If using a scope longer than 35 cm, advance it to full insertion in the descending colon, which is 20–30 cm long and relatively fixed to the left paracolic gutter.

11. Begin systematic examination of the colon as you gently withdraw the scope. When you encounter a fold, examine its hidden surface by gently hooking the edge of the fold with the flexible tip and allowing the colonic wall to straighten.

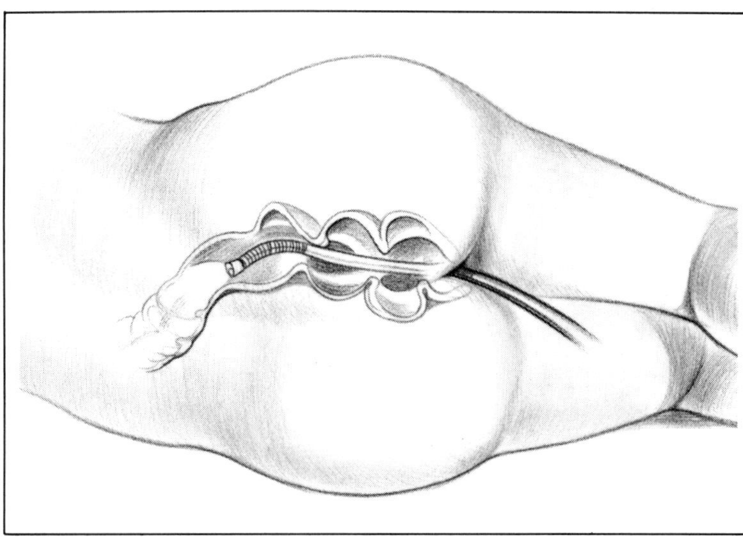

Figure 19-4 Scope has reached sigmoid colon.

12. As you withdraw the scope, do not try to evacuate large blood clots, fecal particles, or foreign objects such as kernels or seeds. Only thin mucus and secretion can be aspirated through the narrow suction channel. During scope withdrawal, use the sigmoidoscopic biopsy forceps or brush to perform a biopsy of any lesions or suspicious areas. This can help avoid a second intubation. Do not use cautery on any lesion unless a complete bowel preparation has been done because of the hazard of potentially explosive bowel gas that may be present. Just before removing the scope, aspirate all the air you introduced into the colon for visualization.

13. Carefully document in the patient's record all the findings of the examination, including the following:

- The indications for performing the examination
- Type and adequacy of bowel preparation
- Findings of digital and anoscopic examinations
- Insertion technique and ease of insertion
- Findings of full visual mucosal inspection
- Depth of scope insertion
- Anatomic site of lesion
- Appearance and depth of lesion
- Sites of biopsy or photographs
- Patient's tolerance of the procedure

Instrument Care

Clean the instrument promptly after each use before secretions dry out. Wash the shaft, suction and biopsy channels, and biopsy instruments in a solution of surgical soap; rinse alternately with a 30% alcohol solution and clean tap water. Do not immerse the ocular head of the scope or the controlling knobs and levers; wipe these parts clean with disinfecting alcohol. To disinfect the shaft of the scope, immerse the head. Gas sterilization is advisable following use in a patient with hepatitis or AIDS.

Suggested Readings

Eddy D: American Cancer Society: Guidelines for the Cancer-Related Checkup: Recommendations and Rationale. *Ca* 1980;30(4):194-240.

Hunt RH, Waye JD (eds): *Colonoscopy: Techniques, Clinical Practice, and Colour Atlas.* Chicago, Year Book Medical Pubs Inc, 1981.

Morgenstern L, Lee SE: Spatial distribution of colonic carcinoma. *Arch Surg* 1978;113:1142-1143.

Rodney WM, Felmar E: Flexible sigmoidoscopy: A "how-to" guide. *Your Patient and Cancer* 1984;4(2):57-66.

Shinya H: *Colonoscopy: Diagnosis and Treatment of Colonic Diseases.* New York, Igaku-Shoin Medical Publishers, 1982.

20

Rubber Band Ligation of Hemorrhoids

Timothy Appenheimer, MD

Although ligation of hemorrhoids predates Hippocrates, only in the past three decades have methods and technologies emerged that make it a practical and effective office treatment of internal hemorrhoids.

Recent studies suggest that hemorrhoids result from downward displacement of small masses of somewhat erectile tissue called anal cushions. These cushions represent congregations of the hemorrhoidal venous plexus. Usually three anal cushions are located just above the pectinate line; they are thought to facilitate complete anal closure. Straining at stool engorges these vascular cushions, and repeated straining may cause downward displacement, producing internal hemorrhoids. The downward displacement may be accompanied by discomfort and bright red bleeding from ruptured engorged capillaries. When an internal hemorrhoid is pushed outside the anal canal, it is said to be prolapsed.

Application of constricting elastic bands to mucosa overlying or just proximal to the internal hemorrhoid results in fibrosis that fixes the anal cushion in position and may decrease its vascularity. This relieves discomfort and bleeding while preserving the function of the anal cushion.

While hemorrhoids can cause discomfort and a great deal of anxiety, the mere presence of internal hemorrhoids, without signs or symptoms, does not justify intervention.

Indications

- Prolapse of internal hemorrhoids
- Persistent bleeding
- Rectal itching
- Fecal soiling

Contraindications

- Active local infection
- A history of inflammatory bowel disease, a clotting disorder, or chronic liver disease (in which case portal vein pressure may be increased)
- The presence of an anal fissure or other rectal pathology

Caution: Ligation is not the appropriate treatment for external hemorrhoids (those originating below the pectinate line). Sensitive dermal nerve endings in external hemorrhoid tissues make this procedure extremely painful.

Materials

- Anoscope (a fenestrated model of the Hinkel-James type is preferred)
- Water-soluble lubricant such as K-Y Lubricating Jelly or Surgilube
- Hemorrhoidal ligator (McGivney) with appropriate rubber bands (This is a modification of earlier instruments designed by Blaisdell and Barron.)
- Forceps (Allis, McGivney, or alligator)
- Hemostat
- Surgical scissors
- Adjustable proctologic table (optional)

PROCEDURE

Always have a barium enema study done, and perform or order flexible sigmoidoscopy before you make a firm decision to ligate. These precautions will allow you to rule out a lesion higher in the rectum, which could be obstructing venous return and causing the hemorrhoids to become symptomatic. Surgery in that setting would probably be the treatment of choice, obviating the need for ligation. The technique assumes adequate digital examination before ligation. Bowel preparation is seldom necessary, but the bowel should be emptied voluntarily or by phospho-soda enema (Fleet) before the procedure to avoid the need for defecation in the first 24 hours following ligation.

1. Load one or preferably two rubber bands onto the ligator by attaching the cone to the ligator ring and sliding the bands over the cone until they are seated on the ligator ring (Figure 20-1). Remove the cone. Two bands are suggested so that one would remain in place if the other should rupture.

2. Place the patient in the jackknife position on a proctologic table or in the knee-chest position on a standard examining table.

3. Apply lubricant to the fenestrated anoscope, and insert the scope. Remove the obturator and slowly withdraw the anoscope to identify

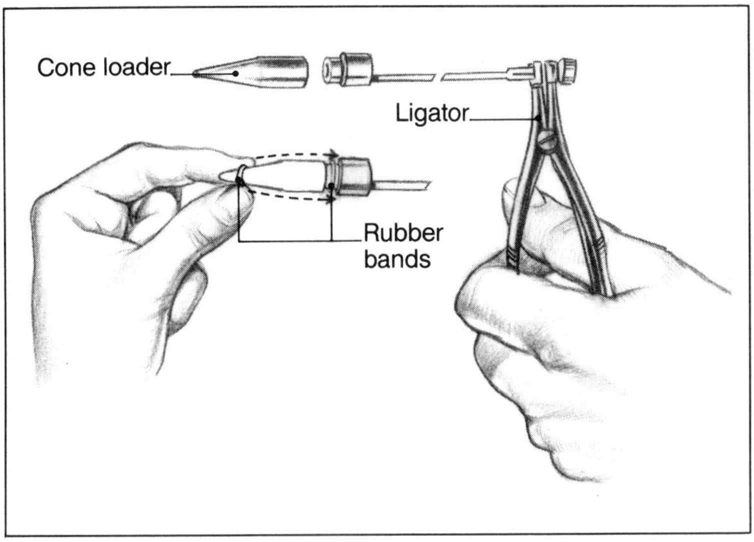

Figure 20-1 Attach cone to ligator ring and slide two rubber bands over the cone onto the ring. *Note:* Loading two rubber bands at a time provides a back-up should one of the bands break.

enlarged hemorrhoidal cushions. Normally, you'll find hemorrhoids in fields of redundant rectal mucosa. Identify the most prominent hemorrhoid.

4. Remove the anoscope, replace the obturator, and reinsert the anoscope with the fenestration in the direction of the most prominent hemorrhoid.

5. Again slowly withdraw until redundant hemorrhoidal mucosa protrudes into the anoscope. Have the patient perform Valsalva's maneuver to make the protrusion more pronounced.

6. With an assistant holding the anoscope in position, place the loaded ligator ring over the bulging mucosa. Insert forceps through the ring and gently grasp the leading portion of mucosa (Figure 20-2). If the patient feels marked pain at this point, the tissue is probably below the pectinate line. Discontinue the procedure.

7. If the patient feels little or no pain, pull the mucosal protrusion through the ligator ring.

8. Carefully push the ligator ring against the rectal wall and relax traction on the hemorrhoid to protect the rectal mucosa against the sudden shearing force exerted at the base of the hemorrhoid when you release the bands.

9. Squeeze the ligator handle to release the rubber bands onto the base of the mucosal mass (Figure 20-3), and remove forceps, ligator, and anoscope.

Complications

- When rubber band ligation is done properly, most patients experience very little rectal discomfort. Pain immediately following the procedure indicates poor placement of the rubber bands and

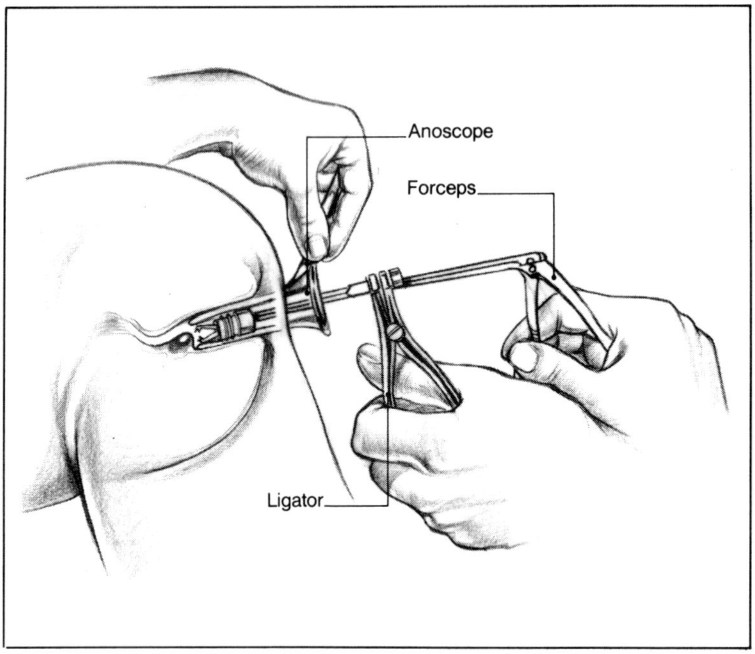

Figure 20-2 Have an assistant hold the anoscope in position. Insert forceps through the ligator ring and grasp the mucosal bulge.

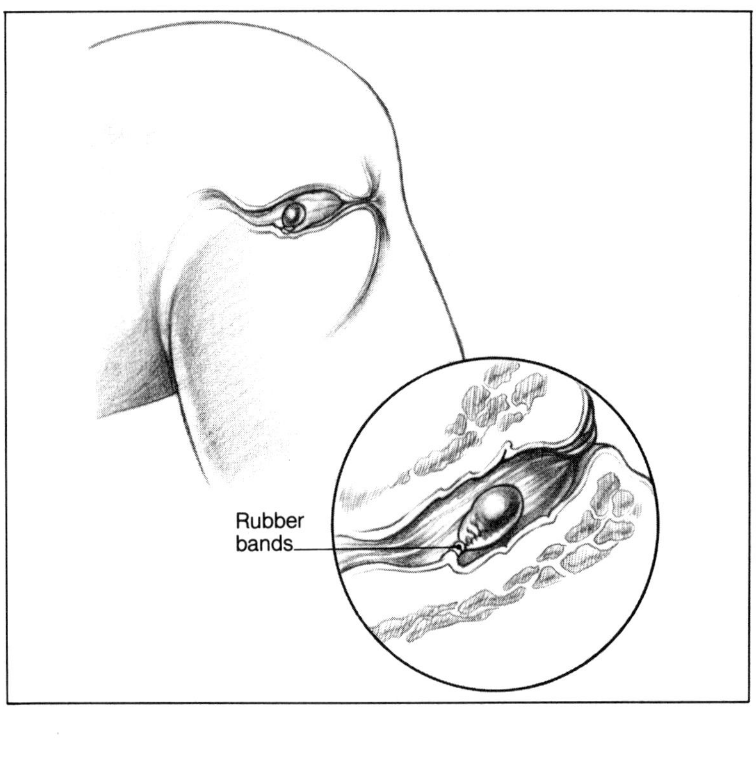

Figure 20-3 Squeeze the ligator handle to release a rubber band onto the base of the mucosal mass.

prompts removal, using a hemostat and surgical scissors as needed.

- If the patient has pain that begins after he or she leaves your office, recommend a nonprescription analgesic. Instruct the patient to phone again if this fails to provide relief. Persistent pain can indicate infection, sphincter spasm, or perianal hematoma, and always warrants reexamination.
- Be sure to alert the patient to the light bleeding or mucus discharge he will probably experience 4–8 days after the ligation. Assure him that this is the normal process of events, as the necrotic tissue separates from the rectal wall.

Follow-up Care

- Patient education is key in preventing further hemorrhoidal development. Advise the patient that hemorrhoids are likely to recur if constipation continues. Emphasize the importance of adequate dietary fiber intake, and supplement the diet with psyllium-containing bulking agents such as Metamucil or Syllact if necessary.
- Most patients remain ambulatory after the procedure and can return to work the same day. It is not unusual for a patient to require two or more rubber band ligation procedures for complete relief of symptoms. After you treat the most prominent hemorrhoid at the first visit, others may later become more symptomatic. Schedule a follow-up examination at 2–3 weeks to determine whether additional ligation will be necessary.
- While some experienced operators routinely band two separate hemorrhoid sites 180 degrees apart during a single ligation session, you will probably have better results and certainly better patient tolerance if you treat one hemorrhoid at a time. If symptoms persist, three or four repeat procedures at four-week intervals may be needed.
- Patient satisfaction after ligation is about 88–92%, only slightly less than after surgical hemorrhoidectomy.

Suggested Readings

Alexander-Williams J, Crapp AR: Conservative management of hemorrhoids. Part I: Injection, freezing and ligation. *Clin Gastroenterol* 1975;4:595-618.

Dennison AR, Wherry DC, Morris DL: Hemorrhoids: Nonoperative management. *Surg Clin North Am* 1988;68:1401-1409.

Smith LE: Hemorrhoids: A review of current techniques of management. *Gastroenterol Clin North Am* 1987;16:76-91.

21

Paracentesis and Peritoneal Lavage

Leslie E. Weber, MD

Abdominal paracentesis is simple, safe, and easy to perform. It provides useful diagnostic information as well as therapeutic results. Concomitant peritoneal lavage, which has largely replaced the four-quadrant abdominal tap, increases the accuracy of the information obtained.

Indications

- To evaluate the need for emergency laparotomy in a trauma patient, particularly when he or she was known to have sustained a blunt blow to the abdomen.
- To assess trauma victims for other abdominal calamities, such as a possible splenic rupture.
- To help determine the cause of ascites and relieve its discomfort by removing fluid.

Note: Avoid frequent therapeutic paracentesis because fluid generally tends to reaccumulate rapidly.

- To help assess the conditions of pancreatitis or peritonitis. In such cases, the concomitant use of peritoneal lavage may provide some relief. For a simple diagnostic tap, 0.9% NaCl (normal saline) is good. Otherwise use a specifically balanced electrolyte solution containing 15 g/L of glucose, 500 USP units of heparin, 1 g kanamycin sulfate (Kantrex, Klebcil), and 100,000 USP units of bacitracin in normal saline, sufficient to make 1,000 mL of lavage fluid.

Contraindications

- Cellulitis of the anterior abdominal wall
- A bleeding disorder or coagulopathy emergencies

Note: In an emergency, patients with a mild to moderate bleeding tendency can be tapped using great caution.

Relative Contraindications

- Scars from a previous laparotomy or abdominal surgery that may have caused adhesion of an underlying bowel loop
- An enlarged liver or spleen that extends into the lower quadrants
- A large, distended urinary bladder

Materials

- Sterile gloves
- Povidone-iodine (Betadine) antiseptic solution
- Sterile drape (optional)
- 5- or 10-mL syringe
- 2-in., 21-gauge needle
- 2% lidocaine HCl (Xylocaine HCl) with or without epinephrine, 2–3 mL
- 50-mL disposable syringe
- Short-bevel, 2-in., 14-gauge needle with stylus
- Sterile 16-gauge polyethylene intraluminal catheter, identical to that used for subclavian puncture
- 1,000 mL normal saline solution (500 mL for patients 50 kg [110 lb] and under)
- 1,000 mL electrolyte solution containing 15 g/L of glucose, 500 USP units of heparin, 1 g kanamycin sulfate (Kantrex, Klebcil), and 100,000 USP units of bacitracin in normal saline
- Specimen tubes
- Gauze pads

PROCEDURE

1. Empty the patient's bladder, by catheterization if necessary, and place him or her supine, with the head of the examining table or bed slightly elevated. Prepare the skin with povidone-iodine solution. Drape the patient if you choose.

2. At a site in the middle about 3 cm (1¼ in.) below the umbilicus, use the 2-in., 21-gauge needle and the 5- or 10-mL syringe to infiltrate the skin with 1–2 mL of 2% lidocaine. Advance the needle to the peritoneum and inject an additional 1 mL of lidocaine.

3. With the stylus in place, insert the 2-in., 14-gauge needle perpendicular to the skin. Advance it up to the hub. If you are concerned about an undue amount of pressure within the abdomen, a Z-track insertion technique can lessen the likelihood of leakage once the procedure is completed. To do this, advance the needle a layer at a time, sliding the tissue as you go. You will often sense a pop as you penetrate the peritoneum. If ascites is present, entry is confirmed by aspiration of ascitic fluid (Figure 21-1).

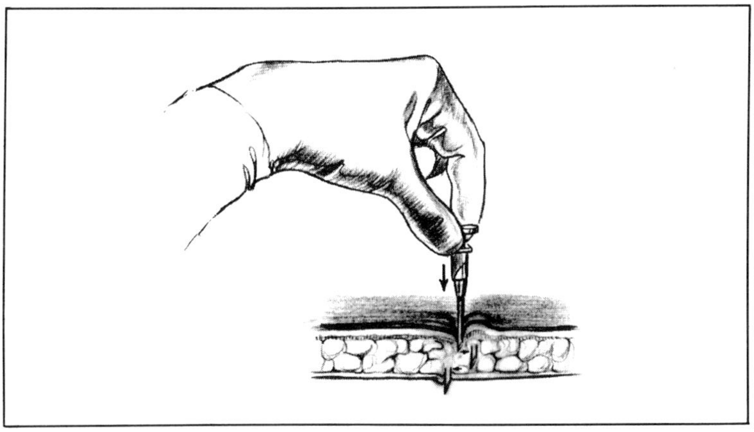

Figure 21-1 With stylus in place, needle is inserted perpendicular to the skin and advanced to the hub. Often there will be a "popping" sensation as you penetrate the peritoneum. If ascites is present, there will be fluid return.

4. Remove the stylus, attach the 50-mL syringe, and aspirate. If you withdraw frank blood, consider the finding positive for significant intra-abdominal injury, and stop the procedure. The patient will need immediate laparotomy. If ascitic fluid is present, you can remove it. But do so cautiously: The removal of more than 1,000 mL of fluid may precipitate hypotension.
5. If you have no return, proceed with lavage. Disconnect the syringe, insert the catheter through the needle (Figure 21-2), and remove the needle (Figure 21-3).
6. Connect the catheter to the bottle of lavage fluid. Elevate the bottle, and allow the solution to run rapidly, wide open, into the peritoneal cavity (Figure 21-4).
7. When the bottle is empty, place it on the floor, and allow it to refill with solution. You may rock the patient slightly from side to side to facilitate the flow (Figure 21-5).

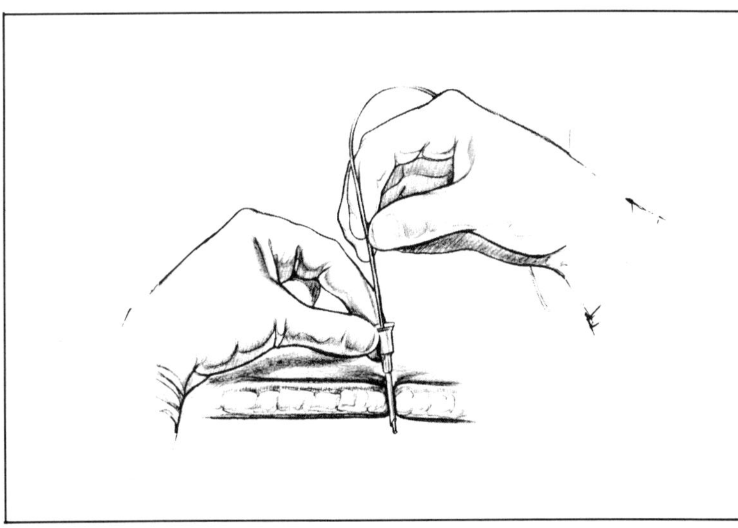

Figure 21-2 To proceed with lavage, disconnect the syringe and pass catheter through the needle.

Figure 21-3 With catheter in place, remove the needle.

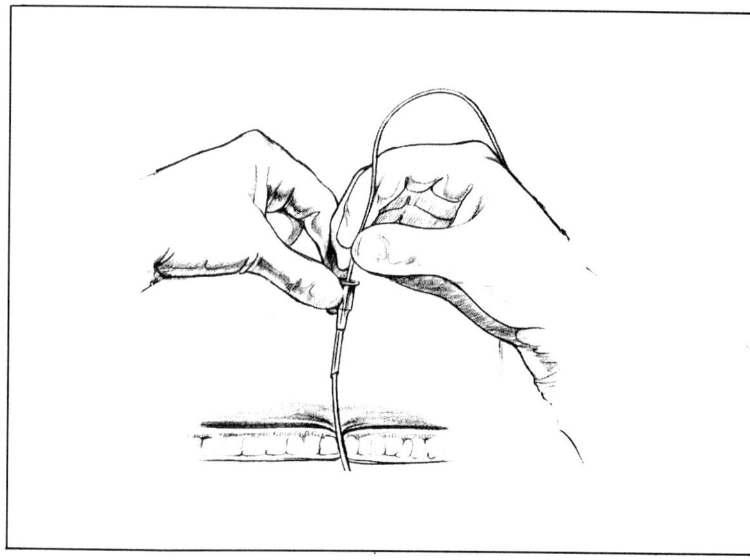

Figure 21-4 Connect catheter to bottle of saline and elevate bottle. Allow solution to run rapidly into peritoneal cavity.

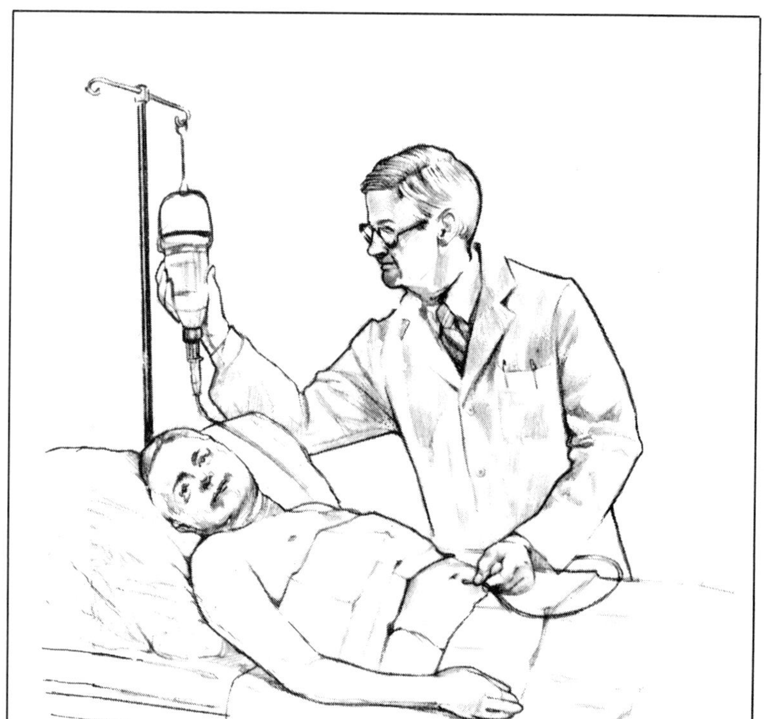

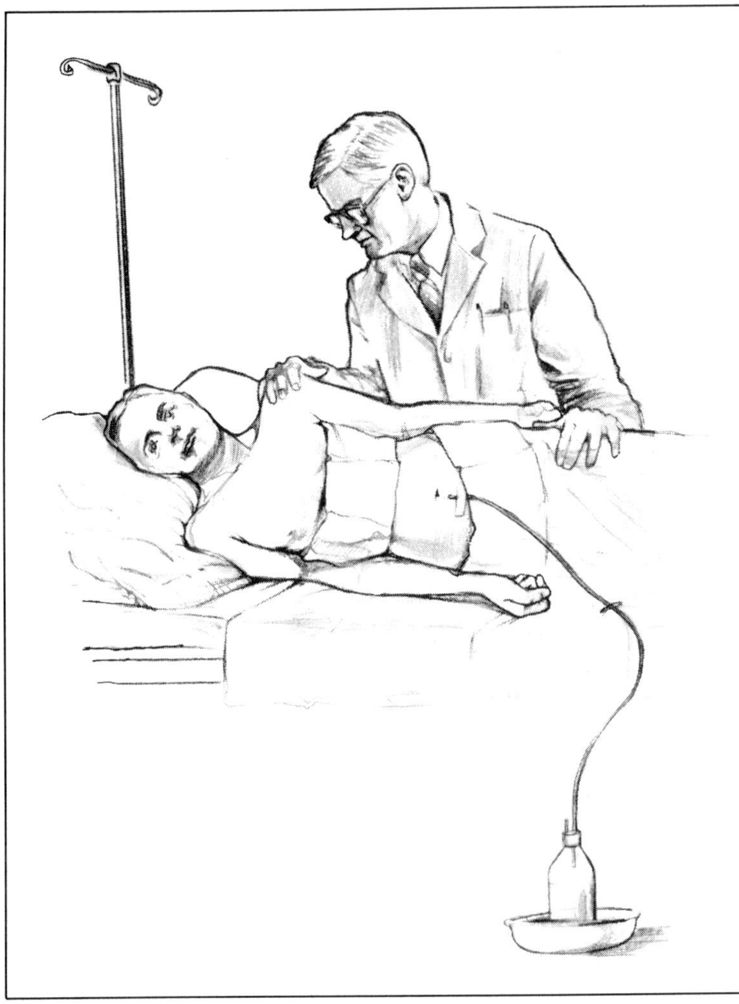

Figure 21-5 Place the empty bottle on the floor to allow the fluid to drain out. Gently rocking the patient from side to side facilitates flow.

8. While the fluid is draining, disconnect the tubing momentarily, and allow some fluid to run onto a white gauze square to see more clearly whether it is blood tinged. This technique lets you detect as little as 0.25 mL of blood; a light pink tint is a positive result.
9. Consider obtaining specimens of the returned fluid for analysis, especially in nonemergency situations. In most abdominal trauma patients, visual examination of the returned fluid is sufficient for initial therapeutic decisions. If you suspect pancreatic trauma, you may choose to analyze the amylase level.
10. Remove the catheter, and cover the skin wound with an adhesive bandage. Virtually all such wounds are self-healing and require no pressure.
11. Observe the patient for hypotension, fever, chills, and abdominal distention or tenderness.

Laboratory Results

- *If the patient has sustained blunt trauma* and the extent of damage is uncertain, an RBC count greater than 100,000 μL or a WBC count greater than 500 μL in the fluid indicates significant injury and the need for immediate laparotomy. With lower counts, you may treat and follow up conservatively.
- *If you suspect pancreatitis*, order a peritoneal fluid amylase level for comparison with the serum amylase level. Peritoneal values several times higher than serum levels are strong evidence of pancreatitis. Unlike serum levels, which often fall quickly after the onset of acute pancreatitis, peritoneal fluid amylase levels tend to remain elevated for several days. This distinction is particularly helpful when serum levels are only slightly elevated.
- *If you suspect peritonitis*, obtain a Gram's stain and culture of the fluid.
- *If ascites is present,* examine the fluid for albumin. Determine the gradient between serum and ascitic fluid by subtracting the ascitic fluid albumin level from the serum level. About 90% of patients with chronic liver disease have gradients of 1 g/dL or more. With a lesser value, portal hypertension is unlikely: The fluid probably arises from an exudative peritoneal lesion.

A cell block can be performed on a centrifuged specimen of ascitic fluid. This specimen should consist of 100 mL or more and can be useful to determine the presence of a malignancy.

Also obtain a WBC count and differential, Wright's stain, Gram's stain, and culture. In some cases, you may also want amylase values and a determination for carcinoembryonic antigen.

Complications

Peritonitis related to the procedure has not been reported. Although other complictions are rare, these are the ones you may find:

- Bowel perforation, especially if the bowel is fixed by adhesion from a previous laparotomy. The perforation almost always heals itself when you withdraw the needle. Leakage is infrequent.
- Bleeding from the puncture site, which can be controlled by applying pressure.
- Bleeding from laceration of an epigastric vessel, which is not likely if you introduce the needle as described: in the midline, below the umbilicus.

Suggested Readings

Bayless TM (ed): *Current Therapy in Gastroenterology and Liver Disease*, 1984-1985. St Louis, CV Mosby Co, 1984, pp 476-477.

Hill GJ II: *Outpatient Surgery*, ed 2. Philadelphia, WB Saunders Co, 1980, pp 105-107.

Ismail A, El Kafafy S, El Kafor AA: The role of peritoneal lavage in diagnosis of abdominal emergencies. *Br J Clin Pract* 1984;38:125-129.

Olsen WR, Hildreth DH: Abdominal paracentesis and peritoneal lavage in blunt abdominal trauma. *J Trauma* 1971;11:824-829.

22

Digital Removal of Fecal Impaction

Holly Hendrickson, MD

Constipation—both straining at stool and less frequent bowel movements—may reflect normal aging, or it may signal a pathologic process such as colon cancer or hypothyroidism. Delay or inhibition of defecation results in stool accumulation in the rectum; when water is extracted, the stool dries; and if the patient is unable to evacuate, impaction occurs.

Fecal impaction must be removed, and the condition is often difficult to recognize. Patients at high risk are those with a history of constipation and impaction. Among the signs and symptoms you may note are abdominal distention, pain, anorexia, nausea, or vomiting. Paradoxical diarrhea and fecal incontinence can occur when liquid mucus and stool seep around the impaction; these patients may also experience urinary retention or incontinence. Low-grade fever, tachypnea, and dysrhythmias may occur, as well as mild leukocytosis, hyponatremia, or hypokalemia. The condition often appears in elderly patients who are confused or agitated. Psychosis and dementia may contribute by preventing patients from following their own urge to defecate or to communicate.

Many medications can cause decreased colonic motility, leading to impaction. Narcotics, tricyclic antidepressants, other anticholinergic drugs, iron, and calcium supplements are often implicated. Long-term use of laxatives, of course, frequently results in laxative dependence.

Immobility, lack of exercise, and a diet low in fiber and fluids contribute to constipation, as can autonomic neuropathy from diabetes. Stroke, multiple sclerosis, Parkinson's disease, and spinal cord lesions can also lead to constipation by requiring anticholinergic medications or by impairing bowel function. Colonic polyps or tumors can obstruct stool; and anal canal fissures and hemorrhoids may cause patients to delay defecation. Such a practical matter as attempting to use a bedpan or toilet that is too high can also contribute to the problem.

To diagnose fecal impaction, do a rectal examination. If you find a hard stool, digital removal is indicated. An X-ray study of the abdomen will reveal stool in the colon and sometimes air-fluid levels in the small bowel. If the rectal vault is empty while obstructive signs are present, the patient may have a high impaction or another process such as tumor, ruptured abdominal viscus, or infection.

Indications

- Hard stool in the rectal vault
- The patient cannot pass the stool on his or her own

Contraindication

- An unstable patient, such as one with acute chest pain, pulmonary edema, or delirium

Relative Contraindications

Extra care is needed to avoid mucosal injury in patients with such problems as these:

- Recent colorectal surgery with fresh wounds and anastomoses
- Friable bowel wall from prostate or colon malignancy
- Inflammatory bowel disease

Preparation

- Mineral oil retention enema. Use 115 mL, and ask the patient to retain 20–30 minutes if possible. If the patient cannot do this, insert with a Foley catheter, and blow up the balloon to hold the enema fluid in.
- Alternatively, have the patient take 30 mL mineral oil orally every hour until oil begins to seep out of the rectum (24–48 hours). Administer while the patient is awake, and up to two hours before he goes to bed.

  Note: Do not use mineral oil in patients at risk of aspiration.
- In a highly anxious patient, premedication with a narcotic may be helpful before trying the digital procedure.
- Explain the procedure to the patient. Have him lie on his left side with the right leg flexed and a protective pad under the buttocks. Drape the patient for comfort and privacy.

Materials

- Gloves
- Lidocaine HCl 2% jelly (Xylocaine 2% Jelly)
- Protective pad
- Bedpan or basin to hold stool fragments

PROCEDURE

1. Apply 1–2 mL lidocaine jelly to the gloved index finger; then apply jelly to the anus and the anal canal as far as the finger can reach.
2. Wait five minutes for anesthesia, reinsert the finger, and use a circular motion to help the anus relax. Keep the finger inserted.
3. Insert the middle finger alongside the index finger, moving slowly to allow the anal sphincter to relax. Using a scissoring action with the fingers, slice the stool into smaller pieces. Remove them one at a time. Work up and around the mass as well as into it until the bulk of the stool is gone.
4. Administer one or two tap water enemas to evacuate the bowel completely.
5. Wash and dry the anal area, and instruct the patient to drink plenty of fluids.

Complications

- Bleeding. This should not occur if the stool is well lubricated with mineral oil or lidocaine jelly.
- Shortness of breath or chest pain. Stop the procedure, and assess the patient. Do not resume until he is stable.

Follow-up Care

- Laboratory studies may be needed to rule out electrolyte imbalances, hypothyroidism, and colonic tumor or stricture.
- Encourage the patient to eat a high-fiber diet, to drink 6–10 glasses of fluids daily, and to increase physical activity.
- Adjust medications, including nonprescription drugs, and discontinue unnecessary ones.
- Encourage good bowel habits, and tell the patient how important it is to establish a regular time to defecate and always obey the urge.
- As indicated, prescribe stool softener or bulking agents: docusate sodium (Colace) or psyllium hydrophilic mucilloid (Fiberall, Hydrocil Instant, Metamucil, etc.), with adequate fluids.
- Recommend glycerin suppositories if the patient does not have a bowel movement at least every three days. If this is not effective,

prescribe magnesium hydroxide (Phillips' Milk of Magnesia) 30 mL by mouth or bisacodyl (Dulcolax, Fleet Bisacodyl) suppositories.

Suggested Readings

Klein H: Constipation and fecal impaction. *Med Clin North Am* 1982;66(5):1135-1141.

Mager-O'Connor E: How to identify and remove fecal impactions. *Geriatr Nurs* 1984;5(3):158-161.

Wrenn K: Fecal impaction. *N Engl J Med* 1989;321:658-662.

23

Skinfold Measurements

Carol Russ, RD
Charles E. Driscoll, MD

Anthropometric measurements are useful in assessing body size, growth, presence of undernutrition or obesity, and changes in body composition resulting from diet or disease. For the most reliable and helpful results, they should be done with some regularity. In adults, the measurements include height, weight, and upper arm circumference as well as skinfolds. In children, head circumference is added.

Skinfold measurements, when properly done, can help estimate the percent of body fat. But remember that the figures derived from these skinfold measurements are approximations only. They are more useful as instruments for evaluating changes in body composition than for determining absolute percentages of body fat (Table 23-1).

TABLE 23–1

Guidelines for Evaluating Percent Body Fat

BODY FAT NORMS*

	Women	Men
Very low	14–17%	7–10%
Low	17–20%	10–13%
Average	20–24%	13–17%
Above normal	24–27%	17–20%
Very high	27–30%	20–25%
Obese	Above 30%	Above 25%

*Norms for female athletes are 13–20% with an absolute minimum of 10%; for male athletes, norms are 4–12%, with an absolute minimum of 3%.

Indications

- To determine approximate percent body fat in any patient
- To monitor changes in percent body fat in obese and malnourished patients

Relative Contraindications

- Skinfold measurements are difficult in extremely obese patients, and results may be unreliable.
- Results may be unreliable in geriatric patients who have significant skin atrophy and loss of subcutaneous fat.

Materials

- Skinfold caliper
- Measuring tape, flexible steel or nonstretchable fiberglass
- Reference tables to use for estimating percent body fat

PROCEDURE

1. Select sites for skinfold measurement as required by the reference tables you are using. The tables given here (see Tables 23-2 and 23-3) call for three measurement sites—chest, abdomen, and thigh for men; triceps, suprailiac area, and thigh for women. Other tables might include subscapular measurement.

Note: Always have the patient stand if possible, and measure on the right side of the body unless otherwise indicated by a reference source you are following.

2. At each site, grasp the appropriate skinfold between thumb and forefinger, taking care to pick up only skin and immediate subcutaneous fat, not muscle:[1]

- *Triceps*: With the measuring tape, locate the midpoint between the acromion and olecranon over the triceps. With the patient's arm hanging relaxed at the side, take a vertical skinfold (Figure 23-1).
- *Subscapular area*: Take an oblique or diagonal skinfold along the inferior angle of the scapula (Figure 23-1).
- *Chest*: Take a diagonal skinfold on a line connecting the anterior axillary fold and the nipple, midway between the two (Figure 23-2).
- *Abdomen*: Take a vertical skinfold approximately 2 cm (¾ in.) lateral to the umbilicus (Figure 23-2).
- *Suprailiac area*: Take an oblique or diagonal skinfold just above the crest of the ilium where the anterior axillary line extends to the ilium (Figure 23-3).
- *Thigh*: With the patient's weight shifted to the left leg and the right leg slightly flexed, take a vertical skinfold on the anterior aspect of

[1]The authors recommend two reliable metal calipers: Lange Skinfold Calipers, Cambridge Scientific Industries, P.O. Box 265, Cambridge, MD 21613 (301) 228-5111 or (800) 638-9566; and Harpenden Skinfold Calipers, British Indicators, Ltd., St. Albans, Hertfordshire, England. Fairly reliable plastic calipers are available from Ross Laboratories, 625 Cleveland Avenue, Dept. 441, Columbus, OH 43216 (614) 227-3333.

TABLE 23–2

Percent Fat Estimates for Women: Sum of Triceps, Suprailium, and Thigh Skinfolds

	AGE TO THE LAST YEAR								
Sum of skinfolds (mm)	Under 22	23 to 27	28 to 32	33 to 37	38 to 42	43 to 47	48 to 52	53 to 57	Over 58
8–10	1.3	1.8	2.3	2.9	3.4	3.9	4.5	5.0	5.5
11–13	2.2	2.8	3.3	3.9	4.4	4.9	5.5	6.0	6.5
14–16	3.2	3.8	4.3	4.8	5.4	5.9	6.4	7.0	7.5
17–19	4.2	4.7	5.3	5.8	6.3	6.9	7.4	8.0	8.5
20–22	5.1	5.7	6.2	6.8	7.3	7.9	8.4	8.9	9.5
23–25	6.1	6.6	7.2	7.7	8.3	8.8	9.4	9.9	10.5
26–28	7.0	7.6	8.1	8.7	9.2	9.8	10.3	10.9	11.4
29–31	8.0	8.5	9.1	9.6	10.2	10.7	11.3	11.8	12.4
32–34	8.9	9.4	10.0	10.5	11.1	11.6	12.2	12.8	13.3
35–37	9.8	10.4	10.9	11.5	12.0	12.6	13.1	13.7	14.3
38–40	10.7	11.3	11.8	12.4	12.9	13.5	14.1	14.6	15.2
41–43	11.6	12.2	12.7	13.3	13.8	14.4	15.0	15.5	16.1
44–46	12.5	13.1	13.6	14.2	14.7	15.3	15.9	16.4	17.0
47–49	13.4	13.9	14.5	15.1	15.6	16.2	16.8	17.3	17.9
50–52	14.3	14.8	15.4	15.9	16.5	17.1	17.6	18.2	18.8
53–55	15.1	15.7	16.2	16.8	17.4	17.9	18.5	19.1	19.7
56–58	16.0	16.5	17.1	17.7	18.2	18.8	19.4	20.0	20.5
59–61	16.9	17.4	17.9	18.5	19.1	19.7	20.2	20.8	21.4
62–64	17.6	18.2	18.8	19.4	19.9	20.5	21.1	21.7	22.2
65–67	18.5	19.0	19.6	20.2	20.8	21.3	21.9	22.5	23.1
68–70	19.3	19.9	20.4	21.0	21.6	22.2	22.7	23.3	23.9
71–73	20.1	20.7	21.2	21.8	22.4	23.0	23.6	24.1	24.7
74–76	20.9	21.5	22.0	22.6	23.2	23.8	24.4	25.0	25.5
77–79	21.7	22.2	22.8	23.4	24.0	24.6	25.2	25.8	26.3
80–82	22.4	23.0	23.6	24.2	24.8	25.4	25.9	26.5	27.1
83–85	23.2	23.8	24.4	25.0	25.5	26.1	26.7	27.3	27.9
86–88	24.0	24.5	25.1	25.7	26.3	26.9	27.5	28.1	28.7
89–91	24.7	25.3	25.9	26.5	27.1	27.6	28.2	28.8	29.4
92–94	25.4	26.0	26.6	27.2	27.8	28.4	29.0	29.6	30.2
95–97	26.1	26.7	27.3	27.9	28.5	29.1	29.7	30.3	30.9
98–100	26.9	27.4	28.0	28.6	29.2	29.8	30.4	31.0	31.6
101–103	27.5	28.1	28.7	29.3	29.9	30.5	31.1	31.7	32.3
104–106	28.2	28.8	29.4	30.0	30.6	31.2	31.8	32.4	33.0
107–109	28.9	29.5	30.1	30.7	31.3	31.9	32.5	33.1	33.7
110–112	29.6	30.2	30.8	31.4	32.0	32.6	33.2	33.8	34.4
113–115	30.2	30.8	31.4	32.0	32.6	33.2	33.8	34.5	35.1
116–118	30.9	31.5	32.1	32.7	33.3	33.9	34.5	35.1	35.7
119–121	31.5	32.1	32.7	33.3	33.9	34.5	35.1	35.7	36.4
122–124	32.1	32.7	33.3	33.9	34.5	35.1	35.8	36.4	37.0
125–127	32.7	33.3	33.9	34.5	35.1	35.8	36.4	37.0	37.6

BD = 1.1093800 − 0.0008267(X_1) + 0.0000016(X_1)^2 − 0.0002574(X_2), where X_1 is sum of chest, abdominal, and thigh skinfolds and X_2 is age in years. Percent fat = (495/BD) − 450. From Baumgartner TA, Jackson AS: *Measurement for Evaluation in Physical Education,* ed 2. Dubuque, WC Brown, 1982, p. 295. Reprinted by permission of W.C. Brown Co., Dubuque.

TABLE 23–3

Percent Fat Estimates for Men: Sum of Chest, Abdominal, and Thigh Skinfolds

	AGE TO THE LAST YEAR								
Sum of skinfolds (mm)	Under 22	23 to 27	28 to 32	33 to 37	38 to 42	43 to 47	48 to 52	53 to 57	Over 58
23–25	9.7	9.9	10.2	10.4	10.7	10.9	11.2	11.4	11.7
26–28	11.0	11.2	11.5	11.7	12.0	12.3	12.5	12.7	13.0
29–31	12.3	12.5	12.8	13.0	13.3	13.5	13.8	14.0	14.3
32–34	13.6	13.8	14.0	14.3	14.5	14.8	15.0	15.3	15.5
35–37	14.8	15.0	15.3	15.5	15.8	16.0	16.3	16.5	16.8
38–40	16.0	16.3	16.5	16.7	17.0	17.2	17.5	17.7	18.0
41–43	17.2	17.4	17.7	17.9	18.2	18.4	18.7	18.9	19.2
44–46	18.3	18.6	18.8	19.1	19.3	19.6	19.8	20.1	20.3
47–49	19.5	19.7	20.0	20.2	20.5	20.7	21.0	21.2	21.5
50–52	20.6	20.8	21.1	21.3	21.6	21.8	22.1	22.3	22.6
53–55	21.7	21.9	22.1	22.4	22.6	22.9	23.1	23.4	23.6
56–58	22.7	23.0	23.2	23.4	23.7	23.9	24.2	24.4	24.7
59–61	23.7	24.0	24.2	24.5	24.7	25.0	25.2	25.5	25.7
62–64	24.7	25.0	25.2	25.5	25.7	26.0	26.7	26.4	26.7
65–67	25.7	25.9	26.2	26.4	26.7	26.9	27.2	27.4	27.7
68–70	26.6	26.9	27.1	27.4	27.6	27.9	28.1	28.4	28.6
71–73	27.5	27.8	28.0	28.3	28.5	28.8	29.0	29.3	29.5
74–76	28.4	28.7	28.9	29.2	29.4	29.7	29.9	30.2	30.4
77–79	29.3	29.5	29.8	30.0	30.3	30.5	30.8	31.0	31.3
80–82	30.1	30.4	30.6	30.9	31.1	31.4	31.6	31.9	32.1
83–85	30.9	31.2	31.4	31.7	31.9	32.2	32.4	32.7	32.9
86–88	31.7	32.0	32.2	32.5	32.7	32.9	33.2	33.4	33.7
89–91	32.5	32.7	33.0	33.2	33.5	33.7	33.9	34.2	34.4
92–94	33.2	33.4	33.7	33.9	34.2	34.4	34.7	34.9	35.2
95–97	33.9	34.1	34.4	34.6	34.9	35.1	35.4	35.6	35.9
98–100	34.6	34.8	35.1	35.3	35.5	35.8	36.0	36.3	36.5
101–103	35.3	35.4	35.7	35.9	36.2	36.4	36.7	36.9	37.2
104–106	35.8	36.1	36.3	36.6	36.8	37.1	37.3	37.5	37.8
107–109	36.4	36.7	36.9	37.1	37.4	37.6	37.9	38.1	38.4
110–112	37.0	37.2	37.5	37.7	38.0	38.2	38.5	38.7	38.9
113–115	37.5	37.8	38.0	38.2	38.5	38.7	39.0	39.2	39.5
116–118	38.0	38.3	38.5	38.8	39.0	39.3	39.5	39.7	40.0
119–121	38.5	38.7	39.0	39.2	39.5	39.7	40.0	40.2	40.5
122–124	39.0	39.2	39.4	39.7	39.9	40.2	40.4	40.7	40.9
125–127	39.4	39.6	39.9	40.1	40.4	40.6	40.9	41.1	41.4
128–130	39.8	40.0	40.3	40.5	40.8	41.0	41.3	41.5	41.8

$BD = 1.0994921 - 0.0009929(X_1) + 0.0000023(X_1) - 0.0001392(X_2)$, where X_1 is the sum of triceps, suprailium, and thigh skinfolds and X_2 is age in years.

From Baumgartner TA, Jackson AS: *Measurement for Evaluation in Physical Education,* ed 2. Dubuque, WC Brown, 1982, p. 296. Reprinted by permission of W.C. Brown Co., Dubuque.

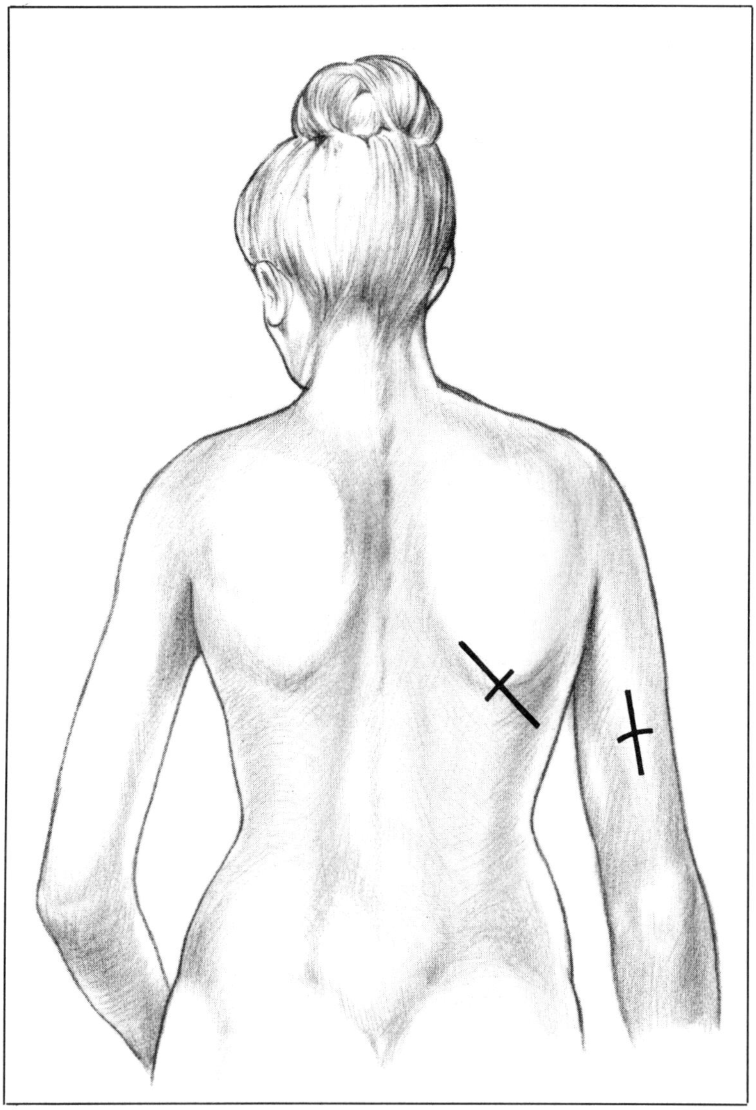

Figure 23-1 Vertical measurement of triceps taken at midpoint between acromion and olecranon. Subscapular area measured at inferior angle of the scapula.

the thigh portion of the right leg midway between the patella and the inguinal fold (Figure 23-2).

3. Maintaining your grasp, place calipers around the skinfold about 5 mm (¼ in.) below your fingers (Figure 23-4). Place the calipers as deep as possible without pinching the muscle.

4. Wait 1–2 seconds after placing the calipers, and read the dial to the nearest 0.5 mm.

5. Repeat the measurement by letting go of the skinfold and picking it up again. If the difference is more than 0.5 mm, take a third mea-

Figure 23-2 Chest: Diagonal skinfold taken medial to anterior axillary line, midway between nipple and axillary line. Abdomen: Vertical skinfold 2 cm lateral to umbilicus. Thigh: Vertical skinfold on anterior aspect of thigh midway between patella and inguinal fold.

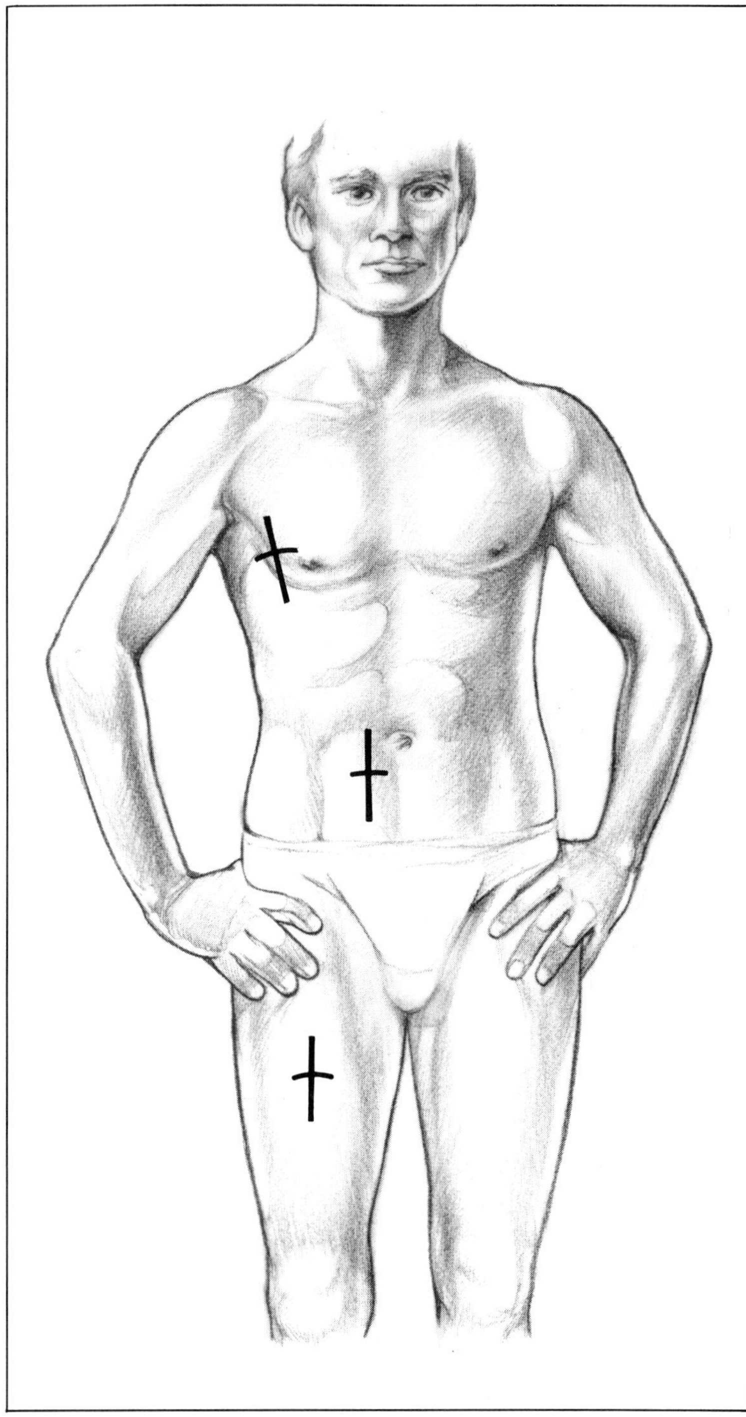

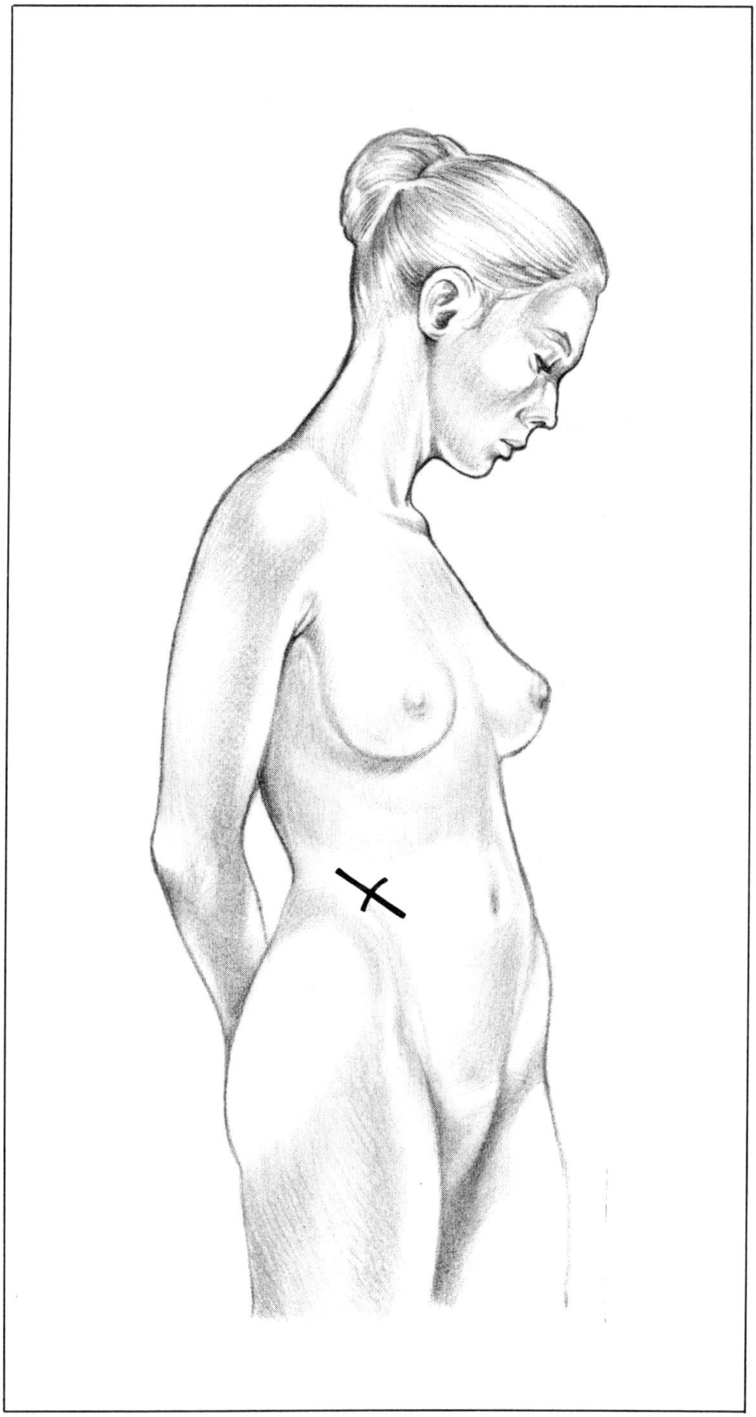

Figure 23-3 Suprailiac area: Oblique or diagonal skinfold just superior to crest of ilium where an imaginary line would descend from anterior axillary line.

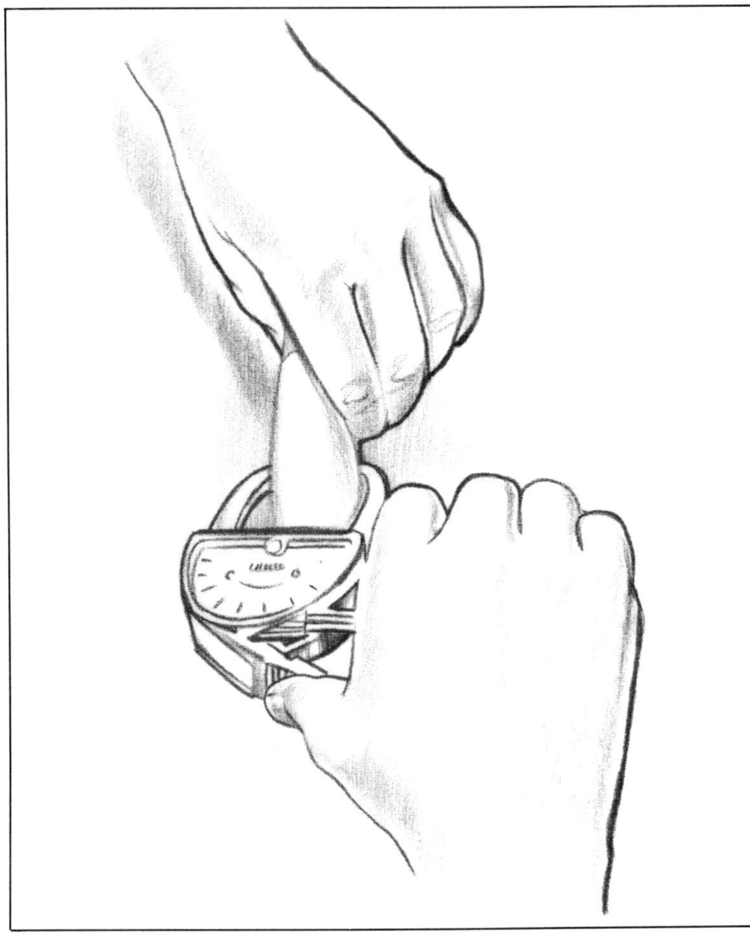

Figure 23-4 Place calipers approximately 5 cm below fingers around skinfold.

surement, and average the two readings closest to one another in value.

Note: If consecutive measurements at a site become smaller with each reading, the fat is being compressed, a situation most often found in "fleshy" patients. Move on to the next site, and return after taking all other measurements. The final value at the problem spot should be the average of the two that appear best to represent the skinfold fat site in the context of the other results.

6. Proceed with skinfold measurements at the remaining sites.

7. Derive an estimate of percent body fat from the sum of several skinfold measurements by consulting one of the accompanying tables as appropriate.

Suggested Readings

Grant A, Dehoog S: *Nutritional Assessment and Support*, ed 3. Seattle, Anne Grant and Susan Dehoog, 1985.

Linder P, Linder D: *How to Assess Degrees of Fatness: A Working Manual*. Cambridge, MD, Cambridge Scientific Industries, 1973.

Simko MD, Cowell C, Gilbride JA: *Nutrition Assessment: A Comprehensive Guide for Planning Intervention*. Rockville, MD, Aspen Systems Corp, 1983.

Storlie J, Jordan HA (eds): *Evaluation and Treatment of Obesity*. New York, SP Medical and Scientific Books, 1984.

IV

MUSCULOSKELETAL/ CONNECTIVE TISSUE PROCEDURES

24

Aspiration and Injection of Joints

Steve A. Wilson, MD
Charles E. Driscoll, MD

The ability to aspirate and inject joints is extremely valuable in the primary care setting for diagnosis and treatment of various arthropathies. Aspiration also may be needed following trauma. The procedures are relatively safe and well tolerated and require no special equipment.

Indications

Therapeutic

- Injecting corticosteroids to suppress inflammation and pain, especially when the patient has been receiving a course of nonsteroidal anti-inflammatory drugs for at least two weeks and it has proved ineffective
- Removing fluid or blood from painfully swollen joints following trauma
- Removing purulent or excessive inflammatory fluid from a joint

Diagnostic

- Obtaining joint fluid when any inflammatory joint disease is suspected, especially if there is swelling or no history of trauma
- Differentiating hemarthrosis from synovial effusion after acute trauma

Relative Contraindications

- Skin infection near the needle entry site
- Previous injection of corticosteroids into the joint—either one injection within the past month or a total of 2–3 previous injections (applies only to corticosteroid injection)

Materials

- Antibacterial skin preparation (povidone-iodine [Betadine] surgical scrub, chlorhexidine gluconate cleanser [Hibiclens], hexachlorophene [pHisoHex])
- Small sterile basin for skin preparation solution
- Sterile 4 × 4-in. gauze sponges
- 70% alcohol solution
- Sterile gloves
- Skin drapes (optional)
- Mask (optional)
- 1% lidocaine HCl (Xylocaine HCl) solution
- 2–3 mL sterile disposable syringe with 1-in., 30-gauge needle; 1½-in., 25-gauge needle (optional)
- Adhesive strip
- *For aspiration:*
  1½- or 2-in. sterile needles, 18-, 20-, and 30-gauge; one or two 20–30 mL disposable syringes; collection tubes: one sterile tube with heparin; one nonsterile tube with heparin or edetate disodium [EDTA]; one nonsterile tube with potassium oxalate; one nonsterile tube without preservative
- *For injection*:
  two 1½-in., 25-gauge sterile needles;[1] corticosteroid for injection

Note: Maintaining sterile conditions throughout the procedure is of utmost importance.

Preparation

1. Have the patient assume a position that is comfortable and provides good exposure to the joint. Determine landmarks (Figures 24-1 through 24-7), and mark the entry point by pressing with your fingernail or the tip of a ballpoint pen with point retracted.
2. Scrub the area with antibacterial skin prep for at least two minutes, then, using gauze sponges, clean with alcohol twice and allow to dry.
3. Wear sterile gloves if you need to palpate the joint further. For additional sterile protection, consider applying skin drapes and donning a mask.
4. For local anesthesia, inject 0.5–1.0 mL of 1% lidocaine through a 1-in., 30-gauge needle with 2–3 mL syringe. (You may want to use a 1½-in., 25-gauge needle to place anesthetic deeper in the tissues in larger joints and to explore the path of entry into the joint space before aspirating with a larger gauge needle.) If the patient is relaxed and you want to aspirate an easily accessible effusion, you may not need a local anesthetic.

[1]A second needle may be needed as a backup if the first one clogs; or you may wish to enter the joint with one needle, leave it in place, detach the syringe, and use the second needle to draw up the drug.

Figure 24-1
Joint: Knee
Position of patient: Supine, knee fully extended
Approach: Anteromedial
Landmarks: Midpatella, medial aspect; medial femoral condyle
Needle insertion depth: 1.0–1.5 cm (3/8–5/8 in.)
Technique: Locate joint space by moving medially from midpatella to point halfway between patella and underlying femoral condyle. Aim needle posteriorly (downward) and laterally to enter.

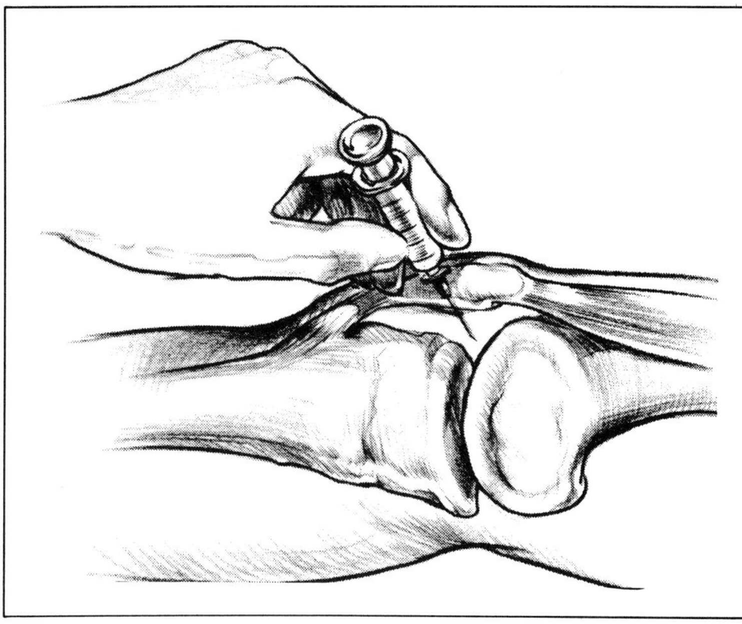

PROCEDURE

1. With a 1½- or 2-in., 18- or 20-gauge needle (30-gauge for finger joints) on a 30-mL syringe, gently enter the joint, directing the needle as indicated in the appropriate illustration. The patient may notice a sharp sensation as the needle pops through the slight resistance of the joint capsule. Withdraw and redirect the needle if you encounter bone or cartilage; be especially careful to avoid scraping the cartilage. Also,

Figure 24-2
Joint: Knee (when patient cannot extend knee)
Position of patient: Sitting, knee flexed 90 degrees over edge of examining table
Approach: Anteromedial or lateral
Landmarks: Infrapatellar tendon, tibial condyle, femoral condyle
Needle insertion depth: 3.5–4.5 cm (1 3/8–1 3/4 in.)
Technique: Locate triangle formed by tendon and condyles. Enter distal to apex of patella medially or laterally to tendon and aim needle slightly cephalad.

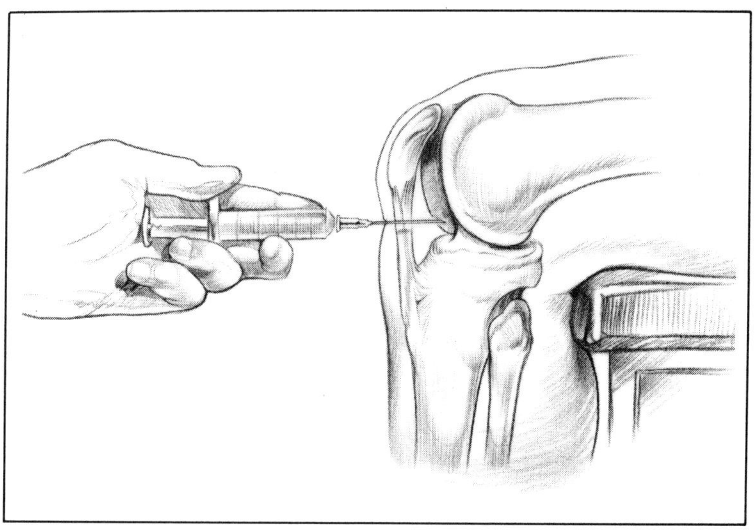

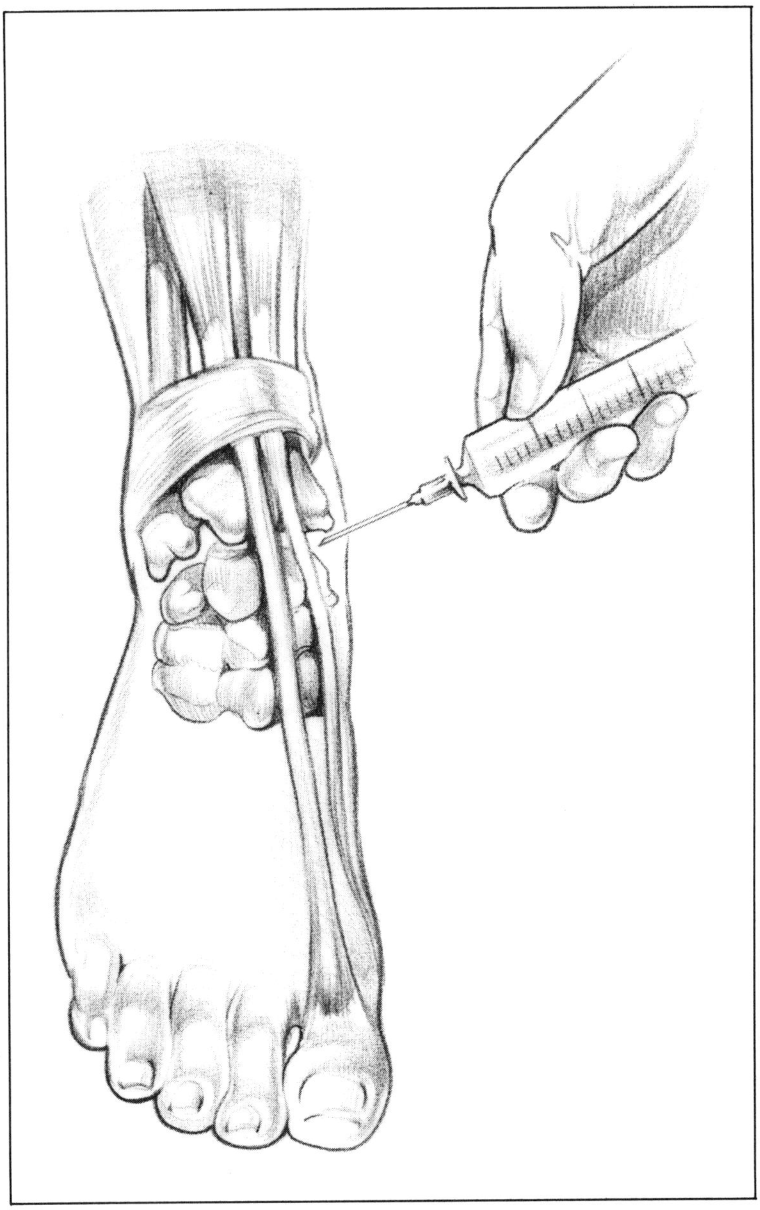

Figure 24-3
Joint: Ankle
Position of patient: Supine, foot in plantar flexion and slight inversion
Approach: Anteromedial
Landmarks: Medial malleolus, extensor hallucis tendon
Needle insertion depth: 3 cm (1¼ in.)
Technique: Locate space between medial malleolus and extensor hallucis tendon. Enter lateral to the medial malleolus, medial to the tendon. Aim needle downward, laterally.

watch for blood entering the syringe in spurts, which indicates tissue trauma.

2. Remove as much fluid as possible, using gentle negative pressure (see step 5). When the fluid stops flowing, try rotating or repositioning the needle slightly and applying mild external pressure on the joint. This may help produce more. If you get a dry tap, you still may be able to gain useful information. Even a small amount of fluid from the

Figure 24-4
Joint: Shoulder
Position of patient: Sitting, arm at side, shoulder rotated externally.
Approach: Anterior
Landmarks: Tip of coracoid process, head of humerus.
Needle insertion depth: 1.5–2.0 cm ($\frac{5}{8}$–$\frac{3}{4}$ in.)
Technique: Locate joint space medial to humerus. Enter inferior to tip of coracoid. Direct needle posteriorly and slightly superiorly and laterally.

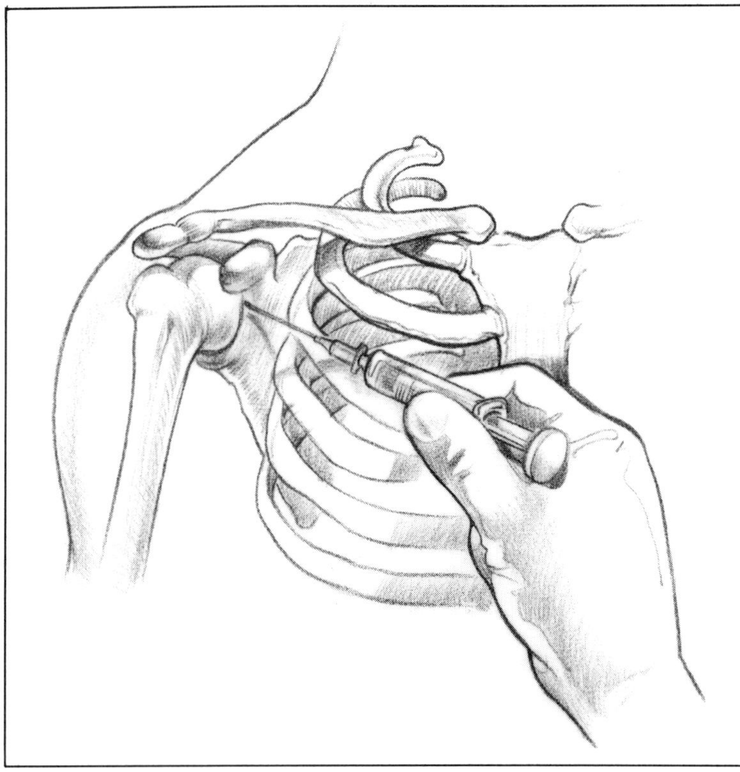

Figure 24-5
Joint: Finger
Position of patient: Hand pronated, traction on finger or finger in slight flexion.
Approach: Dorsolateral or dorsomedial
Landmarks: Proximal and distal aspect of surrounding bones, extensor tendon.
Needle insertion depth: 0.50–0.75 cm ($\frac{3}{16}$–$\frac{5}{16}$ in.)
Technique: Locate articular capsule. Direct needle laterally or medially under extensor tendon.

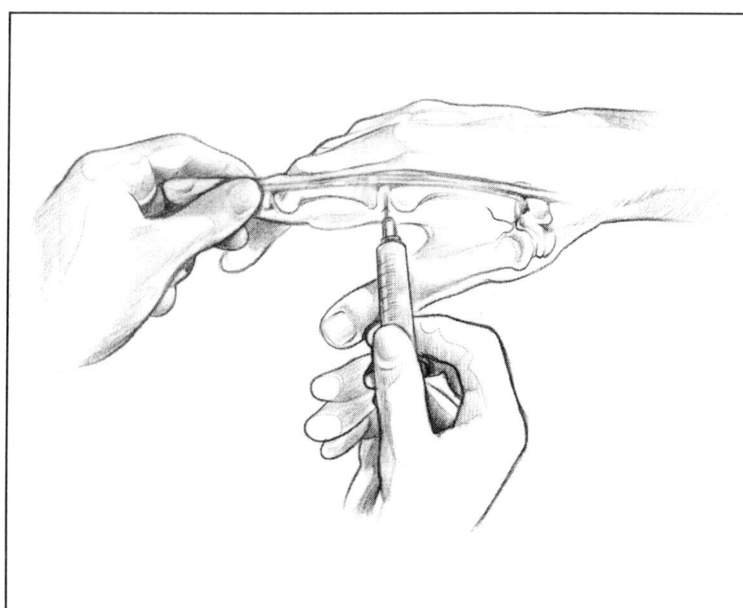

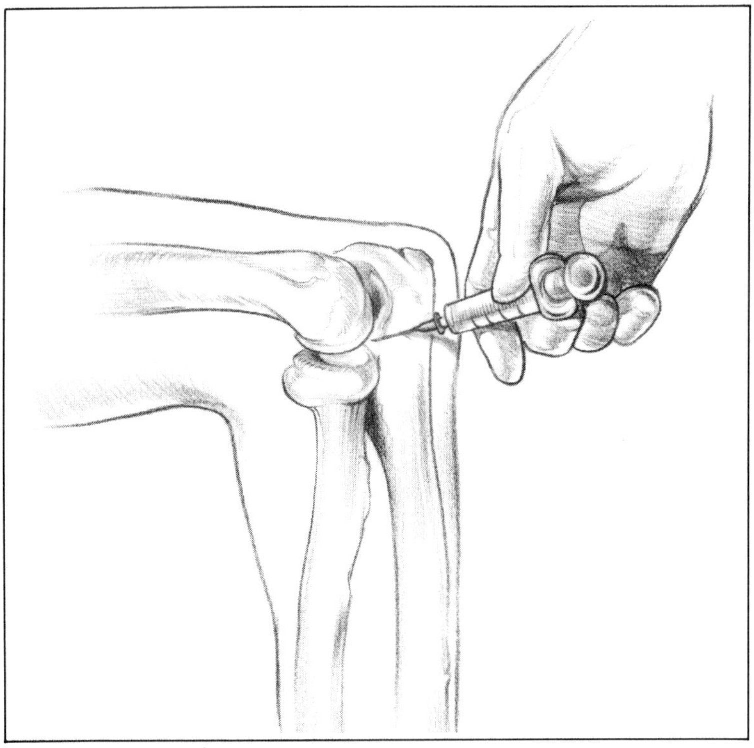

Figure 24-6
Joint: Elbow
Position of patient: Sitting, elbow flexed to 90 degrees, palm pronated on table.
Approach: Posterolateral
Landmarks: Lateral epicondyle of humerus, olecranon process of ulna.
Needle insertion depth: 1.5 cm (5⁄8 in.)
Technique: Locate space between lateral epicondyle of humerus and olecranon process (1 cm [3⁄8 in.] below epicondyle). Direct needle medially and slightly toward hand.

needle can be examined microscopically for the presence of crystals or organisms and possibly cultured.

3. For injection, leave the needle in place and replace the syringe with a 2–3 mL syringe containing steroid medication; inject slowly. The amount of corticosteroid injected is proportionate to the size of the joint and the size of the patient; use the following general dosage guide for prednisolone or equivalent: 2.5–15.0 mg for small joints of the hands and feet; 10–20 mg for wrist and elbow; 20–50 mg for knee, ankle, or shoulder.

4. Remove the needle, apply brief pressure to the site, then cover the site with a sterile adhesive strip. If the joint was injected, gently move it through its range of motion to distribute the medication.

5. Collect fluid as follows:

- Add 2–5 mL of fluid to the sterile heparin tube for culture, and send it immediately to the laboratory.
- Add 2–5 mL of fluid to the nonsterile heparin or EDTA tube for a CBC with white cell differential and morphology studies; immediately shake the tube well to avoid clotting.
- Add 2–5 mL of fluid to the plain nonsterile tube for mucin clot and viscosity studies. Either this tube or the one containing nonsterile heparin or EDTA can be examined for crystals. Save one of them for this examination, making sure the examination takes place within a few days.

Figure 24-7
Joint: Wrist
Position of patient: Sitting, palm pronated, wrist flexed 20–30 degrees over rolled towel with slight ulnar turn.
Approach: Dorsal
Landmarks: Distal borders of radius and ulna, extensor pollicis longus tendon.
Needle insertion depth: 1–2 cm (3/8–3/4 in.)
Technique: Enter distal to line between bony processes of radius and ulna and just lateral to the tendon. Enter perpendicular to skin and direct needle downward.

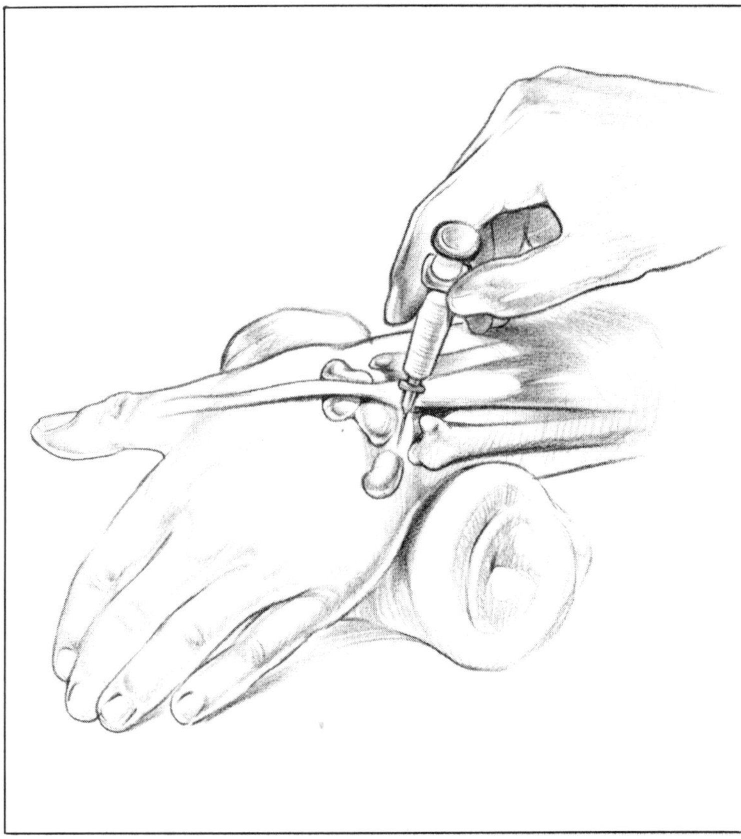

- Add 3–5 mL of fluid to the nonsterile potassium oxalate tube for glucose and other studies as indicated—rheumatoid factor, lupus erythematosus preparation, antinuclear antibody, complement level, and so on. If you are evaluating the complement level, immediately centrifuge the fluid sample and freeze it at −20 °C (−4 °F). To permit proper interpretation of complement level, simultaneously draw a peripheral venous blood sample for evaluation; the same applies if you are doing glucose studies on the fluid sample.

6. Evaluate the results of synovial fluid studies (see Table 24-1).

Patient Instructions

- Tell the patient who receives a corticosteroid injection that he or she may have increased pain in the joint for a few hours or, in rare cases, for a few days. If you inject a weight-bearing joint, have the patient limit activity to preinjection levels for a week to protect the joint and help prolong relief.
- Ask the patient to report any signs or symptoms that suggest bleeding or infection in the joint. These complications are rare with the technique described here.

TABLE 24-1

Synovial Fluid Analysis

Presumptive diagnosis	Appearance	Viscosity	Mucin clot formation	WBC/μL	PMNs* (%)	Protein (gm/dL)	Glucose† (%)	Comments
NORMAL								
	Clear, straw-colored	High	Good	30–150	<20	1–4	90	—
NONINFLAMMATORY (GROUP I)								
Trauma	Clear or turbid, red or xanthochromic	High	Good	750–20,000	<30	1.3–5.0	90	Many RBCs, few cartilage fragments
Osteoarthritis	Clear, straw–e /q/colored	High	Fair to good	1,000–7,500	20–60	2.9–5.5	90	Many cartilage fragments
INFLAMMATORY (GROUP II)								
Systemic lupus erythematosus	Clear or turbid	High	Good	1,000–5,000	<20	1.5–4.0	90	Lupus erythematosus cells
Rheumatoid arthritis	Turbid, greenish yellow	Low	Poor	5,000–100,000	60–95	3–6	80	Latex positive, ragocytes, low complement
Gout	Turbid, white	Low	Poor	1,000–70,000	50–95	2.8–5.0	90	Strongly negative birefringence, sodium urate crystals
Pseudogout	Clear or turbid	Low	Fair	500–80,000	30–95	—	90	Weakly positive birefringence, many RBCs, calcium pyrophosphate crystals
Rheumatic fever	Slightly turbid	Low	Good	300–100,000	60–90	1.5–5.0	90	—
Reiter's disease	Turbid	Low	Fair	700–45,000	>60	2.5–6.0	—	PMNs in macrophages
SEPTIC (GROUP III)								
Bacterial	Turbid, gray or yellow	Low	Poor	5,000–5,000,000 (>75,000)	>90	2.8–6.8	20	Bacteria on Gram's stain, culture positive
Tuberculosis	Turbid, gray or yellow	Low	Poor	2,500–100,000	50	4–6	50	Acid-fast seen on smear (20%); culture (80%) and biopsy (90%) positive

*Polymorphonuclear leukocytes.
†Expressed as a percent of serum glucose levels.

*Adapted with permission from Eknoyan C: *Medical Procedures Manual.* Chicago, Year Book Medical Pubs, Inc., 1981, pp 88-89.

Suggested Readings

Currey HL, Vernon-Roberts B: Examination of synovial fluid. *Clin Rheum Dis* 1976;2:149-177.

Eknoyan G: *Medical Procedures Manual.* Chicago, Year Book Medical Pubs, Inc., 1981, pp 77-94.

Fitzgerald RH Jr: Intrasynovial injection of steroids: Uses and abuses. *Mayo Clin Proc* 1976;51:655-659.

Germain BF: *Synovial Fluid Analysis in the Diagnosis of Diseases of the Joints.* New Orleans, Upjohn Company, 1976.

Miller JA Jr: Joint paracentesis from an anatomic point of view: I. Shoulder, elbow, wrist, and hand. *Surgery* 1956;40:993-1006.

Miller JA Jr: Joint paracentesis from an anatomic point of view: II. Hip, knee, ankle, and foot. *Surgery* 1957;41:999-1011.

Rodnan GP, Schumacher HR (eds): *Primer on the Rheumatic Diseases,* ed 8. Atlanta, Arthritis Foundation, 1983, pp 197-199.

Steinbrocker O, Neustadt DH: *Aspiration and Injection Therapy in Arthritis and Musculoskeletal Disorders: A Handbook on Technique and Management.* Hagerstown, Md, Harper & Row Publishers, 1972.

25

Trigger Point Injection

Ralph H. Knudson, MD

The mechanism action of injecting trigger points is not completely defined. Trigger points are localized areas of waxy degeneration of muscle fibers with associated fibrous destruction, but no surrounding inflammation. They may contribute to a reflex arc that promotes muscle spasm and pain. Injection is believed to cause a reflex trophic circuit activation that may involve the release of endogenous opioids or the release and subsequent depletion of substance P, kinins, or histamines from afferent nerves in and around the trigger points.

Some studies show that needling or injecting trigger points with saline solution alone will relieve pain for two weeks or longer. Injecting lidocaine HCl (Xylocaine HCl) or other local anesthetic such as bupivacaine HCl (Marcaine HCl, Sensorcaine) immediately relieves pain and causes less postneedling discomfort. Another study shows that jet injection of trigger points compares favorably with needle injection for long-term pain relief; patients also report less injection pain with this method.

Among women with chronic pelvic pain, 89% have reported relief after injection of abdominal trigger points. This seems to reinforce the belief that injection of trigger points affects long-term, pain-reinforcing reflex arcs. These arcs can result in unexpected and sometimes confusing patterns of referred pain.

Indications

- Presence of trigger points caused by trauma, muscle tension, fibromyalgia (myofascial syndrome), prolonged or repetitive positions.
- Trigger points must be distinguished from psychogenic rheumatism, subcutis fibrositis, and multiple-site trigger points caused by endocrinopathies (most frequently hypothyroidism, estrogen deficiencies, and pituitary disorders).

Contraindications

- Absolute contraindications are active infection at or immediately adjacent to the trigger point site, bleeding diatheses or anticoagulation, lidocaine or procaine HCl (Novocain) allergy, or other factors making follow-up care and assessment impossible. Among the latter are significant psychiatric disturbance, extremely low pain threshold, or more than 2–3 hours travel time between the patient's home and your office.
- If muscle spasm is so severe that you cannot clearly identify the trigger points, try to reduce the spasm by repositioning, massage, heat, oral benzodiazepines, analgesics, and pain medications before again trying to locate a trigger point and inject it.

Cautions

- If many areas contain trigger points, consider possible underlying endocrinopathy. Most common are hypothyroidism, estrogen deficiency, hypoparathyroidism, hyperparathyroidism, various pituitary disorders, and Cushing's syndrome. Explore and treat these while managing trigger points.
- Be aware that injecting more than one muscle group per treatment session may increase the risk of anesthetic toxicity and the development of excessive and confusing multiple-site, postinjection discomfort.

Materials

- Gauze sponges
- Topical antiseptic (povidone/iodine [Betadine] or benzalkonium chloride [Zephiran])
- Alcohol swabs
- Needles for injection, ranging in size from 3-in. 19 gauge to 1½-in. 25 gauge; smaller, 26–30-gauge needles may be less painful, but may also be less frequently available in physicians' offices, and tend to clog
- Two 10-mL syringes
- 1% lidocaine or other anesthetic
- Ethyl chloride spray

Preparation

- To localize a trigger point, have the patient in a comfortable position with target muscles as relaxed as possible. The patient may be prone or seated with the upper chest and head resting on a table while leaning forward to relax back muscles.
- By systematically palpating muscles of the pain area, probe with the tip of the index or middle finger or both to localize tender

spots. During palpation of a trigger point, the patient will frequently report duplication of the pain or paresthesia over the nearby muscle area. You may also produce involuntary local muscle contraction with the patient actually jumping or flinching. The examining finger may discern a relatively distinct knot of firm muscle tissue.

- Trigger points over the abdomen can be differentiated from internal abdominal pain by palpating when the rectus abdominal muscles are slightly tensed. Do this by having the patient raise both heels off the examining table. Intrapelvic pain, which may be referred to abdominal trigger points, may be identified by palpating the pubic arch, levator, and coccygeal muscles on vaginal examination and by lightly palpating with the forefinger or a cotton applicator in the paracervical areas at about the 3-o'clock and 9-o'clock positions. You can distinguish subcutis fibrositis from trigger points by rolling or pinching the skin without palpating the underlying muscle.
- General locations of the most common sites for trigger points are as shown (for the right-hand side, see Figure 25-1). If you identify multiple trigger points, mark each one with a ballpoint pen, and label the pain intensity with a number from one to 10. Then reexamine to distinguish the most severe sites and the consistency of reported pain.

Figure 25-1

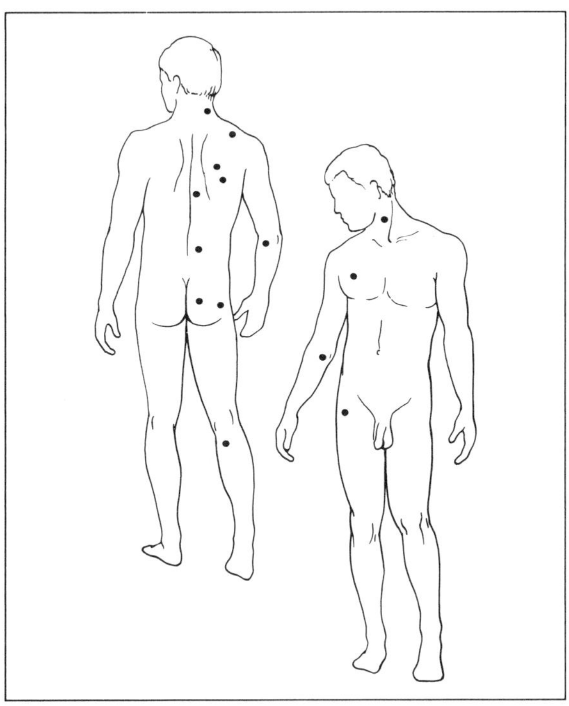

PROCEDURE

1. When you choose a trigger point for injection, make a slight scratch on the skin directly over the site before preparing the skin. This serves as a target during injection, and remains long enough to be a reference point on follow-up examinations.
2. Prepare the skin with gauze swabs and the topical antiseptic solution, then clean with alcohol swabs.
3. Choose the appropriate needle for injection, and affix it to a 10-mL syringe containing 1% lidocaine. A long needle is frequently needed for gluteal tensor fascia areas, medium length needles for upper back and neck, fine needles for sternocleidomastoid, scalene, gluteus, and intercostal muscles.
4. Lightly spray the injection site with ethyl chloride spray to limit skin puncture pain.
5. Insert the needle slowly, talking with the patient, and seek a needle position that most closely reproduces trigger pain.

Note: The angle of insertion varies at different sites. Neck muscles are often approached with the needle from caudal to cephalad; it is often helpful to stabilize the sternocleidomastoid or scalene muscles between finger and forefinger (Figure 25-2). The trapezius is best probed in a cephalad direction while you grasp the muscle body between finger and thumb to avoid inadvertent penetration of the pleura. For the same reason, probe back muscles with the needle inserted at an acute rather than a 90-degree angle to the skin (Figure 25-3). Hamstrings are frequently grasped between thumb and forefinger to avoid inadvertent penetration of nearby major vessels.

Figure 25-2

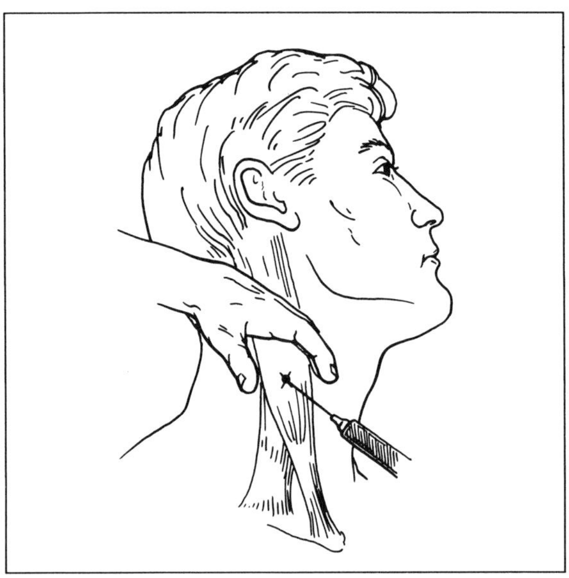

Figure 25-3

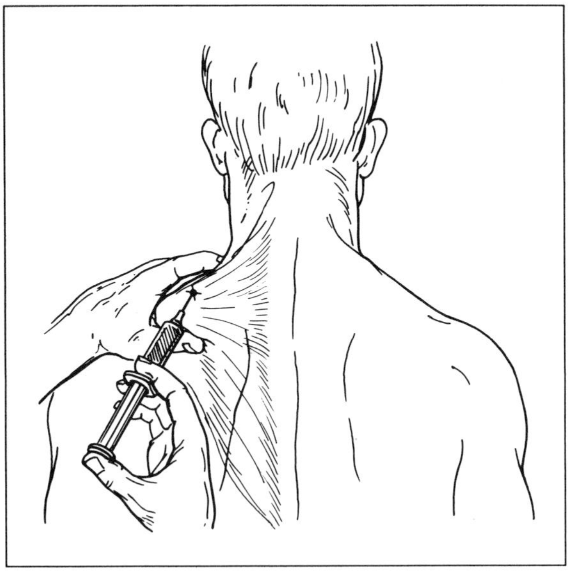

6. Aspirate and slowly inject 2–4 mL of lidocaine into the site.
7. Withdraw the needle to a subcutaneous position, then redirect it to the immediate surrounding areas, seeking other possible trigger points for injection. Explore from medial to lateral in trapezius and back muscles to minimize chances of inadvertent deep injection into the pleura. Use the same technique when injecting trigger points in the buttocks (Figure 25-4).
8. After withdrawing the needle, lightly massage the site of injection and nearby muscles. This often reveals a dramatic relief of muscle tension, with pain reduced or eliminated within minutes.

Figure 25-4

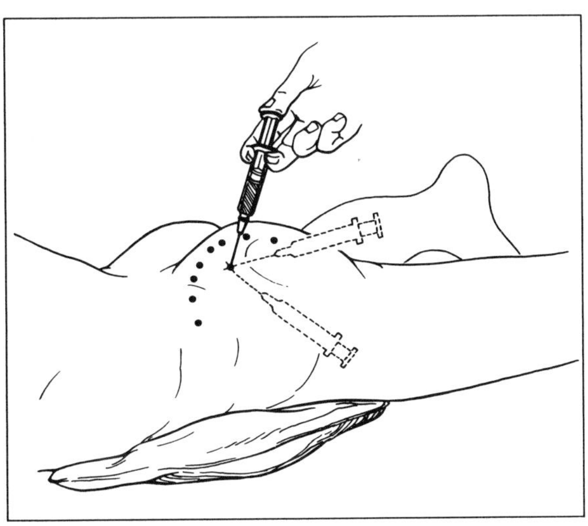

Follow-up Care

1. Instruct the patient to rest the affected area as much as possible, warning him or her that some pain may recur within 2–3 hours after the anesthesia wears off. Even then, the severity of pain should be reduced.
2. Instruct the patient to gently stretch the affected muscle groups daily, using a mist of ethyl chloride spray over the area to reduce stiffness and pain during the movement (Figure 25-5).
3. See the patient in 3–4 days. Reinforce the stretching regimen, inquire about the degree of relief beyond the expected duration of lidocaine anesthesia, and consider reinjection if the patient reports limited relief. As many as four injections may be necessary for complete relief of one site.
4. Consider additional use of nonsteroidal anti-inflammatory medications and tricyclic antidepressants to help manage slowly resolving multifocal trigger point pain.
5. Long-term rehabilitation of muscle groups calls for regular muscle strengthening and stretching exercises under physical therapy guidance.

Complications

Complications are few. Some patients may report increased muscle discomfort secondary to injection trauma, especially if the trigger point was not actually needled. Also reported, but rare, are episodes of lidocaine toxicity, infection, and hematomas at injection sites. Pneumothoraces have occasionally occurred after injection of muscle groups on the thorax.

Figure 25-5

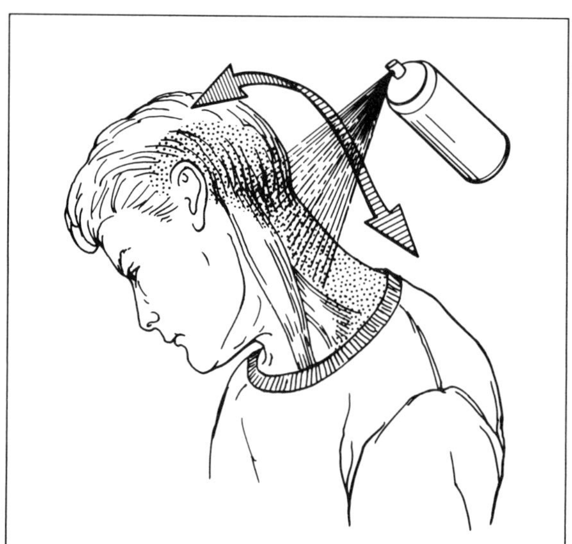

Suggested Readings

Coulehan JL: Primary fibromyalgia. *AFP* 1985;32(3):170-177.

Frost FA, Jessen B, Siggaard-Andersen J: A controlled, double-blind comparison of mepivacaine injection versus saline injection for myofascial pain. *Lancet* 1980;1:499-501.

Hameroff SR, Crago BR, Blitt CD, et al: Comparison of bupivacaine, etidocaine, and saline for trigger-point therapy. *Anesth and Analg* 1981;60:752-755.

Kraus H: Trigger Points, in Kraus H (ed): *Diagnosis and Treatment of Muscle Pain*. Lombard, Ill., Quintessence Publishing Co Inc, 1988, pp 39-50.

Ready LB, Kozody R, Barsa JE, et al: Trigger point injections vs. jet injection in the treatment of myofascial pain. *Pain* 1983;15:201-206.

Slocumb JC: Neurological factors in chronic pelvic pain: Trigger points and the abdominal pelvic pain syndrome. *Am J Obstet Gynecol* 1984;149:536-543.

26

Management of TMJ Dislocation

Dan Heslinga, MD
Charles E. Driscoll, MD

Acute dislocation of the temporomandibular joint (TMJ) can usually be managed by primary care physicians with minimal effort and risk. The TMJ is a sliding joint controlled by the muscles of mastication. At rest, the mandibular condyle sits in the middle of the mandibular fossa of the temporal bone (Figure 26-1). With opening of the mouth, the mandibular condyle slides forward and downward along the articular eminence of the temporal bone.

Sometimes movement continues anterior to the articular eminence without causing difficulty. But in many patients, this excessive forward motion results in dysfunction with muscle spasm and locks the condyle anterior to the articular eminence (Figure 26-2), probably through excessive and prolonged stretching of the capsular ligament and connective tissues of the TMJ. Dislocation can occur during yawning, certain dental procedures, endotracheal intubation, and other situations involving stretching.

The patient with acute TMJ dislocation is typically in excruciating pain, and efforts to close the mouth increase the pain. He or she is usually extremely apprehensive, with muscles of mastication in spasm and no control over saliva. He may have a history of other episodes of jaw dislocation.

Three management techniques are recommended in primary care. In order of preference, they are the extraoral, intraoral, and anesthetic approaches. The extraoral method is successful in most patients, keeps your fingers out of harm's way, and is simple enough that the patient can self-administer it if he suffers recurrent dislocations. The intraoral method can be held in reserve, with the anesthetic method serving as a last resort.

Indication

- Dislocation of the TMJ

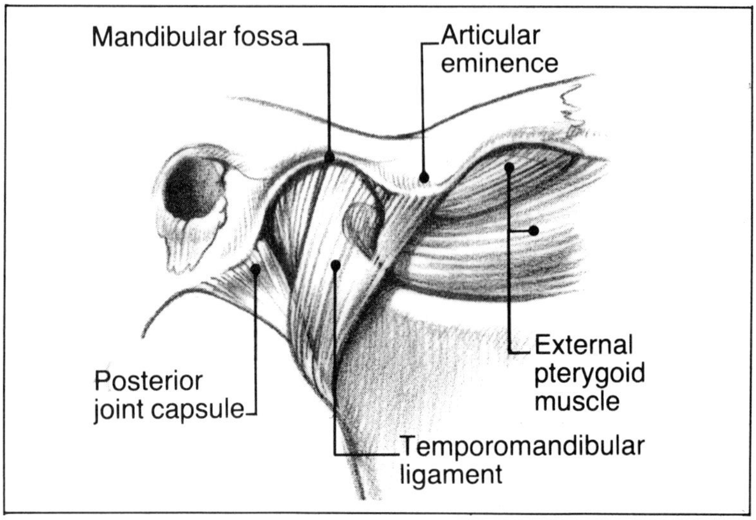

Figure 26-1 Illustration of temporomandibular joint at rest.

Relative Contraindication

- Significant trauma to the jaw. While TMJ dislocation can usually be managed in the office or emergency department, if it is the result of significant jaw trauma, as in a car accident, immediate referral to an oral or ENT surgeon is in order.

Materials

Extraoral and intraoral techniques require no equipment; the anesthetic technique requires the following:

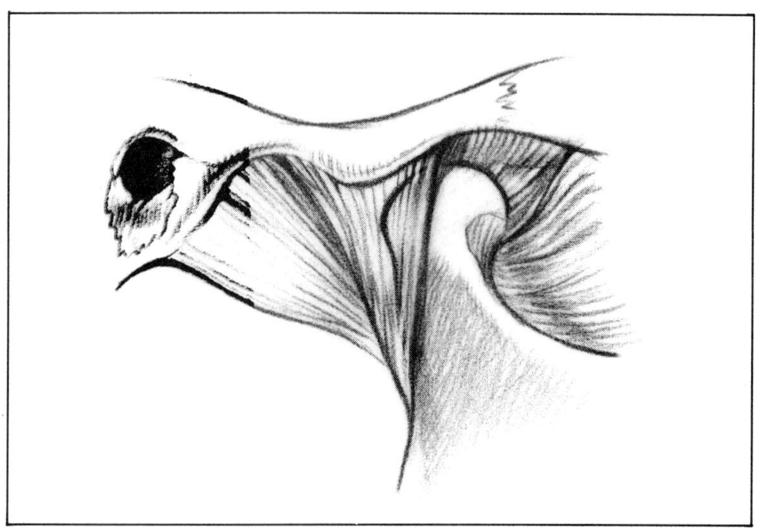

Figure 26-2 Illustration of the condyle locked anterior to the articular eminence.

- Sterile gloves
- Topical disinfectant
- Intraoral syringe with 25-gauge, 1⅞-in. needle
- 2% lidocaine HCl (Xylocaine), 1.8-mL dental cartridge (Carpule)

PROCEDURE

EXTRAORAL

1. At the outset, reassure the patient that simple measures will very likely bring prompt relief.
2. Stand behind the seated patient, and place your fingers on the lateral and superior aspects of the mandibular condyles, easily palpated 2–3 cm (¾–1¼ in.) anterior to the tragus of the ear.
3. With your fingers, apply a light downward force bilaterally over the condyles. As the condyles move, change the direction of the applied force so that it is directed more and more posteriorly (Figure 26-3). Continue the rotating movement, gently sliding the condyles in an inferior and posterior direction until you feel them return to the mandibular fossa.

INTRAORAL

1. Stand in front of the seated patient and place your thumbs in his mouth on the lower molars, your fingers under his chin.
2. Exert downward pressure on the molars while pressing upward on the chin until you feel the condyles return to the mandibular fossa (Figure 26-4).

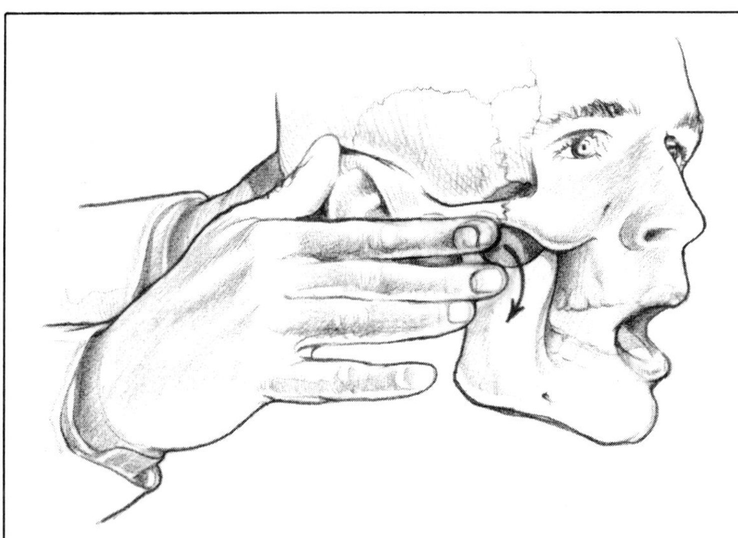

Figure 26-3 Extraoral technique of managing dislocation. Fingers rest on the lateral and superior aspects of the mandibular condyles. Apply light downward pressure bilaterally. As you feel the condyles move, change direction of force more posteriorly.

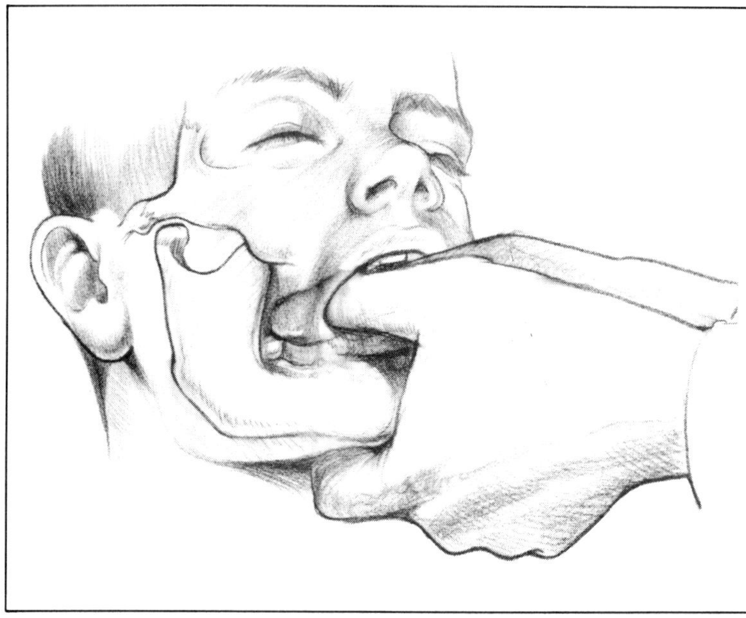

Figure 26-4 Intraoral technique. Exert downward pressure with thumbs on molars, while rest of hand presses up against chin.

Note: Some physicians also exert a posterior force to bring the condyle back over the articular eminence, but excessive pressure of this nature can damage the condyle or articular cartilage of the joint.

ANESTHETIC

1. Prepare either the right or left periauricular area of the face with topical disinfectant; even with bilateral dislocation you need inject only unilaterally.
2. With a gloved index finger, palpate the mandibular fossa. This is relatively easy to locate because the heads of the condylar processes are locked anterior to the eminences in the articular plane.
3. Load the 1.8-mL dental cartridge of lidocaine into the breech of the syringe. Insert the needle into the subcutaneous tissues of the mandibular fossa and direct it medially and slightly anteriorly toward the condylar head, injecting anesthetic solution slowly as you advance the needle (Figure 26-5).
4. When the needle touches the posterior slope of the eminence or the head of the condylar process, withdraw it slightly, aspirate to make sure the needle is not in a vein, and inject the remaining anesthetic solution into the tissue surrounding the mandibular fossa (Figure 26-6). Withdraw the needle. The injection should produce spontaneous reduction without manipulation.

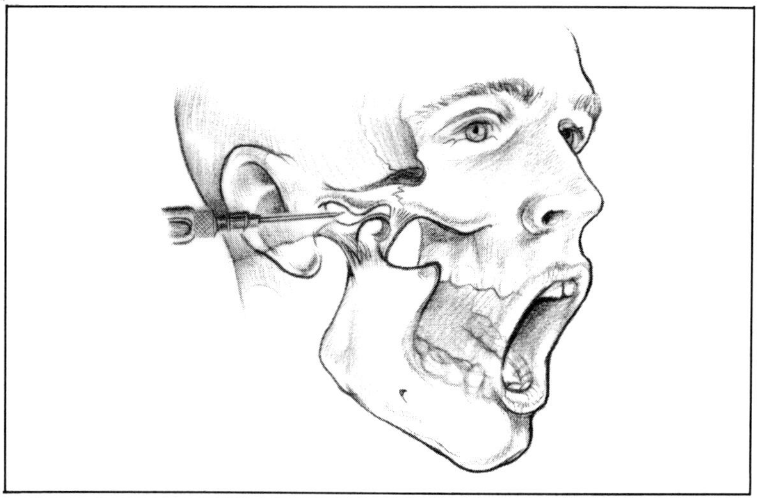

Figure 26-5 Insert needle into the subcutaneous tissue of the mandibular fossa and direct it medially and slightly anteriorly toward the condylar head, slowly injecting anesthetic as you advance the needle.

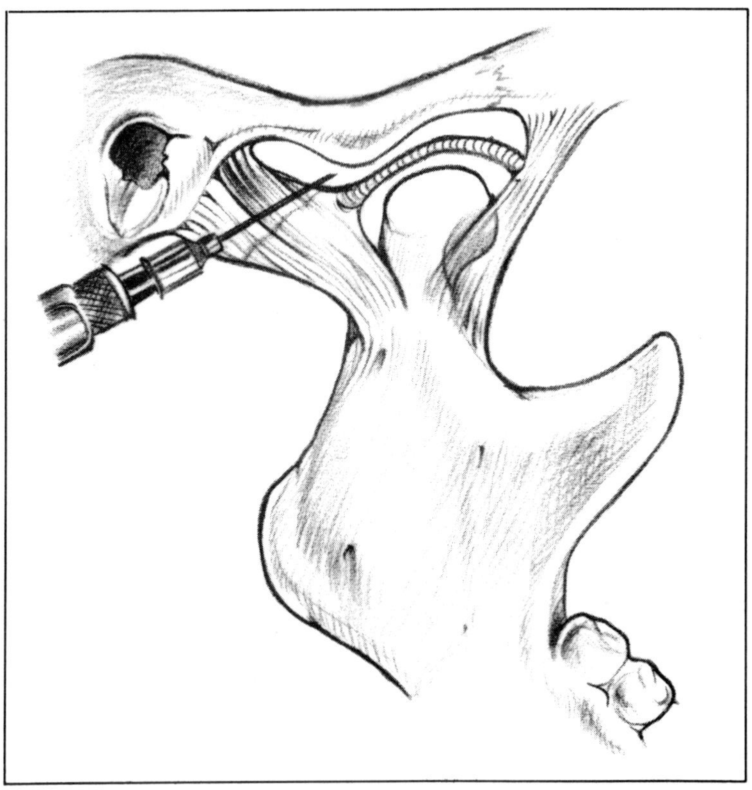

Figure 26-6 When you feel the needle touch the posterior slope of the eminence or the head of the condylar process, withdraw it slightly. Aspirate to check that you are not in a vein, then inject the remaining anesthetic.

Suggested Readings

Littler BO: The role of local anaesthesia in the reduction of long-standing dislocation of the temporomandibular joint. *Br J Oral Surg* 1980;18:81-85.

Vincent JW: Reduction of luxation of the temporomandibular joint: An extraoral approach. *J Prosthet Dent* 1980;44:445-446.

27

Compressive Ankle Splinting

Charles D. Huss, MD

Several methods of treatment for ankle sprains are available, some using compressive dressings and others immobilization. This method incorporates the benefits of both approaches. Compression helps control swelling in the acute postinjury period, and plaster splinting provides immobilization, an important element for pain control.

Indications

- Moderate-to-severe ankle sprains
- Stable, closed fractures of the foot or ankle when a temporary measure is desired. In the early postfracture period, this technique provides immobilization without risk of neurovascular complications that can be associated with circumferential casts when extreme swelling occurs. This method is particularly useful when surgical treatment of a fracture of the foot or ankle will be delayed.

Contraindication

- Unstable fracture

Materials

- Twelve 5 × 30-in. plaster splints
- Rolls of 6 × ¾-in. cotton sheeting
- Rolls of 6-in. stretchable gauze (Kerlix or SOF Band)
- 6-in. elastic bandages
- Plaster bucket with water (temperature according to individual preference)
- Crutches

PROCEDURE

1. Have the patient sit with legs hanging over the edge of the table or patient cart.

2. Roll the cotton sheeting circumferentially around the foot, ankle, and lower leg, starting at the toes and moving proximally. Be sure the sheeting lies flat and extends from the toes to about 5 cm (2 in.) below the popliteal crease. The applied wrap should be one to two layers thick.

3. Roll the stretchable gauze circumferentially over the cotton sheeting, again moving proximally (Figure 27-1). Apply enough tension to mildly compress the underlying cotton wrap. Be sure you apply tension uniformly to avoid creating ridges in the compressive wrap.

4. For positioning, lay dry plaster splints (approximately 12 for an adult) over the gauze wrap from the posterior aspect of the lower leg to the plantar aspect of the foot and the tips of the toes. Tear the splints to length or trim them with shears or a knife.

5. Place the patient's ankle in a neutral position between plantar flexion and dorsiflexion or with the sole of the foot at an angle of about 90 degrees to the lower leg. Maintain this ankle position with an assistant's help if necessary as you proceed.

6. Stack the 12 plaster splints and dip them into the plaster bucket until they are thoroughly wet, then remove them and strip off the excess water. The stripping also works moistened plaster into the gauze mesh wrappings of the splints. Apply the wet splints to the

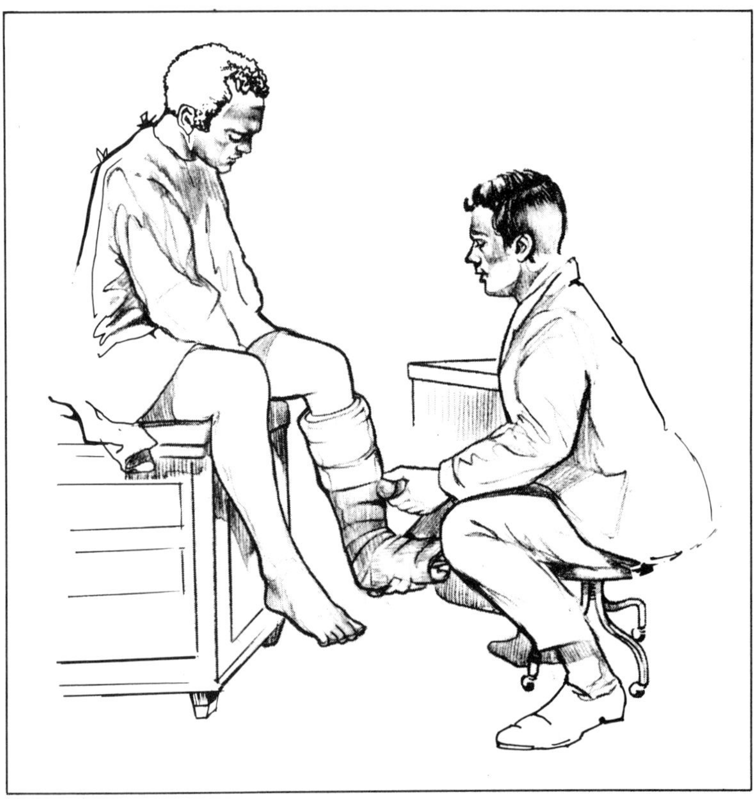

Figure 27-1 With the patient seated and the affected leg hanging off the table, wrap cotton sheeting circumferentially around the leg from toes to below the popliteal crease. Roll stretchable gauze circumferentially over the sheeting with enough tension to smoothly compress the sheeting against the leg.

compressive wrap from the plantar surface of the toes up along the posterior aspect of the leg (Figure 27-2). Be sure the ankle remains in a neutral position during this application.

7. To finish the procedure, roll a 6-in. elastic bandage circumferentially over the foot, ankle, and lower leg to cover the gauze and splints.

8. Stabilize the joint manually, or have your assistant do so, while the plaster begins to harden. Then have the patient elevate the leg on a pillow for final hardening, an overall period of 15 minutes. Be careful not to make ridges in the plaster.

9. After the plaster has hardened, fit the patient for crutches, and demonstrate their use. Urge the patient to keep weight off the splinted region and to avoid exposing the splint to water. Schedule a follow-up visit in 3–5 days. See the patient earlier if the splint becomes soft.

Follow-up Care

At the second office visit, remove the splint by unwrapping the elastic bandage and cutting gauze along the dorsum of the foot and anteriorly

Figure 27-2 Apply wet splints to the compressive wrap from the plantar surface of the toes up along the posterior aspect of the leg.

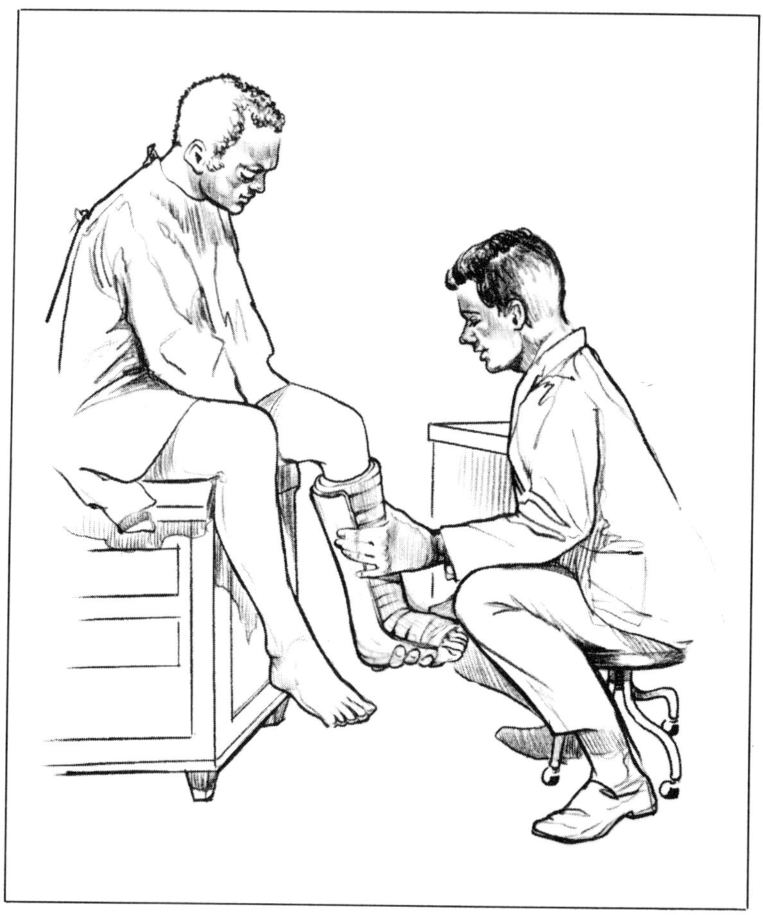

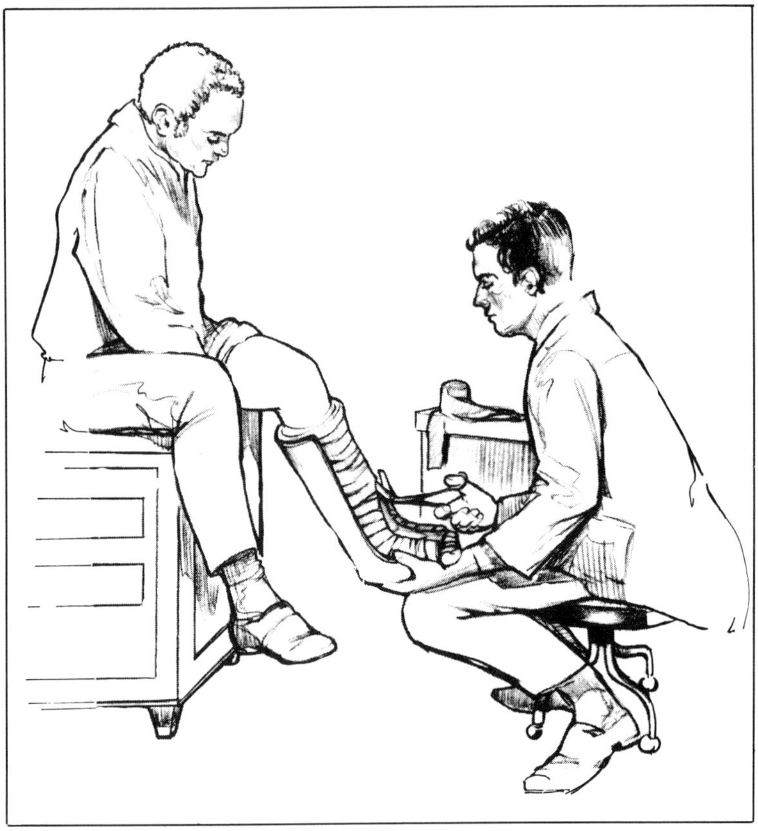

Figure 27-3 Remove the splint by cutting the gauze along the dorsum of the foot and anteriorly up the leg. Separate the underlying cotton sheeting along the same path.

up the leg (Figure 27-3). Separate the cotton sheeting along the same line. If the patient is still unable to bear weight comfortably, you may reapply the same splint.

Suggested Readings

Iverson LD, Clawson DK: *Manual of Acute Orthopaedic Therapeutics,* ed 2. Boston, Little Brown and Co, 1982, pp 45-51.

Shaw DC, Heckman JD: Principles and techniques of splinting musculocutaneous injuries. *Emerg Med Clin North Am* 1984;2(2):391.

28

Immobilizing Clavicular Fractures

Charles E. Driscoll, MD

The incidence of clavicular fracture, one of the most frequent fractures in the general population, appears to be rising—largely due to burgeoning automobile and recreational sports-related accidents. Clavicular fracture in the neonate is a well-known complication of passage through the birth canal; and at the opposite end of life, heavy falls on an outstretched hand often cause this injury in the elderly.

Fractures of the middle third account for at least 80% of all clavicular fractures, followed by those of the lateral and then the medial thirds. In children, medial- and lateral-third fractures carry the risk of injury to the growth plate.

Clavicular injury produces a predictable type of fracture. Direct force on the middle third usually results in a transverse fracture at the junction of the outer and middle thirds (Figure 28-1). A force on the top of the shoulder near the acromioclavicular juncture forces the clavicle down against the first rib, usually resulting in a spiral fracture of the middle third (Figure 28-2). Indirect force—as from falling on the outstretched hand with the arm abducted and flexed—also usually produces a spiral fracture of the middle third by transmitting the force along the shaft of the humerus with the stenoclavicular joint as a counterpoint (Figure 28-3). Palpate this joint in all clavicular fractures to rule out joint injury. A careful neurovascular examination of the afflicted arm is also important.

Fractures of the lateral third may be complicated by ligamentous injury to the coracoclavicular ligament or the articular surface. When the acromioclavicular and coracoclavicular ligaments remain intact (Type I fractures), displacement is minimal, and treatment is relatively easy by external means. With ligament injury, however, the distal fragment tends to remain anchored to the acromion while the proximal fragment rides up and backward. This creates marked, noticeable displacement, and this Type II fracture may require surgery.

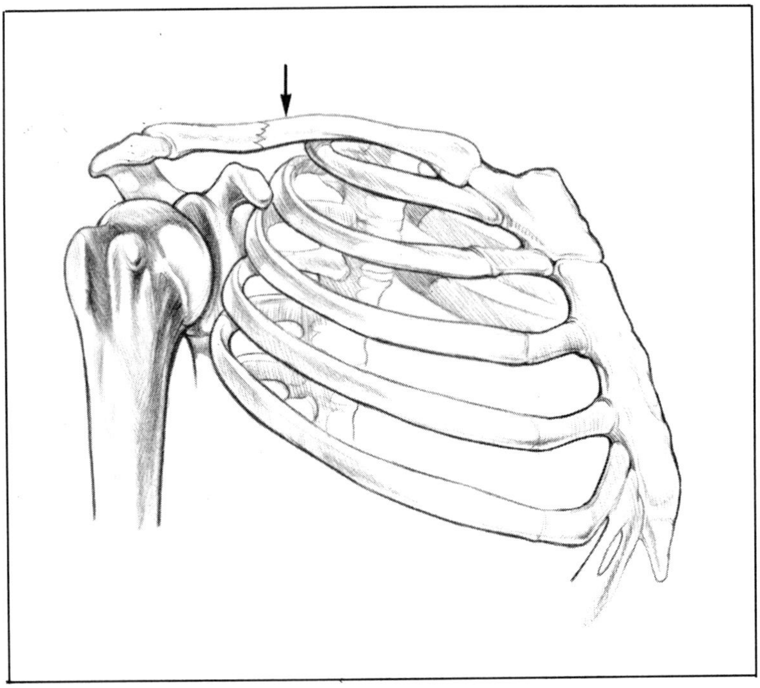

Figure 28-1 Direct force on the middle third of the clavicle usually results in a transverse fracture at the junction of the outer and middle thirds.

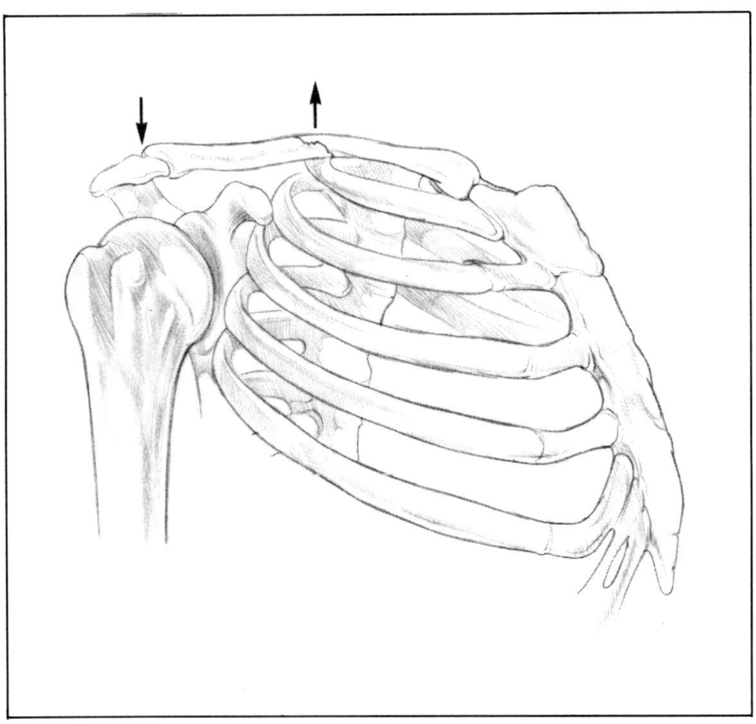

Figure 28-2 Spiral fracture of the middle third.

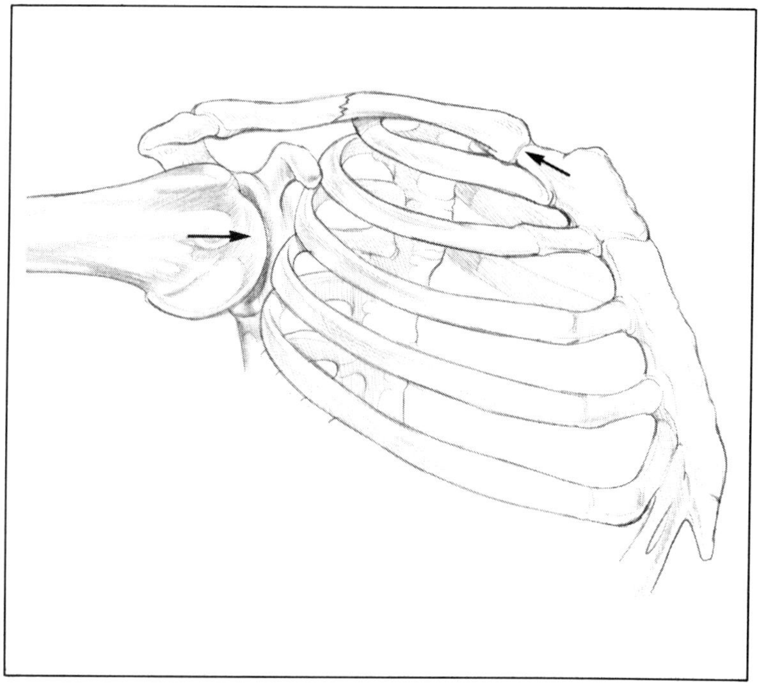

Figure 28-3 Spiral fracture of the middle third from indirect force, such as falling on outstretched hand.

The patient's age is the principal determinant of treatment and follow-up. Newborns require little more than pinning the sleeve of the baby's long-sleeved cotton undershirt to the trunk of the shirt as a sling for 2–3 weeks. Remodeling of the clavicle is excellent, and deformity rarely persists.

For simple, nondisplaced, subperiosteal fractures in children, use only a sling; it should be tied across the opposite shoulder to support the weight of the arm under the elbow. In moderately displaced fractures, use a padded figure-of-8 bandage or commercial clavicle strap to maintain alignment.

In adults and adolescents with little or no displacement, use the soft stockinette, figure-of-8 dressing; a sling may be needed for comfort. For more serious displacement, the fracture should be immobilized with a plaster dressing. In the elderly, a sling is almost always the safest treatment.

Indications for Immobilization by External Methods

- Fractures of the middle third of the clavicle with minimal or moderate displacement (less than 15 mm)
- Type I lateral fractures (proximal to the acromioclavicular and coracoclavicular ligaments)

Contraindications to External Immobilization

- Fractures of the middle third, which usually compromise neurovascular structures
- Type II or III lateral clavicular fractures involving the articular surface
- Fractures with much dislocation of fragments
- Fractures with shortening, usually indicated by gross deformity and wide separation of the ends of the fracture site
- Fractures in patients with multiple chest injuries and an unstable shoulder girdle
- Fractures with symptomatic, confirmed nonunion

When external immobilization is contraindicated, the patient is a candidate for referral or surgical intervention.

Materials

- 100-mL syringe with 1.5-in., 21-gauge needle and 1% lidocaine HCl (Xylocaine HCl) for anesthesia
- Povidone-iodine (Betadine) swabs or alcohol pads
- 20–30 ft of 3-in. stockinette
- Foam rubber or felt padding
- Cotton batting
- 4-in. plaster, several rolls
- Large safety pins
- 3½–4 ft length of 1-in. dowel or a discarded broom handle
- Triangular sling bandage
- As an alternative, commercially produced clavicle straps or a canvas arm sling, though these are more expensive. For the treatment of Type I fractures, the Kenny-Howard sling may be preferable.

PROCEDURES

REDUCTION Conservative measures are usually quite adequate in treating clavicular fractures. Open reduction is rarely indicated, except as noted earlier, and may result in scarring or a higher incidence of nonunion. Most patients do not need manipulation or replacement of fracture fragments.

With displacement and overriding of fragments, however, reduction is necessary to restore the normal length of the clavicle. It should be done before immobilization, as follows:

1. Sterilize the skin with povidone-iodine or alcohol swabs, and inject 3–5 mL of 1% lidocaine HCl into the fracture hematoma.

2. When the patient is satisfactorily anesthetized, seat him or her on a stool, and put a hand on each shoulder from behind. Pull the shoulders upward, backward, and outward simultaneously while applying counterpressure in the midscapular area, usually by placing your knee in the middle of the patient's back (Figure 28-4). This maneuver usually realigns the fracture fragments. (A well-muscled adult may need plaster casting to maintain the reduction.)

3. Have the patient maintain this position by hooking both arms over a dowel or broom handle held horizontally across the back about level with the lower scapula borders (Figure 28-5) as you prepare the bandage for immobilizing the fractures.

APPLYING FIGURE-OF-8 IMMOBILIZATION Use the stockinette bandage invaginated into itself in triple thickness; the single thickness has too much stretch to maintain good positioning.

1. Approximate the length of stockinette for the bandage by placing the end at the middle of the patient's back and looping forward under the right axilla, over the top of the shoulder on the right, down to the middle of the back, looping under the axilla on the left and over the top of the left shoulder, returning to the middle of the back (Figure 28-6). Triple this measurement, and cut the stockinette.

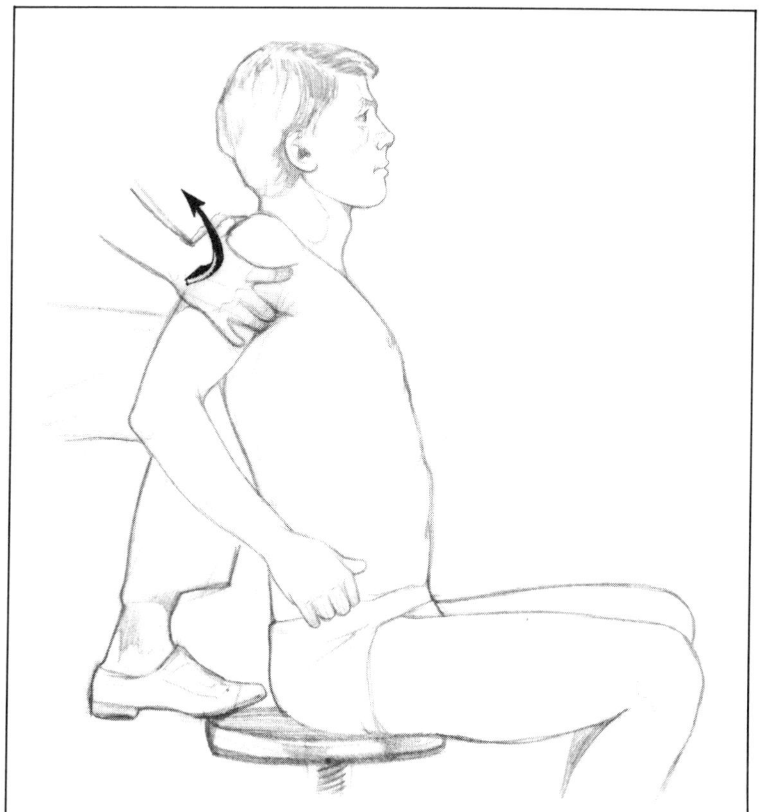

Figure 28-4 Pull shoulders up, back, and out while applying counterpressure against the back with knee.

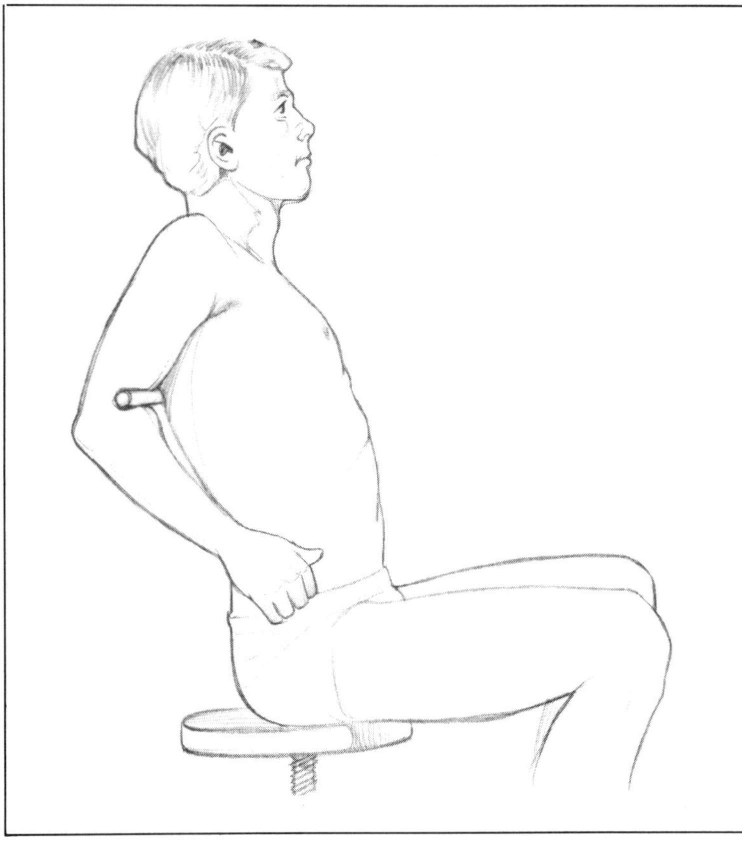

Figure 28-5 Arms hooked over dowel maintains reduction during bandage preparation.

2. To invaginate the stockinette into itself, mark off one third of the material, and hold it at that point with one hand. Reach through the entire length with the other hand, grasp the end, and pull that third back through itself, leaving about two thirds of the original length.
3. Visually divide this portion in half, mark that division with one hand, and reach the other hand through the doubled-up segment. Grasp the loose, single-thickness end, and pull it back through the double thickness to produce the desired triple thickness.
4. Position the patient, keeping the dowel or broom handle in place.
5. Envelope two large pieces (about 3 × 6 in.) of felt or foam rubber in a single thickness of stockinette, and position them in the axillae for padding. Or you can make a slit at each end of the padding and thread the stockinette through to hold it in place (Figure 28-7).
6. Apply the figure-of-8 dressing in the same way you took the initial measurements, place the loose ends of the dressing in the middle of the patient's back, and pin them together with a large safety pin.
7. Remove the dowel or broom handle, and inspect the patient's shoulders for proper alignment. They should be held up, outward, and backward with proper length and alignment of the clavicle restored and maintained by the weight of the arms over the axillary pads.

Figure 28-6 Determining length of stockinette for immobilization.

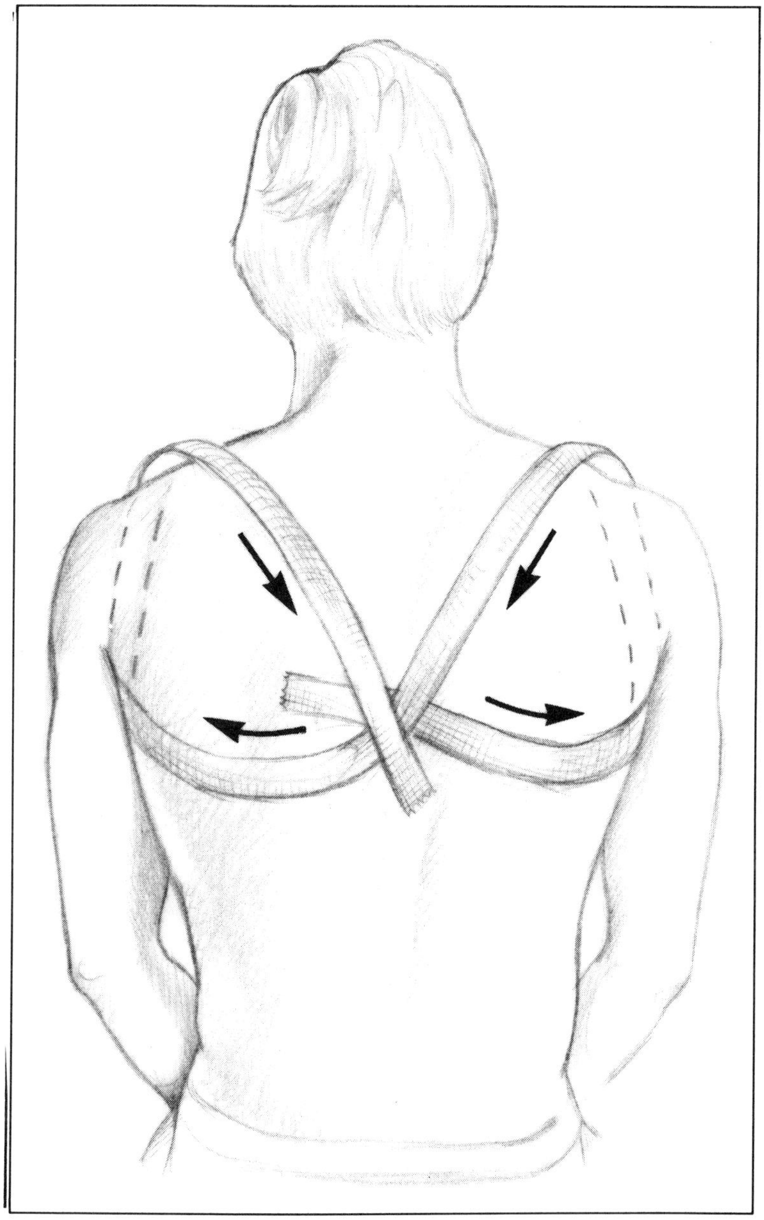

Note: When there are overriding fracture fragments and marked displacement, the stockinette dressing may not be enough. A plaster figure-of-8 dressing is necessary. Follow steps 4 through 7, with these adjustments:

- While maintaining the appropriate shoulder position, first pad the patient with five or more turns of cotton batting in a posterior figure-of-8 dressing.

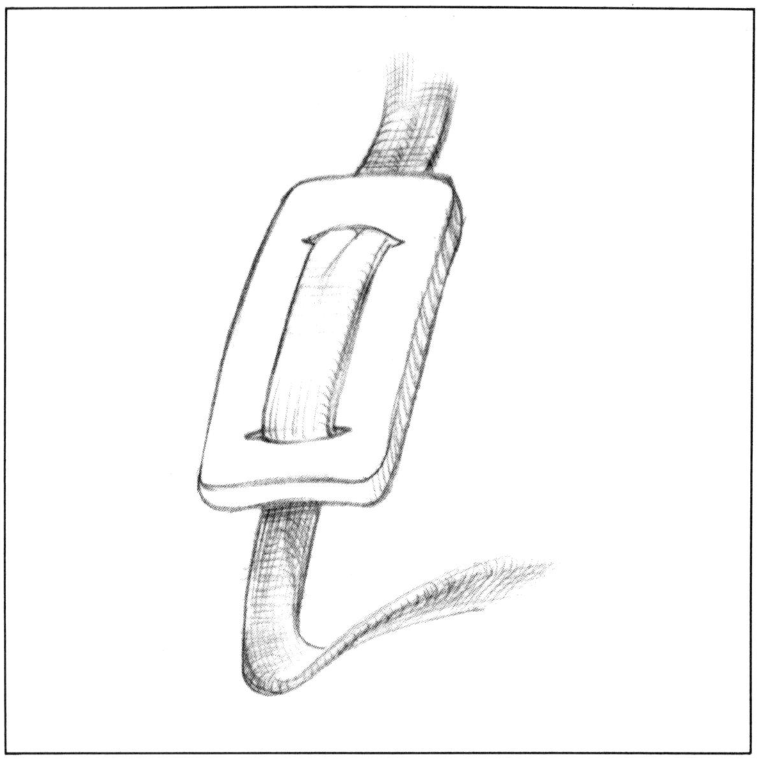

Figure 28-7 Foam rubber padding threaded over stockinette.

- Hold the axilla pads in position while wrapping 10 to 12 turns of a 5-in. plaster bandage in a posterior figure-of-8 dressing.
- When the plaster is firmly set, check immobilization by X-ray, and maintain this for 6–8 weeks until a callus forms and fragments are stable.

Note: To treat Type I fractures of the lateral third, you may prefer the Kenny-Howard sling. The shoulder strap applies downward pressure over the padding and holds the end of the clavicle down while the arm portion of the sling supports the forearm and maintains the acromion in an elevated position (Figure 28-8). An across-the-chest halter pulls the shoulder and sling portions of the brace inward toward the contralateral axilla, which helps to hold the fracture in place. The sling must be worn for 4–6 weeks.

Follow-up Care

- Healing takes 3–4 weeks in children and 4–6 weeks in adults.
- In adolescents and adults with moderate displacement and a soft stockinette figure-of-8 dressing, follow-up should be completed in 6–8 weeks. After four weeks, stability usually allows switching to a simple sling for the remaining 2–3 weeks of healing.

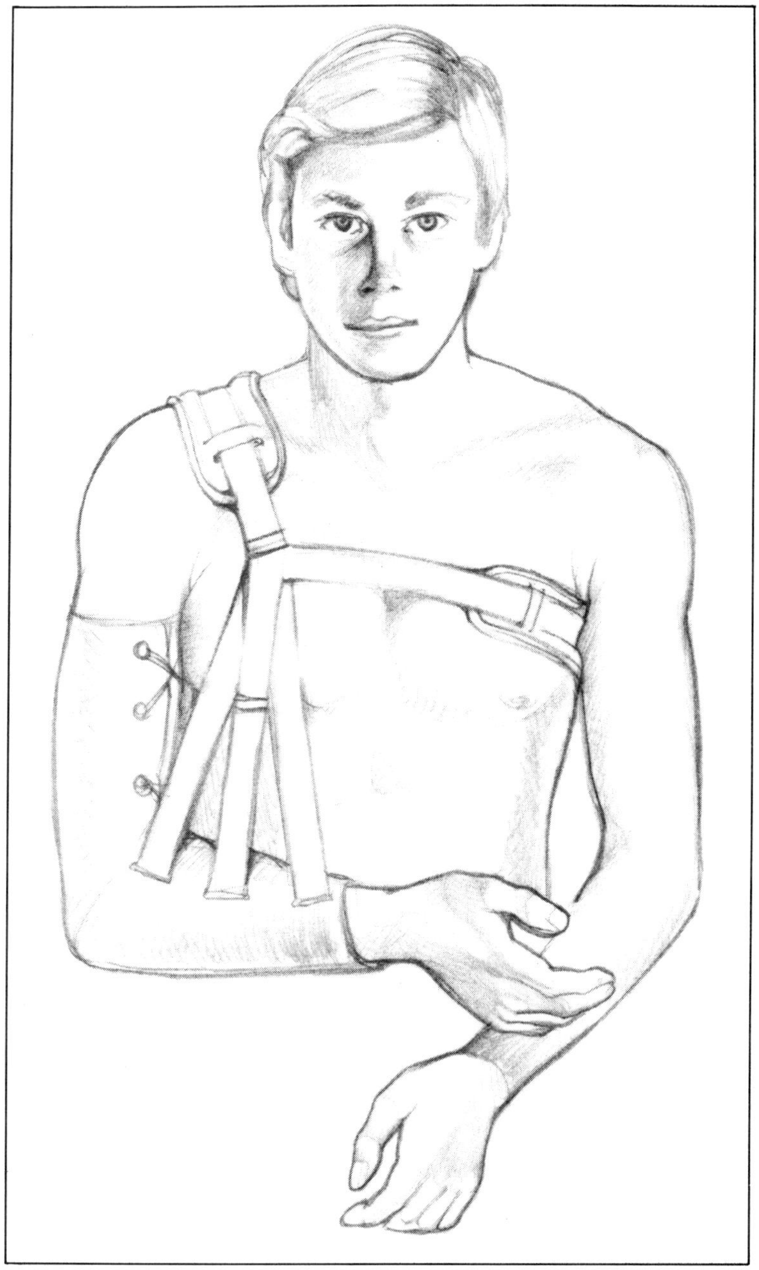

Figure 28-8 The Kenny-Howard sling provides downward pressure on clavicle and maintains the acromion in elevated position.

- In patients with a more serious displacement and a plaster figure-of-8 dressing, determine stability with an X-ray.
- In elderly patients, particularly those with fragile skin and very little subcutaneous tissue for padding, a sling is safer and quite adequate for pain relief and immobilization during healing.

Suggested Readings

DePalma AF: *Surgery of the Shoulder*, ed 3. Philadelphia, JB Lippincott Co, 1983, pp 348-362.

Eskola A, Vainionpaa S, Myllynen P, et al: Outcome of clavicular fracture in 89 patients. *Arch Orthop Trauma Surg* 1986;105:337-338.

Kessel L: *Clinical Disorders of the Shoulder*. New York, Churchill Livingstone Inc, 1982, pp 109-124.

V

GENITOURINARY PROCEDURES

29

Suprapubic Bladder Tap in Infants and Children

Elizabeth A. Burns, MD

Performing a suprapubic bladder tap is an easy way to obtain an uncontaminated urine specimen from an infant or child younger than 4 years of age who is not a candidate for urethral catheterization and who cannot void on command. It provides accurate information on the presence of organisms in the urine and is a helpful adjunct to the physical examination. It is also an integral part of the workup for sepsis in a newborn and for fever of unknown origin or suspected urinary tract infection in young children.

Some physicians use a local anesthetic before performing the tap, but this is seldom necessary, and the injection is probably as uncomfortable and upsetting to the child as the actual procedure.

Indication

- To obtain an uncontaminated urine specimen from an infant or a child younger than 4 years of age

Materials

- 5- or 10-mL syringe
- 23-gauge, 1½-in. needle
- Alcohol or povidone-iodine (Betadine) swabs
- Adhesive strip

PROCEDURE

Note: Postpone the bladder tap for an hour or so if the child has recently voided or if preparing the skin for the tap initiates reflex voiding.

1. Place the child in a supine position; have an assistant ready to control the extremities if necessary during the procedure. (Some physicians prefer a frog-leg position with an assistant providing gentle restraint.)
2. Prepare the suprapubic skin using alcohol or povidone-iodine solution. If you use alcohol, cleanse with an alcohol swab, let the area air dry, then repeat with another swab, and let that dry.
3. Palpate the symphysis pubis. Small children often have a crease in this area that you can use as a conveniently located landmark (Figure 29-1).
4. Attach a 23-gauge, 1½-in. needle to a 5- or 10-mL syringe, and insert it in the midline above the superior pubic border, pointing the needle approximately toward the infant's coccyx (Figure 29-2).

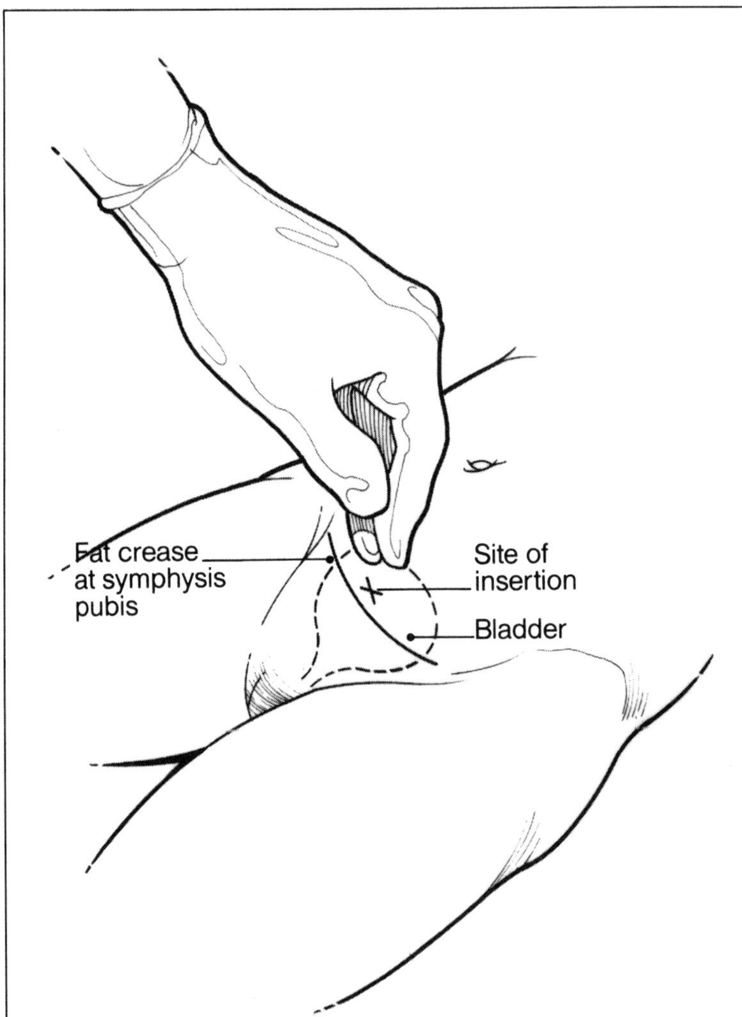

Figure 29-1 To determine the site of needle insertion, place the child in supine position and palpate the symphysis pubis.

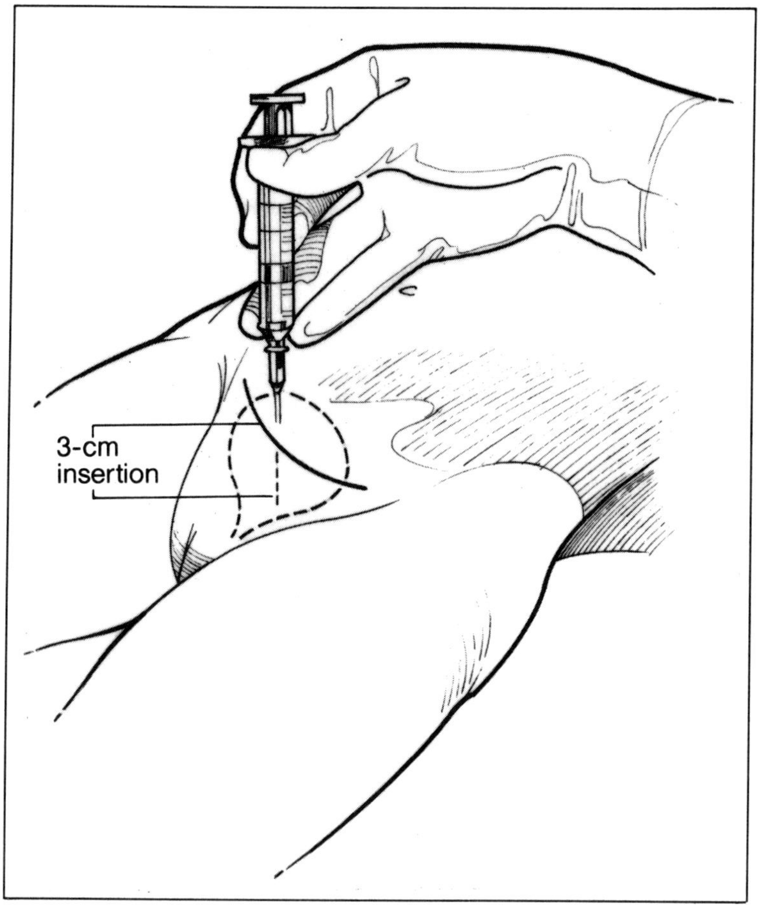

Figure 29-2 Insert the needle in the direction of the coccyx to a depth of 3 cm.

5. Withdraw the plunger slightly to provide slight negative pressure, and advance the needle slowly until urine appears in the syringe.

Note: If you advance the needle 3 cm (about 1¼ in.) with no evidence of urine, assume that you have a dry tap, and withdraw the needle.

6. When urine enters the syringe, collect the amount needed for culture and tests, then withdraw the needle.

7. Apply an adhesive strip over the insertion site if needed.

Suggested Readings

Cloherty JP, Stark AB (eds): *Manual of Neonatal Care.* Boston, Little, Brown & Co, 1980.

Reece RM (ed): *Manual of Emergency Pediatrics,* ed 3. Philadelphia, WB Saunders Co, 1978, p 664.

30

Newborn Circumcision with the Gomco Clamp

Paul S. Williamson, MD

While the American Academy of Pediatrics has declared that there are no absolute medical indications for circumcision of the male newborn,[1] controversy and argument about the advantages and disadvantages of the procedure abound. The majority of American newborn boys continue to be circumcised with cleanliness given as the most common reason parents desire the procedure. Data do not support such traditional reasons as the prevention of cervical or penile cancer, association with sexually transmitted diseases, and psychological reasons. Recent reports of an association between urinary tract infections and uncircumcised male infants are the strongest medical indication for newborn circumcision.[2] Opponents of circumcision feel that the foreskin is nature's protective covering and that daily hygiene after the skin is retractable at 2 to 3 years of age is a perfectly acceptable alternative. Currently the decision to circumcise or not is made by the parents based on what they feel is best for their son.

Contraindications

- Circumcision should not be performed on an infant less than 24 hours old, as it is essential that the newborn have this time to stabilize to the external environment.

---

[1]Thompson HC, et al: Report of the AdHoc Task Force on Circumcision. *Pediatrics* 1975;56:610.

[2]Ginsburg CM, McCrackin GH: Urinary tract infection in young infants. *Pediatrics* 1982;69:409.

- In a premature baby, defer the procedure until he is ready to leave the hospital.
- Any evidence of illness or suspicion that the infant is harboring an active infection.
- A congenital anomaly such as hypospadias (in which foreskin is needed for reconstructing the urethra), incomplete foreskin, shortened penile shaft skin, or a family history of hemophilia.

Materials

- Infant restraint board with adjustable hook and loop tape (Velcro) straps
- Light source
- Warming light
- Sterile gloves
- Sterile towel drapes
- 4×4 in. gauze sponges
- 1 mL 1% lidocaine HCl (Xylocaine HCl) without epinephrine and 1-mL syringe with 27-gauge $\times$ 1.2 cm needle
- Antiseptic skin prep material such as povidone-iodine solution (Betadine)
- Three mosquito clamps
- Suture scissors
- Blunt malleable probe
- Scalpel with blade
- 1×9-in. petrolatum-impregnated gauze dressing
- 1.1 and 1.3 Gomco circumcision clamps

PROCEDURE

The Gomco clamp method of circumcision is preferred over the Plastibell or Sheldon methods because the Gomco technique carries less risk of complications during surgery and fewer subsequent complications. With the Gomco technique, more of the membranous prepuce—the critical area for cancer risk—is excised. The Gomco technique occasions less risk of injury to the glans penis than the guillotine technique of the Sheldon clamp that often leaves "dog-ears" or "corner flaps" at the lateral edges of the preputial incision. With the Plastibell method, hemorrhagic problems may arise if there is loosening of the ligature holding prepuce to the bell; retention of the plastic ring may also cause complications.

1. The infant should not be fed 2–3 hours before surgery. Have in position a diaper-padded restraint board on a waist-high table, a light, all the sterile instrument packs, and a warming light.
2. Before donning sterile gloves, place the infant supine on the restraint board and close the straps over his extremities.

3. Do a 1-minute povidone-iodine surgical scrub of the genital area, concentrating on the penile shaft; wipe off excess with a 4 × 4-in. gauze sponge. Drape the infant with sterile towels.
4. Inject 1% lidocaine without epinephrine (0.2–0.4 mL, depending on the weight of the infant) on each side of the penile shaft over the dorsal penile nerves to block them locally. The anesthetic technique, as developed for infants by Kirya and Werthmann,[3] involves stabilizing the penile shaft in one hand, the piercing the skin of the penile shaft at a 25-degree angle at the 10 o'clock and 2 o'clock positions, 1 cm distal from the pubic bone, inserting the needle no more than 0.25–0.5 cm. Take care to enter the subcutaneous space, avoiding surface veins (Figure 30-1). Wait about 3 minutes for the anesthetic to take effect.
5. Identify the lumen of the prepuce; clamp the dorsal edge of skin with a mosquito hemostat and lift it. If the infant cries, release the clamp and wait a little longer; in some rare cases, you may have to wait 6–8 minutes for the anesthetic to take effect.
6. Insert a second clamp (closed) through the preputial space to the dorsal base of the glans at the corona and open the clamp to dissect the prepuce laterally (Figure 30-2). Use a blunt malleable probe to

Figure 30-1 Penile dorsal nerve block. Stabilize the penile shaft with one hand, then inject 1% lidocaine *without epinephrine* to the depth of 0.25–0.5 cm at 10 o'clock and 2 o'clock, 1 cm distal from the pubic bone.

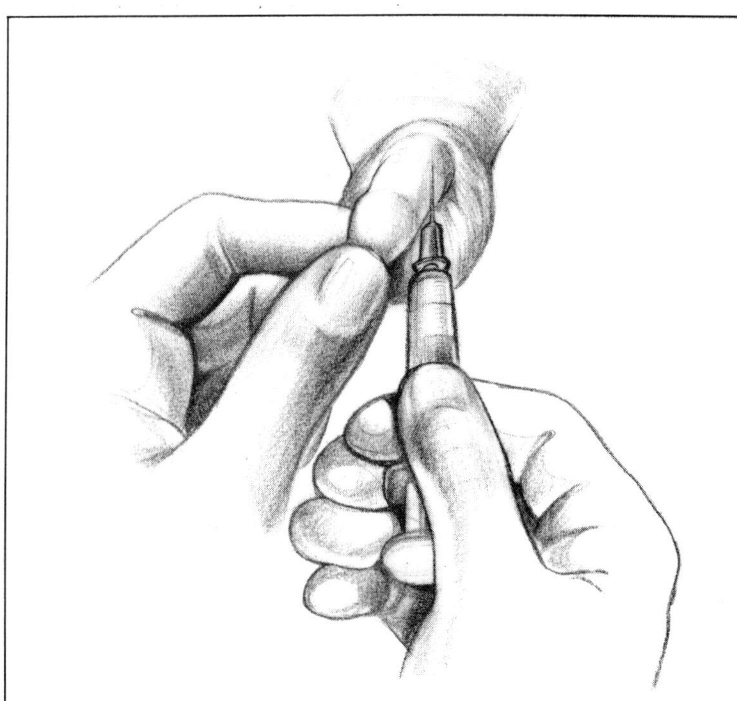

[3]Kirya C, Werthmann MW Jr: Neonatal circumcision and penile dorsal nerve block—A painless procedure. *J Pediatr* 1978;92:998-1000.

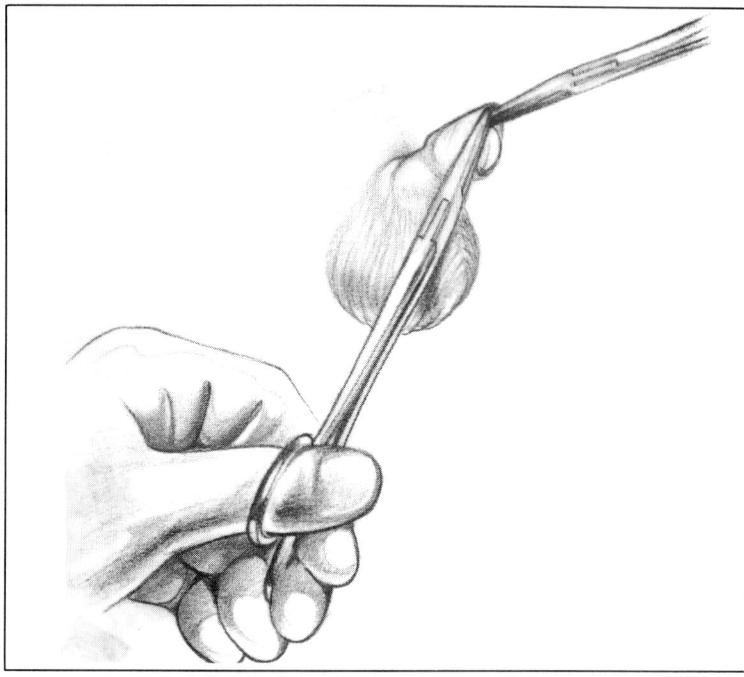

Figure 30-2 Lift the dorsal edge of the prepuce with a mosquito hemostat. Insert a closed hemostat through the preputial space to the dorsal base of the glans at the corona. Open the clamp to laterally dissect the prepuce. Note: If application of initial clamp to lift the prepuce elicits pain response, remove the clamp and wait 6–8 minutes for anesthetic to take effect.

complete dissection of the prepuce from the glans while continuing to elevate the prepuce with the first mosquito clamp.

7. Carefully slide an opened clamp over the dorsal midline of the prepuce to 1 mm from the distal edge of the corona, keeping the point beneath the prepuce elevated to avoid trauma. Close the clamp to crush the dorsal prepuce (Figure 30-3), and keep it closed for 5 seconds. The crush will maintain hemostasis after you divide the prepuce down the middle of the crush.

8. Still holding the edge of the prepuce with a clamp adjacent to the crush line, insert the opened scissors along the crush line with the blunt side beneath the prepuce elevated to avoid trauma. Divide the prepuce down the center of the crush with the scissors to just above the coronal sulcus (Figure 30-4).

9. With a clamp at either edge of the slit in the prepuce, peel back the corners (Figure 30-5). Take care to include both the skin and mucosal layers in the tissue you clamp and peel back; if you don't, the surface of the glans will not be completely exposed. If the initial blunt probing did not fully dissect the glans-prepuce plane, use a 4 × 4-in. gauze sponge to peel back the remainder of the membranous portion until you see the coronal sulcus and the glans exposed in its entirety. You will know you have achieved the correct plane and depth of dissection if you see a slight amount of smegma exposed in the coronal sulcus. After full dissection, bring the prepuce back up over the glans.

10. Select a 1.1 or 1.3 Gomco bell according to the size of the infant's penis, and insert it into the plane just dissected; it should easily

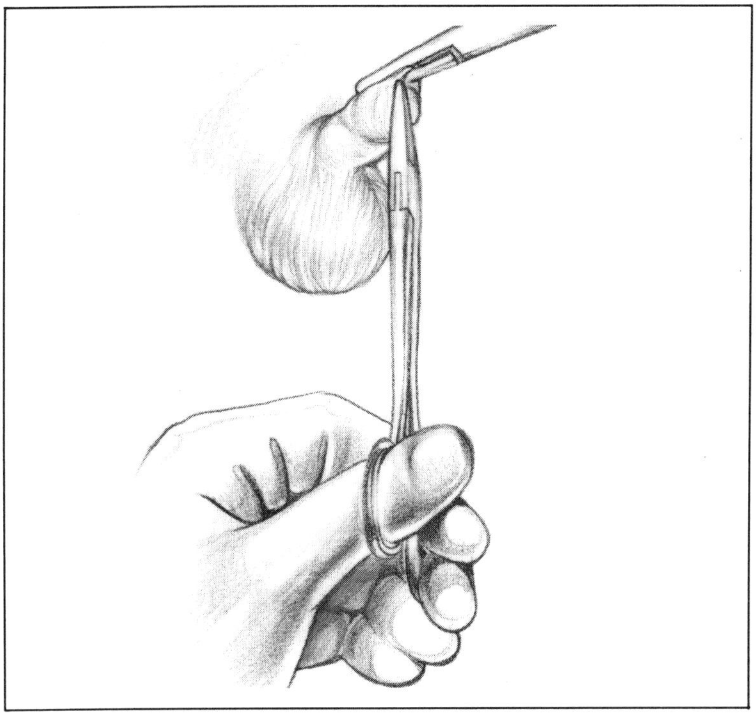

Figure 30-3 To maintain hemostasis as you divide the prepuce, place a clamp at the dorsal midline 1 mm from the distal edge of the corona and hold it shut for 5 seconds to crush the dorsal prepuce.

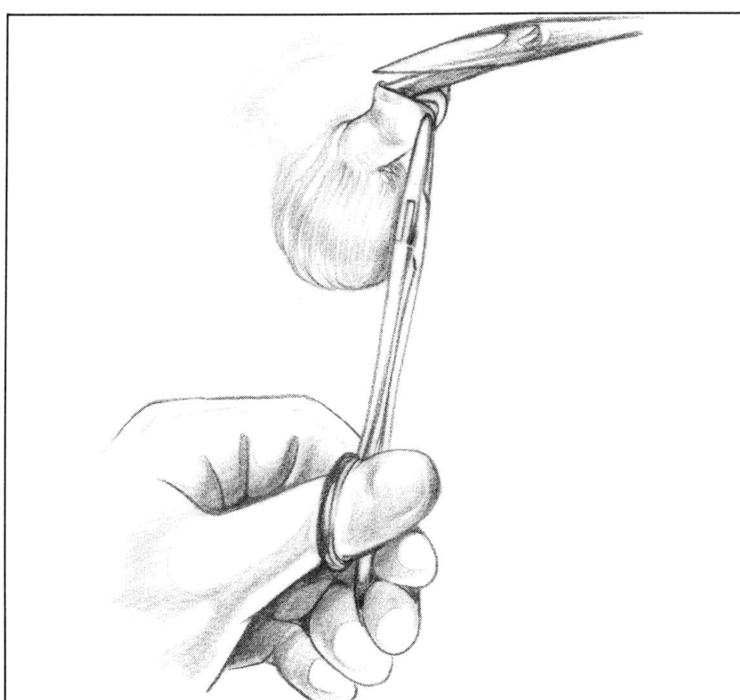

Figure 30-4 To divide the prepuce, insert open scissors along the crush line with the blunt side down to avoid trauma. Slit the prepuce down the crush line to a point just above the coronal sulcus.

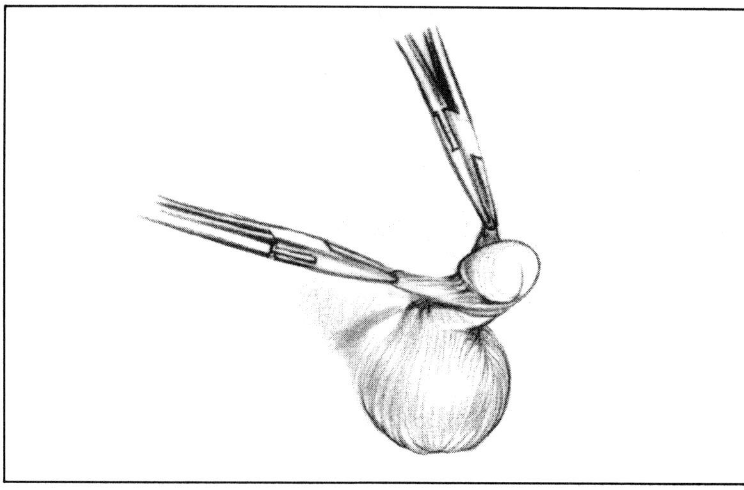

Figure 30-5 Clamp both edges of prepuce and peel back. **Note:** Be sure to peel skin *and* mucosal layer to fully expose glans. Full dissection is achieved when the coronal sulcus is clearly visible. After full dissection, bring the prepuce back up over the glans.

reach as far as the coronal sulcus. Bring the two edges of the dorsal slit up around the shaft of the bell and cross clamp this incision with the third clamp (Figure 30-6). Remove corner clamps.

11. Place the open ring of the Gomco circumcision clamp plate over the shaft of the bell. Use a mosquito clamp to reach through the ring opening and parallel clamp the dorsal slit so you can remove the cross clamp without losing either edge of the prepuce (Figure 30-7).

12. Fully loosen the thumbscrew knob of the Gomco clamp to allow the crossbar of the bell shaft to fall into the grooves of the clamp arm (Figure 30-8).

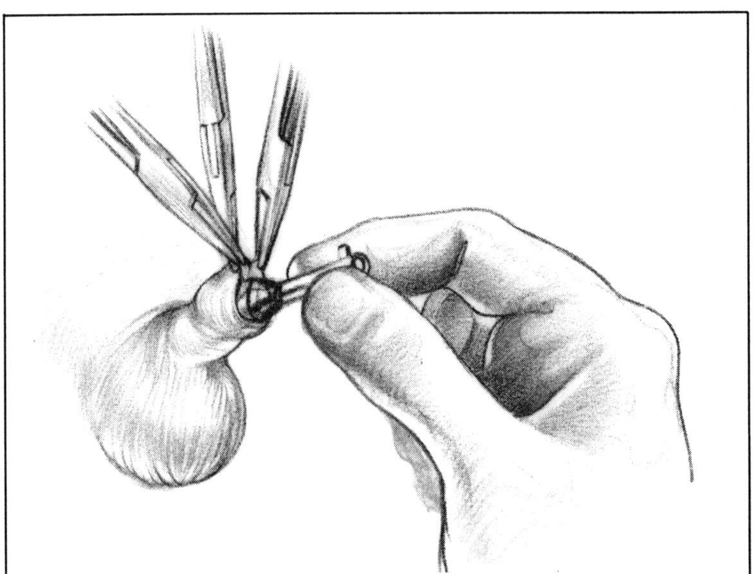

Figure 30-6 Third hemostat cross-clamps the prepuce up around the Gomco bell.

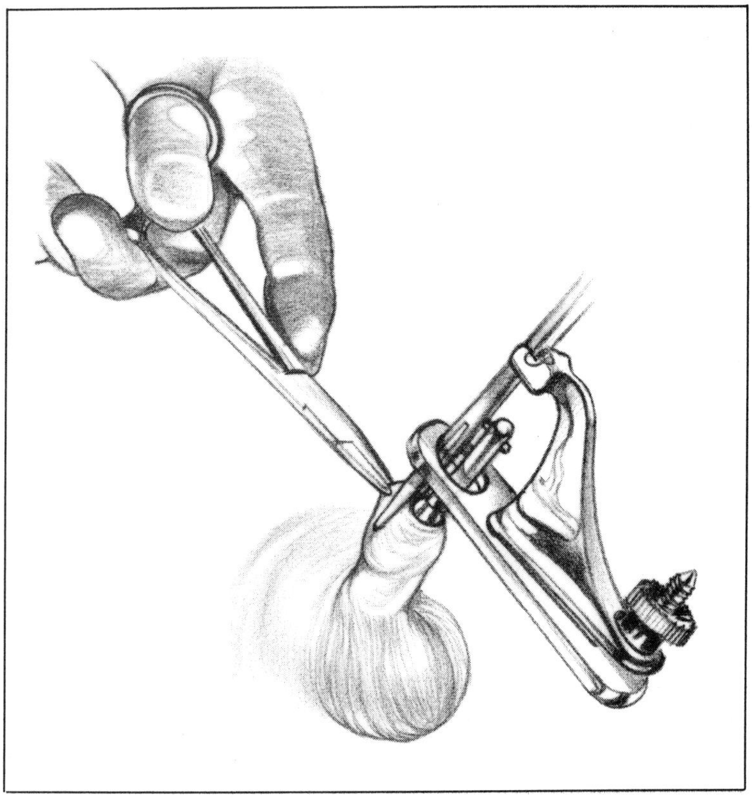

Figure 30-7 With the two side clamps removed, place the open ring of the circumcision clamp plate over the shaft of the bell. Place a mosquito clamp through the ring and parallel clamp the dorsal slit so you can remove the cross-clamp without losing the edge closure.

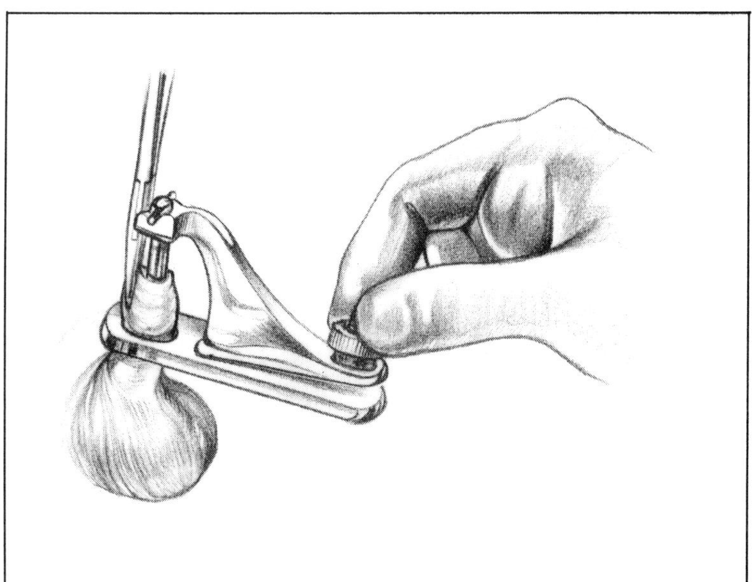

Figure 30-8 Loosen the thumbscrew until the crossbar of the bell shaft falls into the grooves of the clamp arm.

13. Hold the plate of the Gomco clamp horizontally and stretch about 0.75–1.0 cm of the prepuce onto the bell.

Important: If you stretch the prepuce too tightly, too much skin will be removed; if too loosely, too little skin will be removed. This means pulling about as much skin through the ring as you leave below it. Take some time to adjust the skin so the clamp will make a symmetric crush around the prepuce.

14. When you are sure of the placement of the skin over the bell, tighten the thumbscrew of the Gomco clamp to produce a symmetric ring crush through the foreskin at the corona level. Leave the clamp in place 5 minutes for good hemostasis.

15. With the Gomco clamp still in place, trim the prepuce with a cold scalpel blade at the upper plate edge against the bell (Figure 30-9).

16. Loosen the thumbscrew, remove the clamp, and carefully loosen the bell from the incised edge of the penile skin. Wrap a petrolatum-impregnated gauze dressing around the raw edge of the incision to keep diapers from sticking to the area.

Follow-up Care

Keep the circumcised infant under observation for 24 hours for signs of bleeding or infection. Have the diapers changed promptly as needed and the incisional margins cleansed with warm water and mild soap at each diaper change. A light petrolatum coating should be applied around the incisional margin at each diaper change for about a week or until the incision is healed. Instruct parents to report promptly

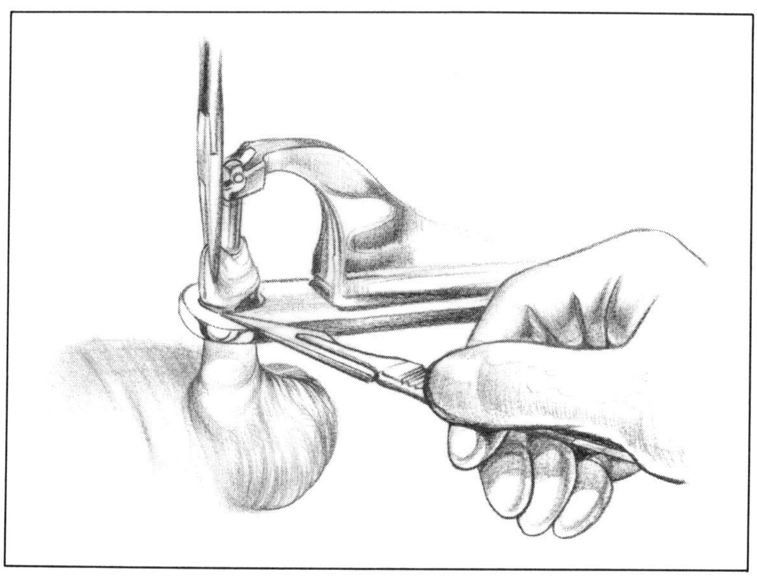

Figure 30-9 Trim prepuce at the upper plate edge with a cold scalpel blade.

fever, swelling, skin redness around the incision, and any bleeding that is more than a slight spotting.

Complications

Circumcision is not a minor procedure. Meticulous technique must be observed to avoid complications:

- Slight hemorrhage at the incision is the most common problem and can be controlled by direct pressure, or by a silver nitrate stick.

Caution: Never use electrocautery because total sloughing necrosis of the penis has occurred with this technique. If a vessel is open and these minor adjustments don't control bleeding, ligate the vessel at the margin of the incision. Most bleeding can be prevented by leaving the Gomco clamp on for a full 5 minutes before trimming the prepuce. Some minor spotting is to be expected after the procedure, and spotting may be observed in the diaper for the first day.

- Infection is the second most common complication. It is usually minor and local—and nearly always controlled by topical antibiotic ointment applied to cover the raw incision. Antibiotic ointment may be used in place of petrolatum for one week. In rare cases, major infectious complications can occur, such as Fournier's syndrome (a gangrenous infection of the penis, scrotum, and inguinal area), septicemia, or necrotizing fasciitis of the abdomen. Use of systemic antibiotics at the first sign of infection beyond the incision is mandatory for the prevention of these rare but serious occurrences.
- Surgical trauma can occur—usually as a result of careless dissection of the glans-prepuce plane or overdenudation of the penile shaft. Inadequate removal of the prepuce produces later adhesions and can also give the appearance of noncircumcision. Urethral fistulas have been produced by kinking the urethra into the Gomco clamp or freehand sewing of the incisional margin too deeply into the urethra. Bivalving of the glans and scrotal lacerations have also been reported.

Suggested Readings

Gee WF, Ansell JS: Neonatal circumcision: A ten-year overview: With comparison of the Gomco clamp and the Plastibell device. *Pediatrics* 1976;58(6):824.

Kirya C, Werthmann MW: Neonatal circumcision and penile dorsal nerve block—A painless procedure. *J Pediatr* 1978;92(6):998-1000.

31

Passing a Urinary Catheter

Elizabeth Loeb, MS, MD
Robert E. Rakel, MD

Because of the risks involved, the decision to order urinary catheterization should be made only after careful consideration of the alternatives. Unless aseptic technique is scrupulously followed, catheterization can introduce bacteria into the bladder, possibly causing cystitis or sepsis in any patient or epididymitis in males. The danger of such infection increases in elderly or debilitated patients, women in the puerperium, or patients with diabetes or large volumes of residual urine. Long-term indwelling catheters can cause formation of urinary calculi as well as changes in the urinary bladder as a result of inflammation. Excessive pressure at the penoscrotal angle from an indwelling catheter can cause urethral fistulas in the male patient.

Among other reasons to consider the patient's situation carefully before ordering urinary catheterization are the following:

- Catheterization can be painful in patients with degenerative hip disease
- A demented or delirious patient could traumatize the urethra by pulling out an indwelling catheter with the balloon still inflated.

Indications

FOR TEMPORARY CATHETERIZATION

- To relieve temporary urethral obstruction or inability to void
- To obtain a sterile urine specimen from patients who cannot perform a clean-catch void because of weakness, obesity, or other medical complications
- To collect sterile urine from asymptomatic women with pyuria or bacteriuria on clean-catch specimens
- To determine residual urine volume or serve as an access route for the injection of contrast medium or normal saline for urologic studies such as cystometrography, cystoscopy, or delineation of the urethral anatomy

FOR INSERTING AN INDWELLING CATHETER

- To monitor urine output in critical care or comatose patients
- To relieve anatomic or physiologic obstruction following urethral or prostatic surgery
- To alleviate persistent incontinence, which is especially beneficial in patients experiencing tissue breakdown or decubitus ulcers in the perineal and anal areas

Contraindications

- Partial or complete rupture of the prostatic urethra
- Acute urethral or prostatic infection
- Inability to pass the catheter without using force

Materials

- Adequate lighting
- 3-in. adhesive tape
- Povidone-iodine solution (Betadine)
- Safety pin
- Urine collection basin
- Kelly clamp
- Sterile catheterization tray or kit containing:
- Straight catheter or retention (Foley) catheter with 10-mL balloon (usually No. 14 or No. 16 French catheter)
- Drapes, including waterproof underpad and fenestrated drape
- Gloves
- Cotton balls (at least five)
- Forceps
- Water-soluble lubricant
- Specimen container with lid
- 10-mL syringe filled with sterile water (Foley set)
- Flat drainage bag, tubing, and puncture port (Foley set)

Preparation

Note: Having an assistant often facilitates the procedure and helps to maintain aseptic technique, especially when patients are uncooperative, restless, or weak.

1. If the patient is conscious, explain the procedure to him or her. If you are determining residual volume, have the patient void.

2. Provide privacy. Position the patient supine with knees bent, hips abducted, and feet resting 60 cm (2 ft) apart. Consider Sims' position for the patient with contractures of the hips or knees.

3. Drape the patient. Place the sterile catheterization tray in easy reach, generally between the patient's feet, and adjust the light.
4. If you are inserting an indwelling catheter and the drainage set is in a separate package, open it and attach the set to the bed frame near the bottom of the bed.
5. Wash your hands thoroughly, open the tray, and put on sterile gloves.
6. If you are inserting an indwelling catheter, test the integrity of the balloon, using the 10-mL syringe and sterile water.
7. Place a waterproof drape under the patient's buttocks. Place the fenestrated drape (hole in the center) over the perineum, with the labia or penis exposed.
8. Saturate cotton balls with povidone-iodine solution, prepare the specimen container if one is needed, and squeeze lubricant onto the sterile field in an accessible location.

PROCEDURE

FEMALE PATIENT

1. With your nondominant hand, approach the genitalia proximally and expose the meatus by placing your thumb and forefinger between the labia minora, retracting them outward and upward toward the symphysis.

Caution: Consider this hand now contaminated; if it slips during or after cleansing the genital area, prepare the area again.
2. Clean the area of the meatus with cotton balls soaked in povidone-iodine solution: Manipulating forceps with your dominant hand, pick up the cotton balls one at a time. Use each ball to wipe from front to back with a downward pull, and discard each ball outside the sterile field.
3. With your dominant hand, pick up the catheter 8 cm (3 in.) from the tip. Use a Kelly clamp to handle the catheter, if you prefer. Lubricate the first 5 cm (2 in.), being careful not to clog the drainage hole. Check to be sure the other end of the catheter is in the collection basin.
4. With gentle pressure, insert the catheter into the urethra. You may be able to facilitate insertion by having the patient inhale to open the meatus as you advance the catheter. Direct the catheter superiorly and posteriorly into the bladder (about 8 cm) until you obtain urinary return (Figure 31-1). If there is not urinary flow, rotate the catheter. Lack of urine could also indicate misdirection of the catheter into the vagina. If this has occurred, remove the catheter and recatheterize, using a new sterile catheter. If you are using a retention catheter,

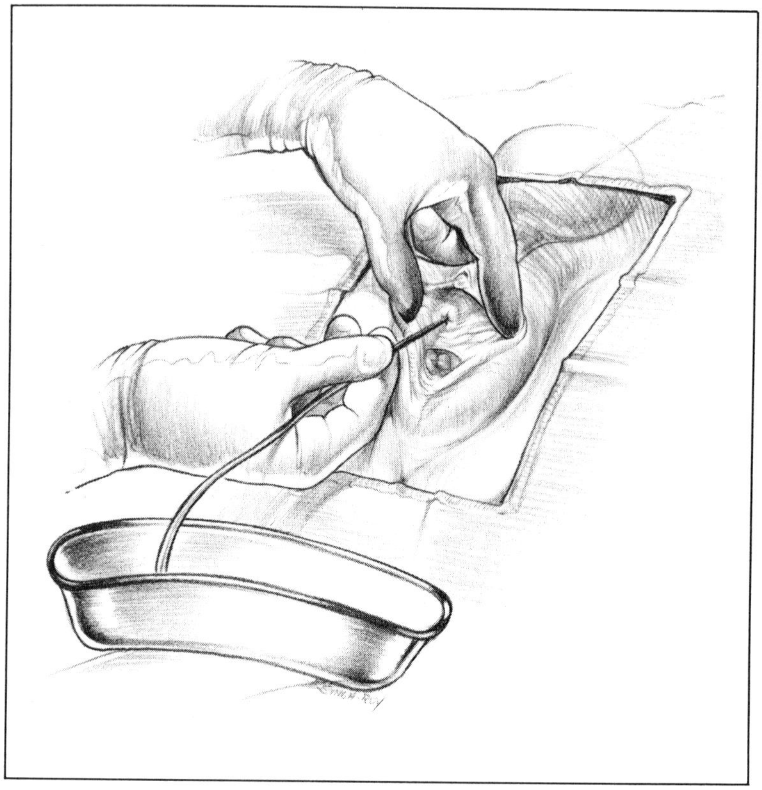

Figure 31-1 Passing a urinary catheter in a female patient. The nondominant hand retracts the labia minora outward and upward toward the symphysis. The dominant hand holds the lubricated tubing approximately 8 cm from the tip and gently inserts it into the urethra until urine return is seen. Be sure to check that the other end of the catheter is in a basin.

insert it 5 cm beyond the point where you obtain urinary return. Release the labia.

MALE PATIENT

Note: If the patient has an enlarged prostate, consider using a No. 12 French or a coude-tip Foley catheter.

1. With your nondominant hand, grasp the penis firmly, directly behind the glans—a light grasp may cause an erection.
2. Holding cotton balls soaked in povidone-iodine solution with forceps manipulated by your dominant hand, start at the glans to cleanse the penis with spiral motion around the circumference of the shaft and 5–7 cm (2–3 in.) down the shaft. In an uncircumcised man, start by retracting the foreskin and wiping off all smegma. Discard cotton balls away from the sterile field.
3. With your nondominant hand, hold the penis at an angle of 60–90 degrees to the patient's body with the meatus toward the patient's head (Figure 31-2).
4. With your dominant hand, pick up the catheter 8 cm (3 in.) from the tip. Use a Kelly clamp to handle the catheter, if you prefer. Lubri-

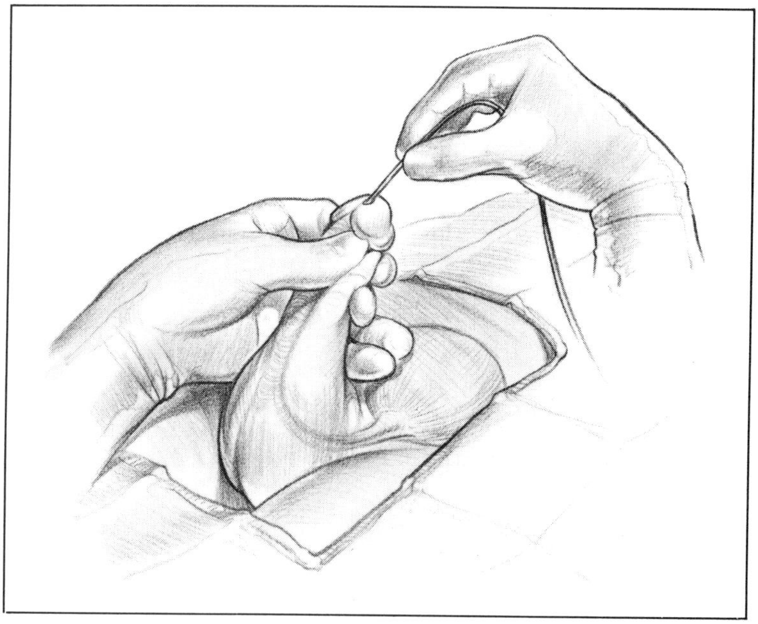

Figure 31-2 Catheter insertion in a male patient. The nondominant hand firmly grasps the penis behind the glans and holds the penis at a 60–90 degree angle to the patient's body. With the dominant hand, gently insert the well-lubricated catheter along the anterior wall of the urethra to a depth of approximately 15–18 cm, or until urine return is achieved.

cate the first 5 cm, being careful not to clog the drainage hole, and lubricate the urethral orifice. Check to be sure the other end of the catheter is in the collection basin.

5. Gently insert the catheter along the anterior wall of the urethra and advance it 15–18 cm (6–7 in.) until urine begins flowing. If you are using a retention catheter, insert it 2.5–5.0 cm (1–2 in.) further.

Caution: Never force the catheter. If you meet substantial resistance, remove the catheter, and squeeze 2–3 mL of lubricant from a sterile, newly opened tube into the urethra before again inserting the catheter.

6. If the patient is uncircumcised, return the foreskin over the glans to prevent phimosis.

Postinsertion Procedure

MALE OR FEMALE PATIENT

1. Holding the catheter in place with your dominant hand, collect a urine sample in the specimen container, if needed. Let the rest of the urine drain into the basin.

2. If the bladder contains a large volume of urine, consider clamping the catheter tubing for 30 minutes after the patient has passed the first 1,000 mL. A controversial theory unsubstantiated by research holds that rapid decompression of the bladder can lead to shock secondary to release of the pressure of pelvic vessels.

3. If you used a straight catheter, remove it when the urine stops flowing. If you inserted an indwelling catheter, start to inflate the balloon once you think you inserted the catheter far enough to get the balloon into the bladder. Inject sterile water through the catheter side arm, observing the patient for pain that would indicate the balloon is still in the urethra. In the absence of pain, complete inflation using 10 mL of sterile water, then gently pull on the catheter to check that the balloon is anchored against the bladder neck. Connect the drainage system to the catheter.

4. Tape the indwelling catheter in place—to the inner thigh, if the patient is female, and laterally, to the dorsum of the thigh, if male. This arrangement in the male patient prevents compression at the penoscrotal angle, which can lead to pressure sores, abscesses, and fistulas (Figure 31-3).

5. Dry the perineum, return the patient to a comfortable position, and remove your gloves. Attach the catheter to the patient's gown with a safety pin.

Complications

Most complications associated with insertion of a urinary catheter, such as false passage, sepsis, and urethral stricture, are uncommon and may be avoided by strict adherence to aseptic technique and by inserting the catheter gently.

Figure 31-3 Indwelling catheters in the male patient should be taped to the dorsum of the thigh to prevent compression at the penoscrotal angle.

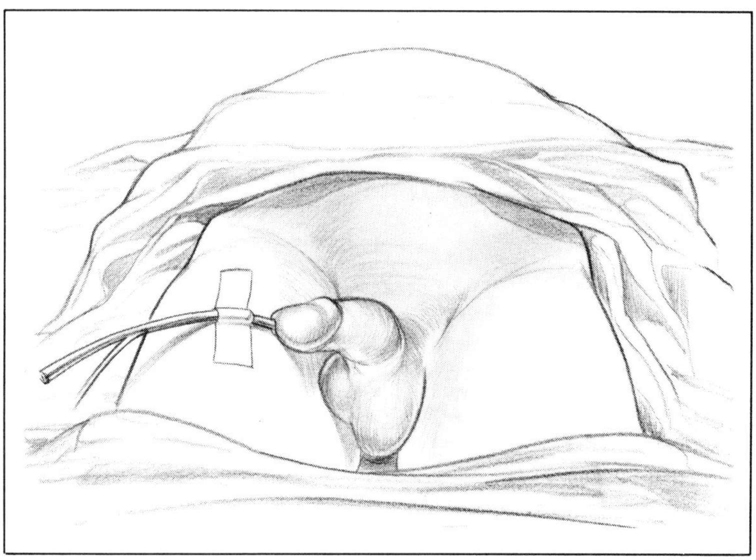

Suggested Readings

Implementing Urologic Procedures. Horsham, Pa, Intermed Communications, Inc, 1982.

Slade N, Gillespie WA: *Urinary Tract and the Catheter.* New York, John Wiley & Sons, 1985.

Smith DR: *General Urology,* ed 11. Los Altos, Ca, Lange Medical Publications, 1984.

32

Emergency Treatment of Priapism: Intracorporeal Aspiration and Irrigation

Charles E. Driscoll, MD

Priapism is a prolonged, painful erection unrelated to sexual desire; it occurs when blood inflow to the penis exceeds outflow. Prompt treatment is necessary to avert short-term complications of infection and urinary retention and the possibility of long-term erectile impotence.

Priapism may be idiopathic or secondary. Typical causes in children and adolescents are sickle cell disease and leukemia that contribute to the condition by sludging and thrombotic episodes. In young adults the cause is often alcohol, marijuana, or other drug addictions. Neurologic disorders, nephrotic syndrome, trauma, and vasculitis are other possible causes in adults of any age. Priapism in the elderly is most likely to be caused by complications from drugs such as antihypertensives, antipsychotics, androgens, anticoagulants, antidepressants, diazepam (Valium), and papaverine HCl injected to treat impotence.

In most cases, prompt aspiration and irrigation will bring about partial or total detumescence so that venous outflow exceeds inflow. Irrigation with alpha-agonists has recently been added to treatment regimens for priapism with good results. The procedure is successful in 75% or more of cases regardless of etiology, but recurrence is more likely in cases secondary to sickle cell disease or leukemia. Such patients may need surgical shunt intervention.

Priapism and its compromised venous outflow may cause local tissue hypoxia and hypercapnia, and increasing pain and longer-lasting priapism are associated with still greater hypoxia and a worse prognosis. Some authorities recommend getting a blood pH and blood gas analysis on the aspirated blood as a guide to the degree of ischemia. Criteria for significant ischemia are these: The condition has persisted for more than 36 hours; pH is lower than 7.25; P_{O2} is less than 30 mmHg; and P_{CO2} is greater than 60 mmHg. In such severe, fortunately rare priapism, surgical shunt is the preferred treatment rather than aspiration and irrigation.

Materials

- Topical antiseptic such as povidone/iodine (Betadine)
- Sponges
- Sterile drape
- Sterile gloves
- 5-mL syringe with 35-gauge needle and 5 mL of 1% lidocaine HCl (Xylocaine HCl) for anesthesia
- 19-gauge butterfly needle
- 20-mL Luer-Lok syringe
- Three-way stopcock
- 1-L bag sterile normal saline
- IV administration set
- Sterile basin
- 5-mL heparinized glass syringe for drawing blood-gas specimens
- Sterile adhesive bandage or dressing

PROCEDURE

1. Obtain informed consent, carefully explaining that impotence is a known complication of priapism.
2. Thoroughly cleanse the penis, and prepare the skin. Wearing sterile gloves, drape the surrounding area to create a sterile field.
3. Locate the 3 o'clock or the 9 o'clock position on the penile shaft, approximately 1 inch from the corona. Avoid the dorsal neurovascular bundle and the ventral urethral areas (Figure 32-1). Overlying the corpus cavernosum, subcutaneously inject 0.5–1.0 mL lidocaine HCl to anesthetize the aspiration site. Because of cross-flow circulation, you need to aspirate only one side of the penis.
4. With the three-way stopcock connected to the 20-mL syringe and the 19-gauge butterfly needle connected to the stopcock, insert the needle into the corpus cavernosum through the anesthetized skin (Figure 32-2).

Figure 32-1

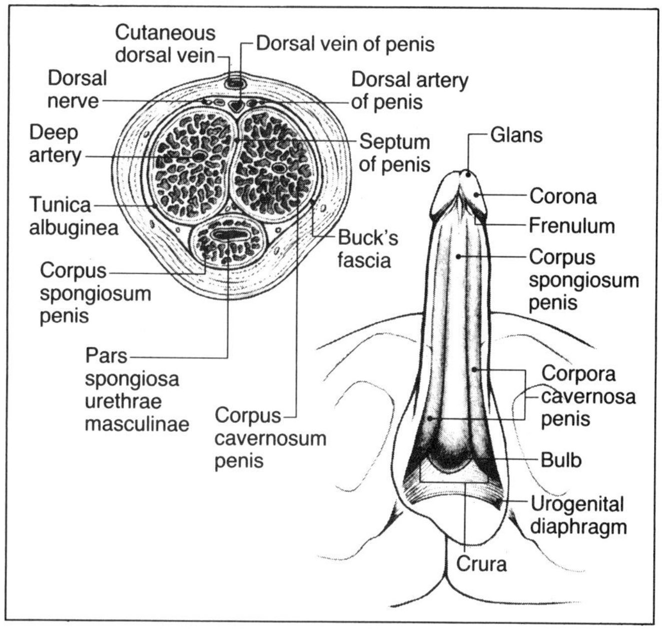

5. Open the stopcock to the needle, and aspirate blood into the 20-mL syringe. The blood will be dark and viscous. (If you want to measure blood gases, use the heparinized glass syringe for the first aspiration, then change to the 20-mL syringe.) Close the stopcock to the needle, open the third portal, and eject the aspirate into the sterile basin. Close the third portal, open the stopcock to the needle, and repeat until all obtainable blood is aspirated. Squeezing or milking the penis may increase the aspiration.

6. When aspiration is complete, begin irrigation. Add 1 mL of epinephrine 1:1000 to the 1-L bag of sterile saline. Attach the IV administration set, run fluid through the tubing, and connect the tubing to the third portal of the stopcock (Figure 32-3).

7. Open the stopcock to the third portal, withdraw 20 mL of the saline-epinephrine mix, close the third portal, and open to the butterfly needle. Slowly inject the solution into the corpus cavernosum.

8. Have a sterile-gloved assistant temporarily remove IV tubing from the third portal, and aspirate the 20 mL back into the syringe. Close the needle portal, opening the third portal, and eject the solution into the basin.

9. Repeat step 8 until you obtain satisfactory detumescence and the blood returned from the penis is bright red rather than dark and viscous.

10. Withdraw the needle from the penis, and cover the aspiration site with a sterile dressing.

Note: If you do not obtain satisfactory results after irrigating with 200 mL of fluid, abandon the procedure, and plan for surgical shunting.

Figure 32-2

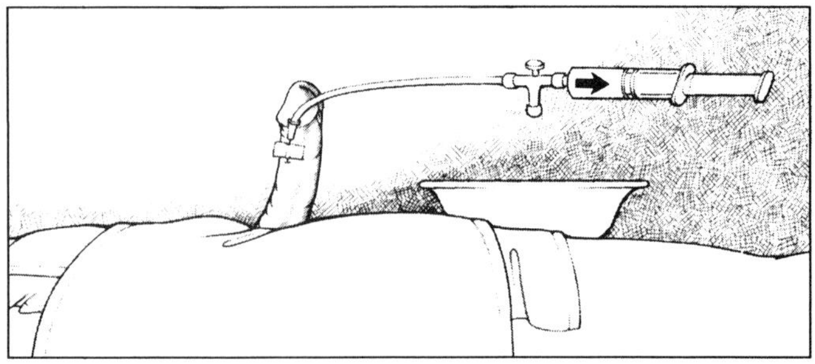

Figure 32-3

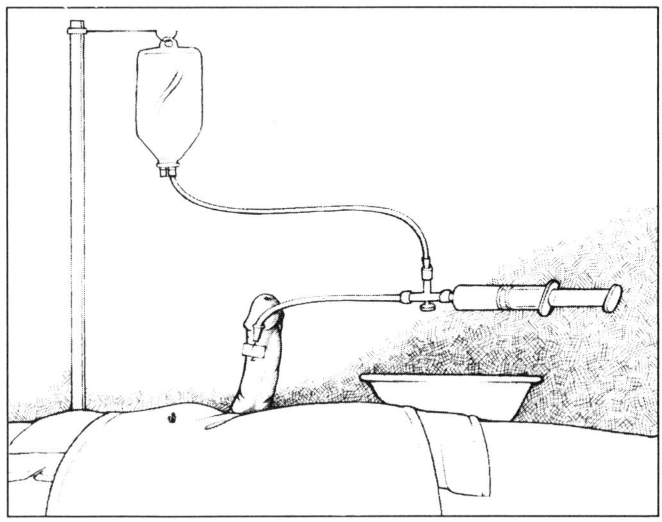

11. Hospitalize the patient for 24 hours of observation to be sure priapism does not recur.

Complications

- Minor hematoma at the aspiration site
- Injury to the urethra or dorsal neurovascular bundle from careless needle placement
- Urinary retention requiring catheter insertion
- Blood pressure or pulse alterations from epinephrine (rare)

Suggested Readings

Fernandez J, Basha M, Wilson G: Emergency treatment of papaverine priapism. *J Emer Med* 1987;5:289-291.

Molina L, Bejany D, Lynne CM, et al: Diluted epinephrine solution for the treatment of priapism. *J Urol* 1989;141:1127-1128.

O'Brien WM, O'Connor KP, Lynch JH: Priapism: Current concepts. *Ann Emerg Med* 1989;18:980-983.

Yealy D, Hogya P: Priapism. *Emer Med Clin North Am* 1988;6:509-520.

33

Examining a Male Patient for Genital Warts

Charles E. Driscoll, MD

Androscopy—colposcopy of the male genitalia—utilizes an acetic acid solution applied to the skin to demonstrate, under magnification, the typical white lesions that may suggest human papillomavirus (HPV) infection. As many as 80% of male partners of women with documented HPV lesions have white changes in the skin of their reproductive organs after application of acetic acid. The lesions may appear on the penis, scrotum, perianal area, and the inner aspect of the thigh (Figure 33-1).

Biopsy of these lesions will reveal characteristic histologic features of HPV infection. Androscopy is essential because these lesions may not be seen by the naked eye. If the lesions go undetected, the patient may continue to transmit infection, and recrudescences may be mistaken for new infection. Male-to-female HPV transmission has been documented, and HPV types 16 and 18 are strongly implicated in cervical cancer.

Indications

Men who have or have had the following:

- Penile warts
- Bowenoid papulosis
- Sexual partners with known HPV infection
- Sex with prostitutes or with 20 or more sexual partners

Contraindications

- None

Materials

- Colposcope
- Gauze sponges, 4 × 4 in.

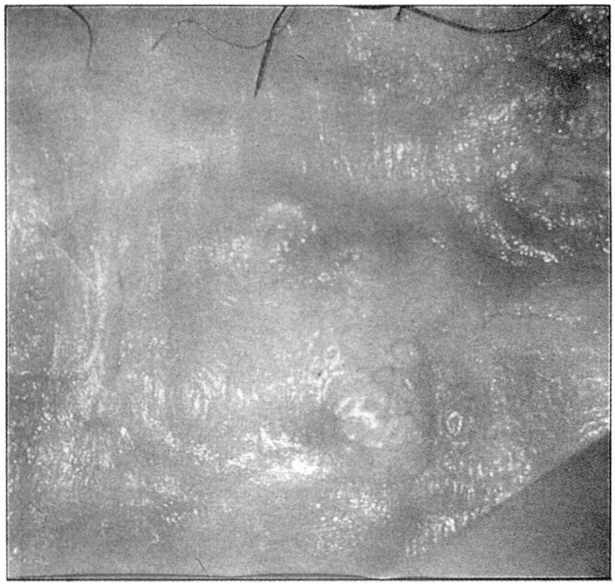

Figure 33-1 Characteristic white lesions appear here on the skin of the reproductive organs after application of 5% acetic acid. As many as 80% of male partners of women with documented human papillomavirus infection show these changes.

- 5% acetic acid solution
- 3-mL syringe, 35-gauge needle attached
- Alcohol swabs
- 1% lidocaine HCl (Xylocaine HCl)
- Colposcopic biopsy forceps, scalpel with a No. 10 blade, or skin biopsy punch
- Topical styptic (Monsel's solution or silver nitrate)
- Specimen jar with 10% formalin

PROCEDURE

1. Examine the scrotal area with the colposcope before staining to identify any lesions. With the supine patient in stirrups in the lithotomy position, examine glans, shaft and scrotal skin, perineal body, and perianal tissues. Use white light at a magnification of 10–15 times. If the patient is uncircumcised, have him hold back the foreskin for glans examination. Look for papillomas or hyperkeratoses.
2. Soak 4 × 4-in. gauze sponges in 5% acetic acid solution, and apply them for about five minutes to the skin areas you want to examine. Weaker solutions, such as 3%, are less effective on keratinized squamous epithelium, but they may be more comfortable for mucosal surfaces such as the glans in an uncircumcised patient.
3. Carefully repeat the colposcopic examination, looking for the white lesions.
4. To obtain a biopsy specimen of the lesions, inject 0.1–0.2 mL of 1% lidocaine HCl (Xylocaine HCl) sublesionally to raise a wheal, then

shave with a scalpel blade, remove by conventional colposcopic biopsy forceps, or take a punch biopsy.

5. Use a topical styptic for hemostasis.

6. Submit biopsy specimens in formalin for histologic examination.

Follow-up Care

- When biopsy reports indicate HPV infection, treat identified lesions with topical application of 80% trichloroacetic acid (Tri-Chlor), cryotherapy, or carbon dioxide laser fulguration.

Note: Recurrence rates may be as high as 10–50% even when treated.

Suggested Readings

Barraso R, De Brux J, Croissant O, et al: High prevalence of papillomavirus-associated penile intraepithelial neoplasia in sexual partners of women with cervical intraepithelial neoplasia. *N Engl J Med* 1987;317:916-923.

Rosemberg SK: Subclinical papillomaviral infection of male genitalia. *Urology* 1985;26:554-557.

Sedlacek T: Evaluating the male partner of the HPV infected patient. *The Female Patient* (suppl), 1990;(15):46-49.

VI

OBSTETRICS AND GYNECOLOGY PROCEDURES

34

Inserting an Intrauterine Device

Elizabeth A. Burns, MD
Martin Bartolac, MD

Only one type of intrauterine device (IUD) is currently available as a contraceptive in the United States. This is an IUD that contains progesterone. The inert devices (Lippes Loop and Saf-T-Coil), and the copper devices (Cu-7 and Tatum-T) are no longer marketed here, but many are still in use. The inert devices can remain in place indefinitely, but the copper IUDs should be removed and replaced three years after insertion.

Progesterone is the mechanism of action in the Progestasert IUD, as it is gradually released into the urinary cavity. This infiltration of progesterone creates a pseudodecidual uterine environment not suitable for embryo implantation.

The theoretic effectiveness of IUDs is 97–99%; their use-effectiveness is 90–96%, depending on such variables as age and frequency of intercourse. Some 50% of pregnancies among IUD users result in spontaneous abortion, prematurity, amnionitis, or gestational bleeding. It has been determined that ectopic pregnancies are more likely to occur in women with an IUD in place than in women who are not using one.

Contraindications

Absolute
- Acute pelvic infection
- Pregnancy

Strong
- Recurrent pelvic infection (gonococcal or chlamydial)
- Multiple sexual partners
- Abnormal uterine bleeding
- History of ectopic pregnancy
- Impaired coagulation from either therapy or a clotting defect

- Postpartum endometriosis
- An abortion within three months

Relative

- Valvular heart disease predisposing to subacute bacterial endocarditis (assess need for prophylactic antibiotics)
- Abnormal Pap smear or cervical neoplasm
- Cervical stenosis
- Small uterus
- Endometriosis
- Leiomyomata or polyps
- Bicornuate uterus
- Dysmenorrhea or menorrhagia
- Anemia
- Inability to check the presence or location of the IUD thread

Materials

- Examining table
- Intrauterine device
- Povidone-iodine solution (Betadine)
- Local anesthetic such as 0.5% lidocaine HCl (Xylocaine)
- Syringe
- 22-gauge spinal needle
- Gloves
- Vaginal speculum
- Drapes
- Bowl for povidone-iodine solution
- Sponges or cotton balls
- Uterine sound
- Cotton swab
- Tenaculum
- Scissors
- Ring forceps or long Kelly clamp
- Silver nitrate sticks

The IUD Candidate

Let the uterine depth, determined by sounding at the time of the initial counseling, guide the choice of an IUD as a contraceptive. Insertion is not recommended unless the uterus sounds between 6 and 10 cm ($2\frac{3}{8}$–$3\frac{15}{16}$ in.)

Progestasert is a good therapeutic choice for the patient with dysmenorrhea or heavy menses.

Timing of IUD Insertion

It is optimal to insert the IUD during the patient's menstrual period when the cervix is soft and dilated. The bleeding that sometimes follows IUD insertion for about one week is not alarming if it is masked by menses. This bleeding, along with the continuing menses, can actually help reassure the patient that she is not pregnant.

Insert an IUD during the remainder of the patient's menstrual cycle only if she has not had intercourse since her last period, was protected during intercourse, or has just finished her period.

Preinsertion Procedure

1. Become thoroughly familiar with the manufacturer's instructions for insertion of the IUD chosen.
2. Explain the concept and the procedure to the patient. Show her the device. Allow sufficient time for her to read the patient information material provided and ask questions.
3. With the draped patient in the lithotomy position on the examining table, don sterile gloves and perform a bimanual examination to determine whether the uterus is anteflexed or retroflexed, to rule out pregnancy, and to detect infection.
4. Reglove with sterile gloves and insert a vaginal speculum to aid in visual examination of the cervix.
5. With sterile materials and sterilized equipment laid out, cleanse the cervix with an antiseptic solution—povidone-iodine solution (Betadine), if the patient is not allergic to it—using a sterile sponge or a cotton ball held by a ring forceps or long Kelly clamp.
6. Administer a paracervical block, if necessary, using a 22-gauge spinal needle and 5–10 mL 0.5% lidocaine HCl (Xylocaine) without epinephrine.

Note: Candidates for local anesthesia are nulliparous women who generally have narrow cervical canals and small uterine cavities, and patients prone to vasovagal activity when experiencing pain. Nonsteroidal anti-inflammatory drugs (such as 250–375 mg naproxen [Naprosyn], or two 275-mg tablets naproxen sodium [Anaprox]) given 30 minutes before IUD insertion may diminish discomfort in these patients.

PROCEDURE

1. Continuing aseptic technique, gently grasp the anterior lip of the cervix with a tenaculum about 1.5 cm (9/16 in.) above the external os.
2. Sound the uterus for direction and depth. With the sound inserted to maximum depth, place a cotton swab at the cervix and remove it with the sound to get an accurate measurement (Figure 34-1).
3. Just before insertion (1–2 minutes, depending on the device), load the IUD into the inserter according to manufacturer's directions.
4. Apply gentle traction of the cervical lip with the tenaculum. If necessary, apply sufficient downward traction to straighten the uterine axis.

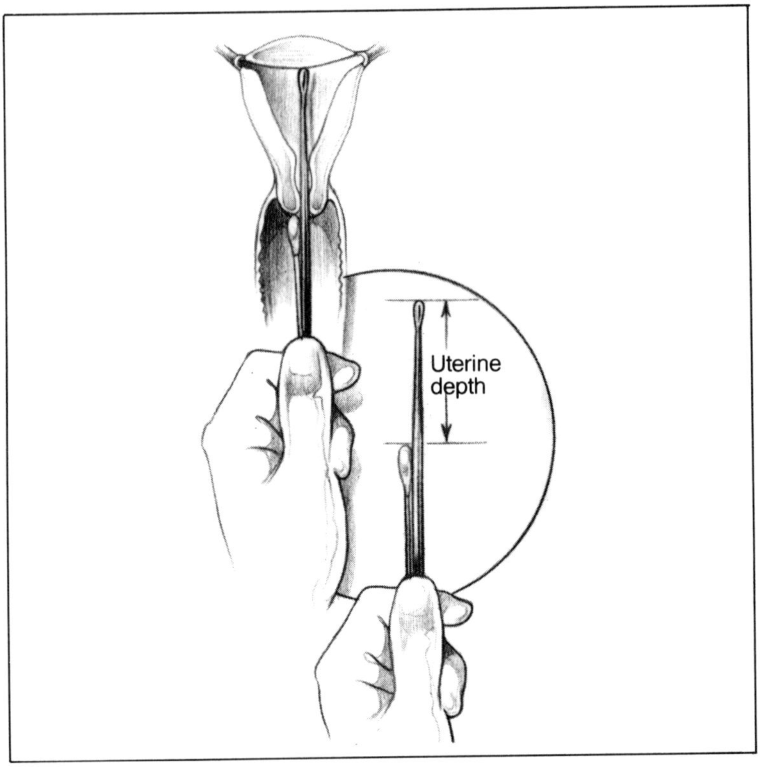

Figure 34-1 Measure depth of uterus by placing swab alongside sound at the cervix and removing them together.

5. Introduce the inserter into the cervical canal and then the uterus, advancing it slowly and gently, checking any indicators provided on the inserter to be sure the device is inserted in the horizontal plane. The arm cocker will slide along the inserter shaft. The number at the base of the arm cocker approximates the uterine depth (in centimeters) and will assist in determining when the fundus is reached (Figures 34-2 and 34-3).
6. To situate the IUD in the fundus, release the thread-retaining plug. This frees the thread and the IUD from the inserter as the inserter is slowly withdrawn (Figure 34-4). To check the position, measure the length of the short indicator thread (Figure 34-5). The depth of the uterus plus the length of the indicator thread should approximate 9 cm for correct placement.
7. Trim the thread of the device at least 5 cm (2 in.) from the cervix; it can always be cut shorter later if desired. Have the patient feel the piece of thread you trim off to familiarize herself with its texture.
8. Observe tenaculum insertion sites. If bleeding persists, use silver nitrate sticks to cauterize the area.
9. After the patient has rested following the procedure, have her feel the thread in her vagina.

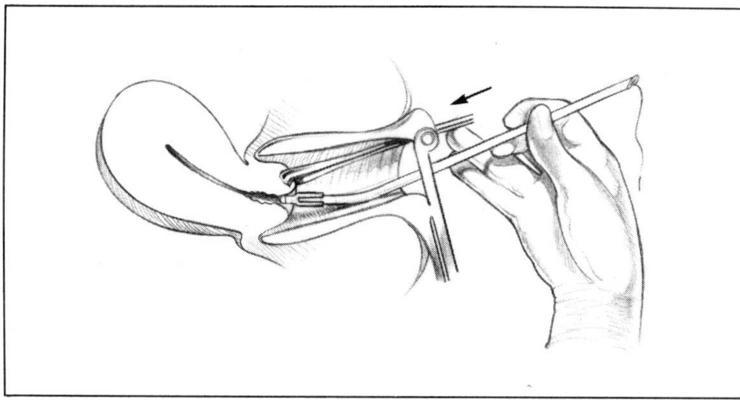

Figure 34-2 Introduce inserter slowly through cervical canal into the uterus, checking to be sure it is in the horizontal plane.

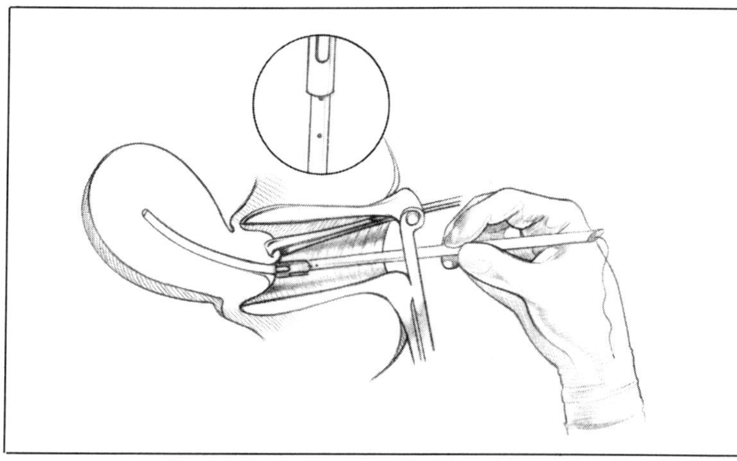

Figure 34-3 Numbers at the base of the arm cocker approximate uterine depth and help determine when the fundus is reached.

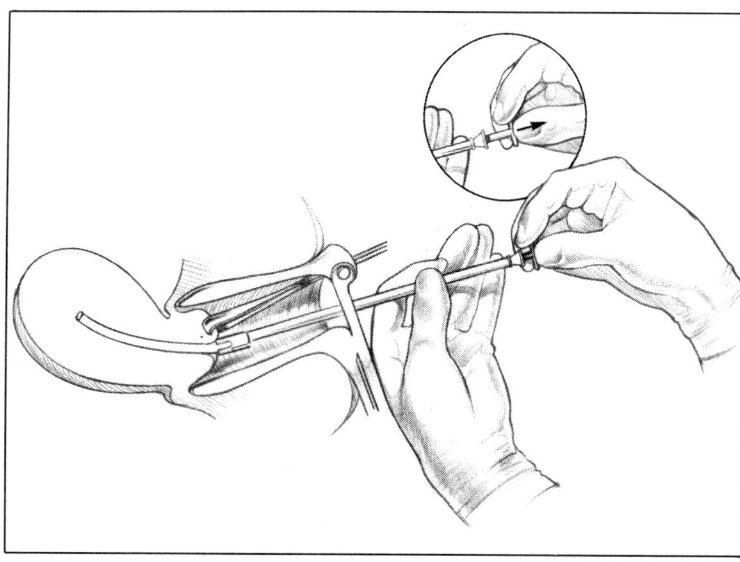

Figure 34-4 Release plug to situate the IUD in the fundus.

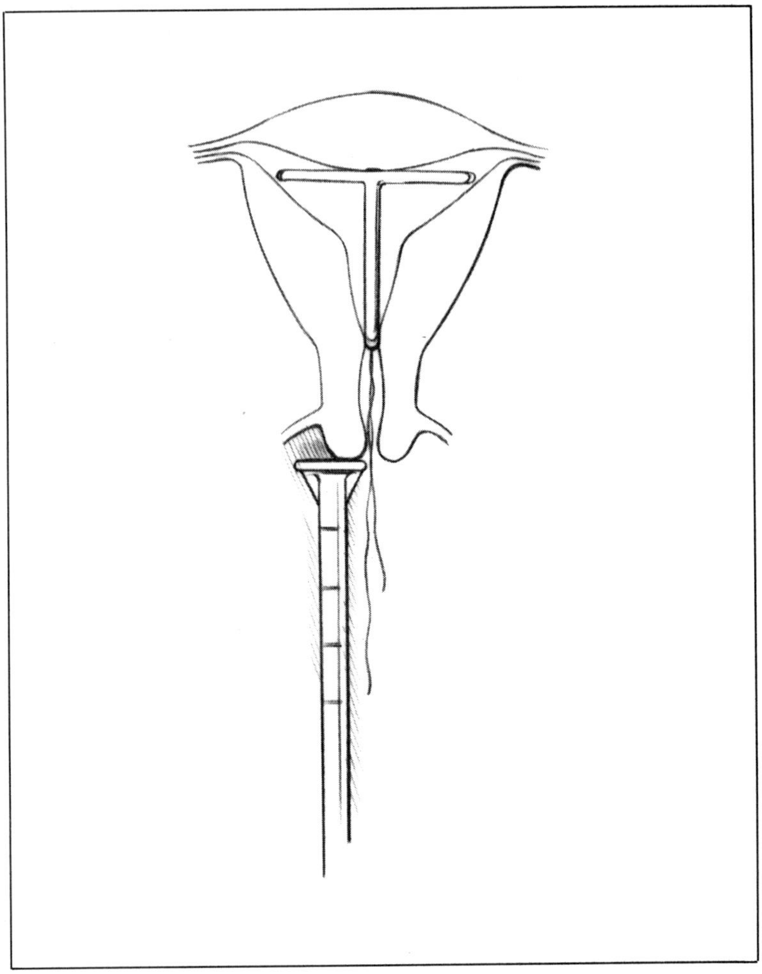

Figure 34-5 To check position of device, measure the length of exposed indicator thread—depth of the uterus plus length of thread should equal approximately 9 cm.

Complications

- *Infection* causes more hospitalization than any other complication of IUD use. Symptoms include pain, fever, and chills. Remove the IUD before treating the patient with antibiotics; an IUD left in place can be a continuing medium for the infecting organism, seeding the endometrium. Treat pelvic inflammatory disease with broad-spectrum antibiotics for 10–14 days. Rule out ectopic pregnancy. Wait 3–12 months before considering reinsertion of an IUD after infection, or recommend another method of contraception if the patient plans future pregnancies. Though a tailless IUD is less apt to cause infection, its status cannot be as easily determined as that of an IUD with a thread.
- *Uterine perforation* occurs in about 1 per 1,000 IUD users and is often asymptomatic. Lowest rates of perforation are reported for

the Lippes Loop and the Cu-7. When symptoms occur, they may include pain, bleeding, gradual apparent shortening of the thread, and symptoms of pregnancy. Ultrasound can detect both metallic and nonmetallic devices effectively. Should the IUD perforate the cervix, you can push the device back in toward the fundus and then remove it through the cervical os. If the device has penetrated the peritoneal sac, laparoscopy or laparotomy is needed to retrieve it.

- *Pregnancy*, uterine or ectopic, is possible with an IUD in place. If uterine pregnancy occurs, remove the IUD if possible. If you can't remove the device, consult with the patient on the option of terminating the pregnancy. Continuing the pregnancy with an IUD in place involves increased risk of spontaneous abortion and increased risk of sepsis. If ectopic pregnancy occurs, treat as you would in a patient not using an IUD.
- *Expulsion* occurs most often in the first two months following IUD insertion and is more common in nulliparous women. The overall rate of expulsion is 5% to 20% per year. Symptoms include discharge, cramping or pain, spotting, dyspareunia in the patient or difficulty with coitus in the partner, and apparent lengthening of the thread. The patient may be able to feel the device when she checks for the thread. You may notice partial expulsion on direct examination or on ultrasonography or radiography. Remove any partially expelled IUD. After determining the probable cause for expulsion, consider changing to a different size or model if indicated.
- *Bleeding* following IUD insertion is common, particularly in the form of heavier or longer menstrual periods or spotting between periods. About 15% of women discontinue IUD use because of this. When a patient presents with these complaints, always consider other causes, such as expulsion of the device, perforation, infection, and causes not related to use, including polyps, neoplasm, and fibroadenoma.

Follow-up Care

- Instruct the patient to check for the thread weekly until she feels comfortable with the checking procedure; then have her check routinely after each menstrual period.
- Recommend that she use an additional method of contraception for the first three months.
- Alert the patient to common side effects of IUD insertion such as pain, bleeding or spotting, and cramps with periods. Ask her to report a late or missed period, abdominal pain, fever, chills, foul smelling discharge, or bleeding with clots.
- Replace a progesterone-containing device every year. Be sure to sound the patient's uterus before inserting a new IUD.

Removal

- Remove the IUD if the patient requests it, if you note endometriosis, if the hematocrit drops five points or below 30%, if the device is partially expelled, or if the device is due for replacement because its stores of copper or progesterone are depleted.
- Removing an IUD usually involves minimal pain. If the device has been in place more than five years, however, narrowing of the cervical canal or embedding of the device in the uterine wall can cause discomfort.
- It's best to remove the IUD during menses, when the os is open. Using aseptic technique, apply slow, gentle, steady traction on the thread with a ring forceps or a long Kelly clamp. If difficulties arise, don't risk breaking the thread. Instead, sound the uterus for 30 seconds, then rotate the sound 90 degrees to dislodge the device. You may want to use a paracervical block (see step 6 in "Preinsertion Procedure").
- Consider dilating the cervix to facilitate removal. You may find exerting downward traction on the cervix with a tenaculum helpful, as well.
- If necessary, remove the device using alligator forceps, uterine packing forceps, a Novak curet, or a hook.
- If the IUD thread is not visible, you can try removing the device in the office using uterine dressing forceps, a hooked uterine curet, or contact hysteroscopy. If necessary, the device can be removed in the hospital using hysteroscopy, dilation and curettage, or suction aspiration.

Suggested Readings

Hatcher RA, Guest FJ, Steward FH, et al: *Contraceptive Technology, 1984-1985,* ed 12. New York, Irving Publishers, 1984, pp 81-89.

Pritchard JA, MacDonald PC: *Williams Obstetrics,* ed 16. New York, Appleton-Century-Crofts, 1980, pp 1021-1028.

Romney SL, Gray MJ, Little B, et al: *Gynecology and Obstetrics: The Health Care of Women,* ed 2. New York, McGraw-Hill Book Co, 1981, pp 831-835.

35

Fine-Needle Aspiration of the Breast

Elizabeth Loeb, MD

Fine-needle aspiration of the breast is a quick and simple procedure of great efficacy. Although surgical biopsy has been the preferred and traditional method of breast tumor evaluation, the currently recommended method is to use examination of cytologic smears from the fine-needle aspiration in conjunction with mammography. This combination has reduced diagnostic errors to 1%.

Note: Do not rely exclusively on mammograms to confirm dysplastic changes because false-negative reports can delay a diagnosis of cancer.

Indications

- To confirm cytologically that vague nodularities and thickenings are benign.
- To diagnose fibroadenoma in young women, allowing postponement of surgery to a more opportune time if desired.
- To confirm cytologically that a cyst is benign and to drain the cyst.
- To distinguish diffuse suppurative disease from neoplasm.
- To establish a positive diagnosis of cancer when considering preoperative irradiation.
- To establish a diagnosis of operable cancer. This helps to convince a reluctant patient of the need for surgery and reduces anesthesia time by eliminating the need for frozen section.
- To analyze the estrogen receptor status of a carcinoma.
- To confirm the diagnosis of an inoperable cancer, such as inflammatory breast carcinoma, for possible irradiation or chemotherapy.

Contraindications

None

Limiting Factors

- A lesion deep in a heavy breast
- Access to a pathologist who is experienced in interpreting cytologic smears

Materials

- Cameco syringe pistol or Aspir-Gun
- 20-mL disposable syringe without Luer-Lok tip
- 22-gauge (0.6–1.0 mm external diameter) disposable needle, 3.8 or 8.8 cm long, with or without a mandrin
- 25-gauge needle
- 3 alcohol prep sponges
- Sterile gauze pads
- Glass microscope slides with frosted ends for labeling
- Spray fixative or a bottle of 95% methyl, ethyl, or isopropyl alcohol to hold slides for immediate fixation of wet smears
- 1% lidocaine HCl (Xylocaine HCl)

PROCEDURE

To prepare for fine-needle aspiration, examine the patient's breast, supraclavicular region, and axilla including the posterior axillary folds. If the mass is difficult to palpate, soap the breast and palpate lightly, asking the patient where the mass is located. Examine any postmastectomy scars carefully for a local recurrence of carcinoma. If you find a tumor eroding the skin surface, use a scalpel to collect the specimen.

1. With the patient supine, attach the syringe to the syringe pistol. By applying light pressure, position the mass between index finger and thumb of your nondominant hand. With your other hand, prep the skin above the mass three times with alcohol prep sponges. If the patient is especially anxious, infiltrate the skin with 1% lidocaine.

2. Position the syringe pistol over the puncture site, insert the needle quickly through the skin, and advance it into the mass (Figure 35-1). The location and nature of the mass may influence your technique in this step:

- If you find skin dimpling, the skin is probably attached to the outer surface of the mass, and you can insert the needle directly through the dimple into the tumor.
- If you find vague, superficial nodules, inflammatory carcinoma, and suspected pagetoid skin, perform a superficial subepidermal aspiration using an angled 25-gauge needle.

Confirm that you have punctured the mass by moving the needle slightly from side to side and feeling the mass move between your fingers.

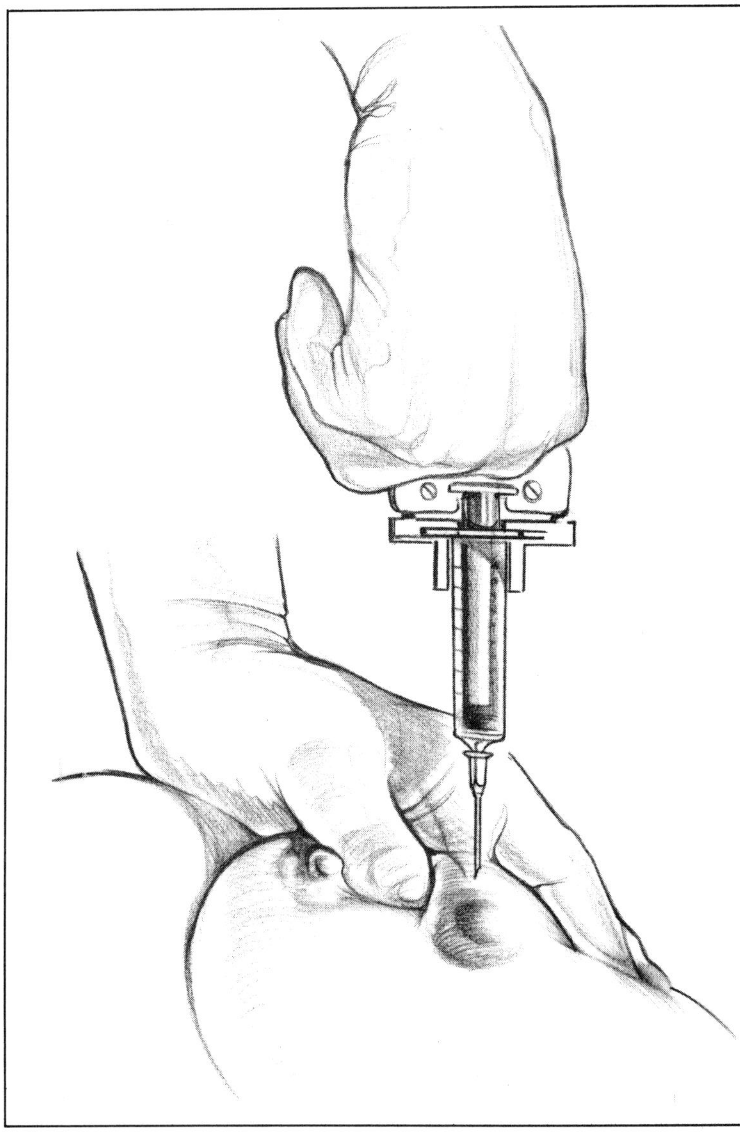

Figure 35-1 Position the mass between the index finger and thumb of the nondominant hand. Position the syringe directly over the mass and insert the needle quickly through the skin and into the mass.

You may have trouble penetrating firm, dense, gritty scirrhous tumors. Grasp the scirrhous mass firmly, especially if it is deep, and use forceful movement with aspiration if necessary to extract tissue; this is often painful to the patient. Benign lesions, especially lipomas, usually offer little or no resistance, depending on the extent of their fibrous stroma.

3. Apply full suction continuously while you move the needle back and forth within the tumor using short, jackhammer-like strokes in slightly different directions (Figure 35-2). Multiple punctures of small nodules give a higher yield of positive material.

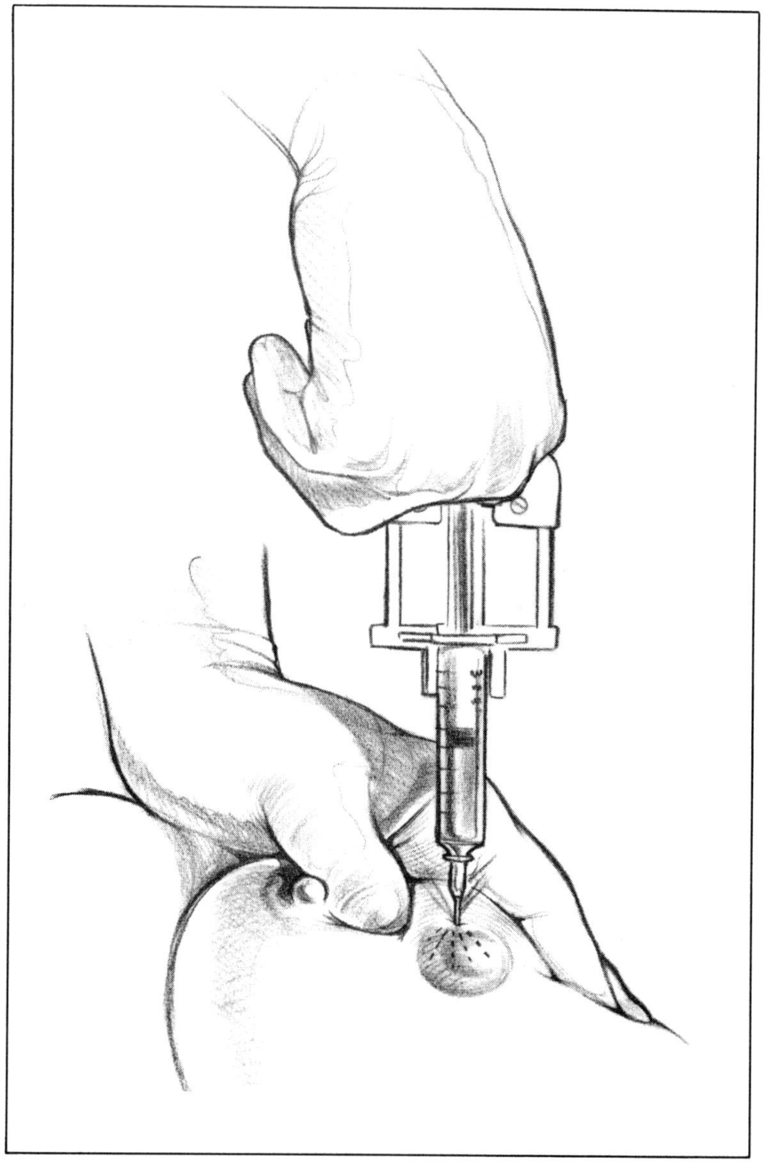

Figure 35-2 Once the mass is entered, apply continuous suction while enacting a jackhammer-like stroke in slightly different directions. When fluid appears at the needle hub, release the syringe pistol to discontinue suction.

4. Watch the needle hub. As soon as you see fluid, release the syringe pistol trigger to discontinue the suction and ensure that you'll obtain good quality cellular aspirates. Negative pressure on withdrawal can cause the specimen to leave the needle and enter the syringe. This ruins the cellular architecture and leads to poor microscopic exam. If you find no specimen in the syringe hub, make 10–12 passes into the tumor to assure good aspiration; some passes may miss a small tumor. If you detect a cyst at this stage, discard clear yellow fluid or fluid devoid of particulate matter and reaspirate any residual mass remaining after fluid removal with a fresh needle.

5. Remove the syringe, and apply pressure to the puncture site with a sterile gauze pad. Blood rapidly appearing at the puncture site suggests a malignancy.
6. Disengage the syringe from the needle, fill the syringe with air, and reattach the needle. Expel the aspirate onto one or several slides. Fix the slide immediately, and submit it with clinical data to the pathology laboratory. Centrifuge any turbid fluid obtained from a cyst, prepare a slide from the particulate matter, and submit that slide to pathology as well.

Complications

The few potential complications are easily averted or controlled:

- Hematoma (controlled by firm pressure)
- Infection (rare)
- Pneumothorax with penetration of chest wall (rare)
- Tumor spread (undocumented with fine-needle aspiration)

Suggested Readings

Frable WJ: *Thin Needle Aspiration Biopsy. Major Problems in Pathology*, vol 14. Philadelphia, WB Saunders Co, 1983, pp 7-73.

Kaminsky DB: Aspiration Biopsy for the Community Hospital. *Masson Monographs in Diagnostic Cytopathology*, vol 2. New York, Masson Publishing USA Inc, 1981, pp 9-77.

Linsk JA, Franzen S (eds): *Clinical Aspiration Cytology.* Philadelphia, JB Lippincott Co, 1983, pp 105-137.

36

Endometrial Biopsy

Elizabeth A. Burns, MD

Well-suited for an outpatient setting, endometrial biopsy by suction curettage provides 95% diagnostic accuracy in the detection of uterine cancer. The technique is also used to evaluate infertility and dysfunctional uterine bleeding. Premedication with nonsteroidal anti-inflammatory drugs and local anesthesia with a paracervical block can improve the patient's comfort and facilitate her acceptance of the procedure.

Indications

- Infertility
- Menstrual disorders, including dysfunctional uterine bleeding
- Postmenopausal bleeding
- Hormone replacement therapy—pretreatment assessment and posttreatment follow-up as indicated
- History of pelvic irradiation, for detection of cell dysplasia
- High risk for endometrial cancer (risk factors include obesity, diabetes mellitus, hypertension, low parity, irregular menses, failure of ovulation, adenomatous hyperplasia, prolonged unopposed estrogen administration, early menarche, and late menopause)

Contraindications

Absolute
- Active infection
- Pregnancy

Relative
- Inadequate pelvic examination
- Cervical stenosis
- Uterine flexion
- Coagulopathy
- Large leiomyoma
- Severe anemia
- Heart disease
- Extreme anxiety

Materials

- Sterile speculum
- Sterile gloves
- Povidone-iodine solution (Betadine)
- Bowl for solution
- Cotton balls or gauze sponges
- 22-gauge spinal needle
- 20-mL syringe
- 0.5% lidocaine HCl (Xylocaine HCl)
- Laminaria or graduated dilators
- Sterile tenaculum
- 4-mm sterile endometrial suction curet with collecting apparatus and vacuum source (Milex Tis-U-Trap)
- Kevorkian-Younge endocervical curet
- Uterine sound (unless curet is designed to serve as a sound
- Preservative (formaldehyde)

PROCEDURE

1. Explain the procedure to the patient, and premedicate if desired about 30 minutes before starting. Set up the suction curettage system (Figure 36-1).

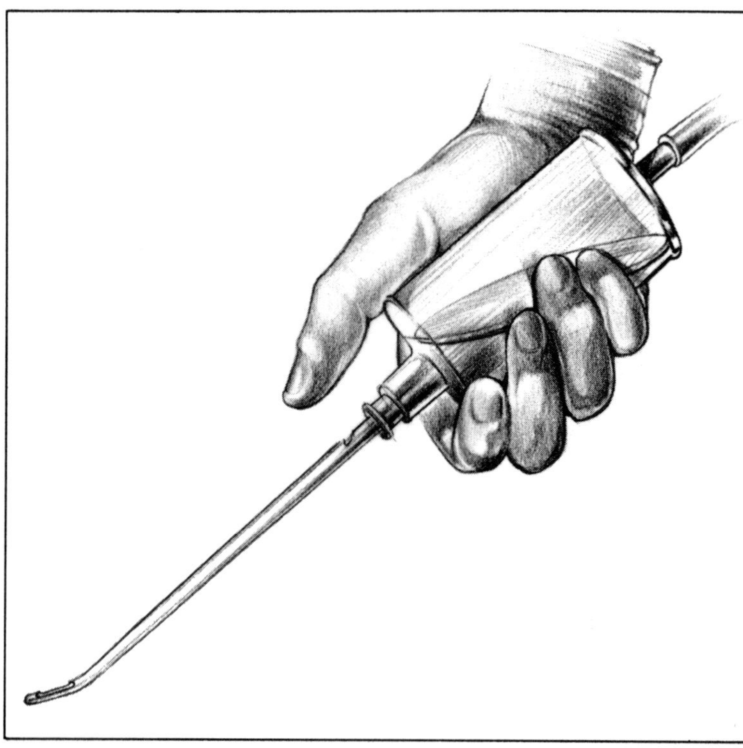

Figure 36-1 Endometrial suction curette with collection container.

2. Perform a bimanual examination to determine the position of the uterus and check for signs of infection.
3. Insert the speculum to inspect the cervix. If you encounter stenosis, you may need laminaria or graduated dilators to complete the procedure. If you use laminaria, delay the procedure to give the cervical os time to dilate. If you use dilators, proceed with step 4, inserting the dilators at step 6.
4. Clean the patient's cervix and vagina with povidone-iodine.
5. If local anesthesia is desired, administer a paracervical block using the spinal needle (Figure 36-2). Inject 10 mL of 0.5% lidocaine at the 9 o'clock and 3 o'clock positions to anesthetize the paracervical ligaments and 5 mL at the 7 o'clock and 5 o'clock positions to anesthetize the uterosacral ligaments.
6. With the tenaculum, grasp the anterior lip of the cervix, and apply gentle traction to straighten the axis of the uterus. You may want to use dilators if the os is stenotic.
7. If endocervical curettage is indicated for postmenopausal bleeding, use a Kevorkian-Younge endocervical curet. Collect the sample on a filter paper or whatever collection vehicle your pathologist prefers, and place it in preservative.
8. Sound the uterus. (Some endometrial curets have centimeter markings and can be used as uterine sounds.)
9. For suction curettage of the endometrium, insert the endometrial curet (Figure 36-3), occlude the suction release opening at the proximal end to let suction build to 51–71 mm Hg pressure (this may take several seconds), and pull the curet out, making small sweeping motions to increase the surface area sampled.

For an infertility evaluation, sample at the 3 o'clock and 9 o'clock positions. For a diagnostic evaluation, curet at all positions of the clock and across the top of the fundus.

Note: To avoid severe cramping, never apply suction while positioning the curet in the uterus.

10. Aspirate some preservative into the system to collect any tissue remaining in the curet, disconnect the collecting chamber, and fill it with preservative. Send the sample to the laboratory for histologic diagnosis.
11. Use silver nitrate cautery if necessary to stop excessive bleeding from the tenaculum site. Have the patient remain recumbent for a few minutes to avert vasovagal syncope.

Complications

- Pain, cramping
- Uterine perforation
- Vasovagal syncope
- Infection
- Drug sensitivity (to povidone-iodine or lidocaine).

Figure 36-2 Paracervical block of 10 mL 0.5% lidocaine at 9 o'clock and 3 o'clock, and 5 mL at 7 o'clock and 5 o'clock. After anesthetizing, tenaculum is applied to straighten the axis of the uterus.

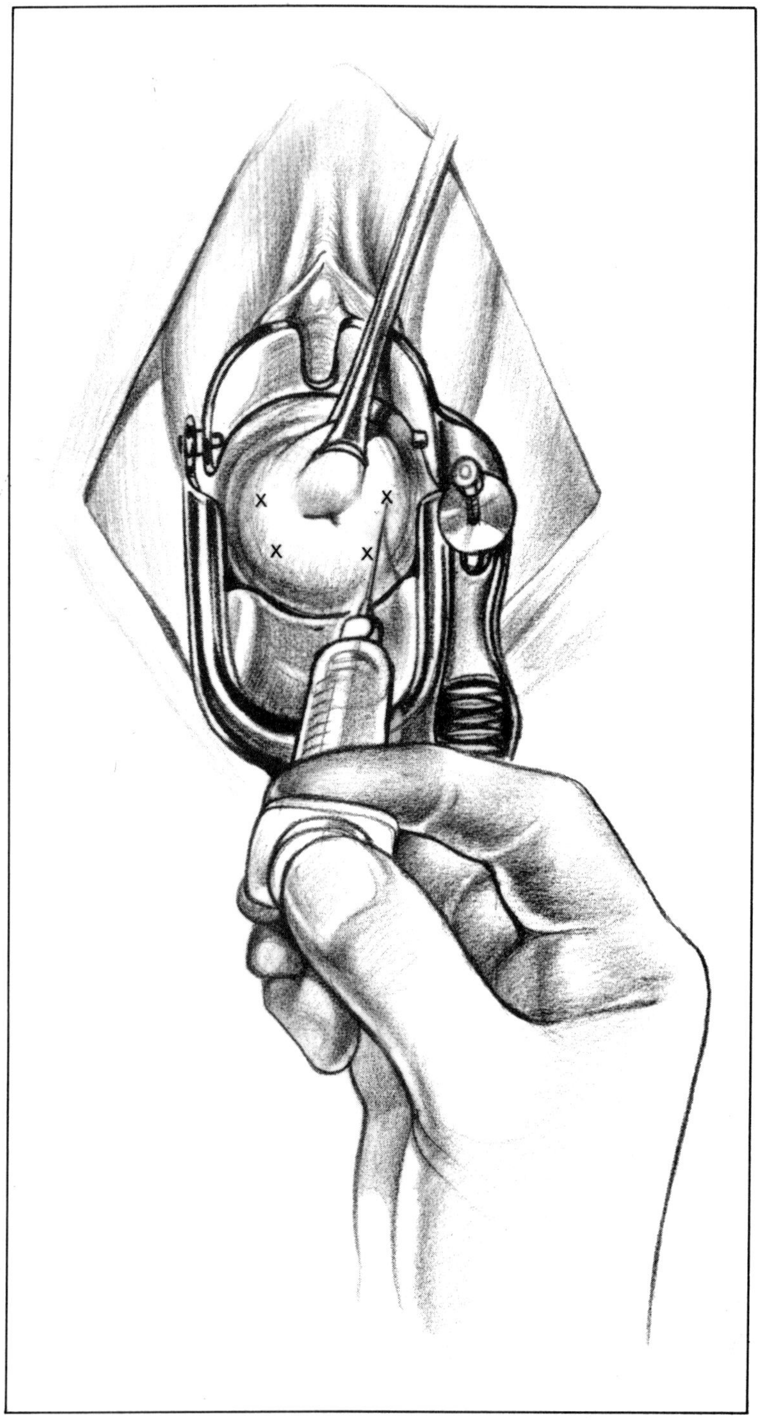

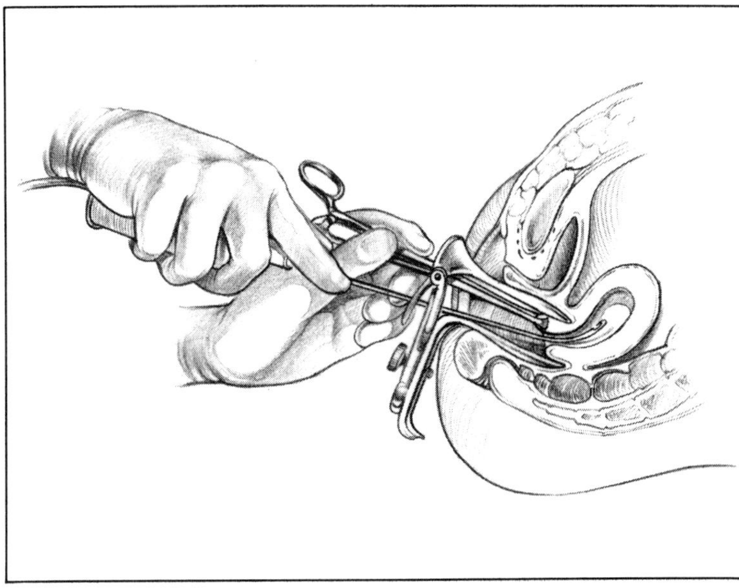

Figure 36-3 Insert the endometrial curette and occlude the suction release opening to allow pressure to build to 51–71 mm Hg. While withdrawing the curette, make sweeping motions to increase the surface area sampled.

Suggested Readings

Fuller AF: Role of the primary physician in the detection and treatment of gynecologic cancer. *Primary Care* 1981;8:111-129.

Hurt WG, Hall DJ: Outpatient endometrial sampling. *J Fam Pract* 1980;10:115-118.

Koss LG, Schreiber K, Oberlander SG, et al: Screening of asymptomatic women for endometrial cancer. *CA* 1981;31:300-317.

Richart RM, Pringle P: Choosing the right biopsy device. *Contemp OB/GYN* (special issue), October 1984, pp 48-57.

37

Biopsy of the Uterine Cervix

R. J. Coble, MD

Although the decline in death rate from carcinoma of the cervix is not completely understood, part of it is due to patient and physician education in early detection and part is due to increased physician awareness of the need for step-by-step evaluation of the patient with an abnormal Pap smear.

When you encounter an abnormal Pap smear (class II or higher), repeat the smear right away to confirm the abnormal cytologic findings and to rule out laboratory error. If the abnormal result is confirmed, proceed to biopsy. While colposcopy with guided biopsy is a superior method, the procedure can be performed without colposcopy.

Indication

- Class II or higher pathology on Pap smear

Contraindication

- Pregnancy, when the lesion is located within the endocervix

Materials

- Colposcope (optional)
- Large-tipped cotton batons and small-tipped cotton swabs
- 3–5% acetic acid solution
- Lugol's solution
- Kevorkian-Younge biopsy forceps or equivalent such as Tischler or Eppendorfer instruments
- Monsel's solution (ferric subsulfate)
- Vaginal speculum
- Specimen jars filled with 10% formalin

PROCEDURE

WITH COLPOSCOPY

1. Explain the procedure, and obtain informed patient consent.

2. With the patient in the lithotomy position, insert the vaginal speculum as you would for a routine pelvic examination.

3. Clean the cervix and vaginal mucosa by wiping away the cervical mucus with a dry cotton baton. Paint the cervical area generously with 3–5% acetic acid solution to help identify abnormal blood vessels, mosaic mucosal patterns, punctate lesions, and white epithelium (Table 37-1).

4. Move the colposcope into place, and focus on the cervical os and surrounding portio.

Note: Anesthesia is seldom necessary, but if you anticipate biopsy of a large area, administer local anesthesia by injecting 1–2 mL of 1% lidocaine HCl (Xylocaine HCl) sublesionally.

5. If you see gross lesions or areas with abnormal patterns, take punch biopsy specimens from these sites with the biopsy forceps. For each specimen, open the biopsy forceps fully, and place the jaws over the entire lesion, including some surrounding normal tissue if possible. If the lesion is large, take one sample at an edge of the lesion to include some normal tissue and a second sample in the center of the lesion. Place each sample in a separate specimen jar labeled to identify the site. Bleeding during the procedure can usually be controlled easily with pressure or Monsel's solution; a hemostatic suture may occasionally be needed.

Note: Remember to send a good clinical history to the pathology laboratory with each specimen to aid in histologic interpretation.

TABLE 37–1

Some colposcopically significant cervical lesions

Lesion	Characteristics	Possible significance
Atypical blood vessels	Well-demarcated areas of vessels markedly irregular in size, direction, shape, and arrangement	Invasive carcinoma
Mosaic mucosal patterns	Well-demarcated areas composed of segments of avascular pathologic epithelium outlined by capillaries	Dysplasia or carcinoma in situ
Punctate lesions	Well-demarcated areas of dilated, elongated hairpin capillaries, often slightly twisted and irregular	Dysplasia or carcinoma in situ
White epithelium	Well-demarcated areas of epithelium that appear white after application of acetic acid	Dysplasia or carcinoma in situ

6. With a cotton baton, apply Lugol's solution as a stain to help identify neoplastic epithelium; normal tissue appears deep reddish brown; dysplastic tissue appears pale yellow. Take biopsy specimens from any areas of apparent dysplasia.
8. No special aftercare of biopsy sites is necessary.

WITHOUT COLPOSCOPY

1. Follow steps 1–3 and 5–6 above, examining the cervix and patterns of staining as closely as possible with the unaided eye. Take biopsy specimens from any suspicious areas.

Figure 37-1 Biopsy samples should be taken at 3, 6, 9, and 12 o'clock on the cervical circumference.

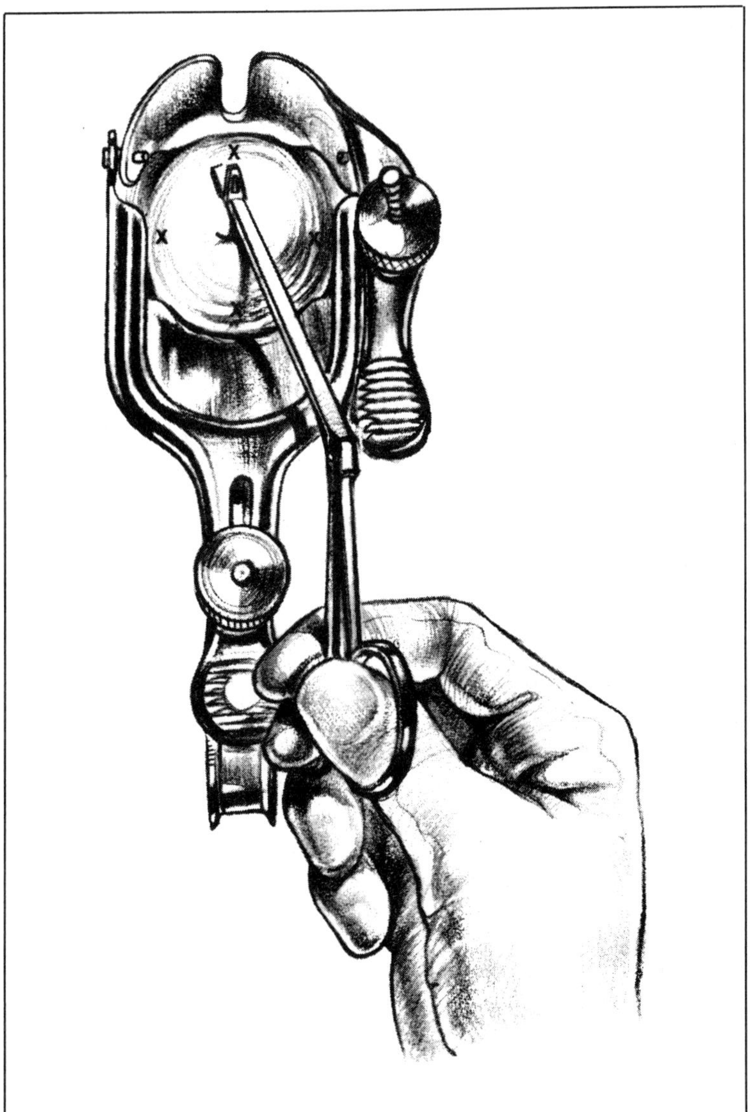

2. If no areas look suspicious even after staining with Lugol's solution, take random biopsy specimens at 3, 6, 9, and 12 o'clock on the cervical circumference (Figure 37-1).
3. No special aftercare of biopsy sites is necessary.

Complications

- Vaginal bleeding more serious than spotting seldom occurs; but if it does, the patient should return for examination.
- Similarly, vaginal discharge or infection rarely occurs, but advise the patient to return if it does.

Follow-up Care

- Follow-up care is dictated by the pathologist's report.
- If examination and biopsy without colposcopy fail to explain the abnormal Pap smear, refer the patient for colposcopically guided biopsy.

Suggested Readings

Duenhoelter JH: *Greenhill's Office Gynecology*, ed 10. Chicago, Year Book Medical Pub Inc, 1983.

Jones HW, Jones GS: *Novak's Textbook of Gynecology*, ed 10. Baltimore, Williams & Wilkins Co, 1980.

Mishell DR, Brenner PF: *Management of Common Problems in Obstetrics and Gynecology*. Oradell, NJ, Medical Economics Books, 1983.

38

Culdocentesis

Thomas A. Francis, MD
Charles E. Driscoll, MD

Culdocentesis, the transvaginal puncture of the pouch of Douglas, is a simple and safe means of collecting peritoneal fluid. It is used most commonly to evaluate hemorrhage associated with ectopic gestations and ruptured ovarian cysts. The knowledge, skills, and facilities to perform culdocentesis would be useful to any physician who provides comprehensive gynecologic care.

The procedure can be extremely helpful in evaluating possible ectopic pregnancy. Indeed, one study found that a positive culdocentesis with a positive serum human chorionic gonadotropin pregnancy test is associated with ectopic pregnancy in up to 99% of cases.[1]

Peritoneal fluid may also provide useful information in other clinical circumstances:

- In infertility investigations, it can show spermatozoa in periovular peritoneal fluid as in vivo proof of sperm migration to the fertilization site.
- It can discriminate between ovulation and a luteinized unruptured follicle through hormonal analysis of the fluid.
- It can be used to detect or follow ovarian cancer, to culture for study in pelvic infections, and to demonstrate intra-abdominal bleeding.

Indications

- Early diagnosis of hemoperitoneum
- Preoperative evaluation of suspected ectopic pregnancy
- Further evaluation of a variety of pathologic and physiologic conditions

Contraindications

- A cul-de-sac obliterated either by adhesions or a palpable mass of unknown type
- A uterus fixed in retroversion, obliterating the cul-de-sac
- Coagulopathies

---

[1]Romero R, Copel JA, Kadar N, et al: Value of culdocentesis in the diagnosis of ectopic pregnancy. *Obstet Gynecol* 1985;65:519-522.

Materials

- 10-mL syringe with a 4-in., 18-gauge or larger spinal needle
- Povidone/iodine (Betadine)-soaked gauze on ring forceps
- Cervical tenaculum
- 10-mL vacuum serum collection tube
- Sterile culture tube
- Bivalve speculum

PROCEDURE

1. After bimanual and rectovaginal examination with the patient in the dorsal lithotomy position, insert the bivalve speculum, and swab the vagina with povidone/iodine-soaked gauze.
2. Grasp the posterior lip of the cervix with the tenaculum (have the patient cough as you do this), and gently pull it anteriorly and forward to expose the posterior fornix (Figure 38-1).
3. Take up the spinal needle with syringe attached, making sure it contains 2–3 mL of air. Holding the needle horizontally, thrust it rapidly through the posterior fornix and into the cul-de-sac about 3

Figure 38-1

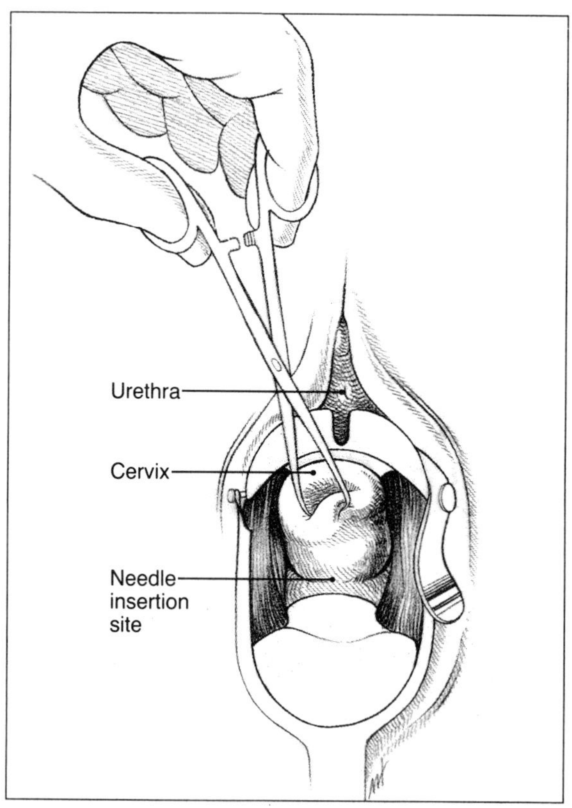

cm along the axis parallel to the posterior wall of the uterus (Figure 38-2). Anesthesia is optional; some experts feel that the injection for anesthesia is as painful as that for the procedure and prefer a single injection to two.

Note: Quick insertion is important; slow entry can push the peritoneum off its underlying connective tissue and make it virtually impossible to enter the cul-de-sac.

4. Inject the air from the syringe. It should flow easily with little pressure on the plunger. If you feel resistance, the tip is in a solid organ, usually the uterus, and should be slightly withdrawn to reposition it.

5. Aspirate the cul-de-sac. If a hemoperitoneum is present, the action of intestinal peristalsis will usually cause local consumption of clotting factors. Residual unclotted blood usually flows easily through the culdocentesis needle into the syringe and does not clot for at least 10 minutes. If you obtain no fluid, try a different angle or puncture site.

6. Inject blood into a stoppered tube for analysis; inject pus into a culture tube, and order a Gram's stain.

Interpretation

- A positive result in culdocentesis is retrieval of 0.5 mL of nonclotting blood. Rapidly clotting blood often indicates blood vessel puncture, but may indicate a briskly bleeding ectopic pregnancy.
- Measure the hematocrit of all blood obtained by culdocentesis. A hematocrit below 15% probably indicates minor bleeding or a

Figure 38-2

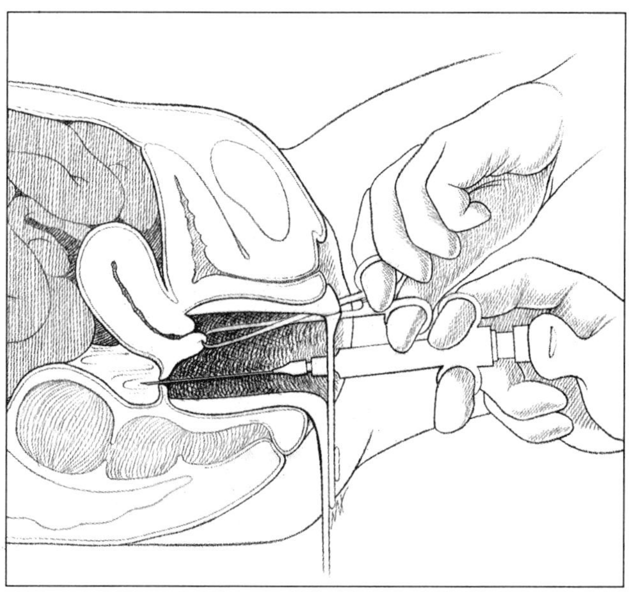

bloody tap. Levels 15% and above are more frequently associated with an ectopic gestation.

- You may aspirate pus or cloudy exudate in pelvic inflammatory disease. Examine this microscopically by Gram's stain and cultures, both aerobic and anaerobic.
- Chocolate-colored material, which represents old blood, may indicate endometriosis; but any cyst that contains old blood, including a long-standing ectopic pregnancy, can produce similar results.
- Clear fluid usually represents ascites, a ruptured ovarian cyst contents, or normal peritoneal fluid.

Note: A tap that yields no fluid should not be considered negative; the needle may have missed the pool of fluid. Try again to obtain fluid.

Complications

Though complications are rare, primary concerns include introduction of bacteria into the peritoneal cavity, rupture of adnexal structures such as pyosalpinx or ovarian cyst, and possible bowel lacerations; the latter are generally of no clinical significance and require no treatment. The best safeguard against rupturing pathologic pelvic structures is careful bimanual examination to be sure the cul-de-sac is free of masses, cysts, or adhesions.

Suggested Readings

Eisinger SH: Culdocentesis. *J Fam Pract* 1981;13:95-101.

Mattingly RF, Thompson JD (eds): *TeLinde's Operative Gynecology,* ed 6. Philadelphia, JB Lippincott, 1985, p 373.

Romero R, Copel JA, Kadar N, et al: Value of culdocentesis in the diagnosis of ectopic pregnancy. *Obstet Gynecol* 1985;65:519-522.

Wiegerinck MA, de Laat WN, Moret E: A new culdocentesis system. *Fertil Steril* 1986;45:434-436.

39

Delivery without an Episiotomy

Elizabeth A. Burns, MD

Delivery without an episiotomy is often mentioned in Lamaze and other childbirth classes as an alternate approach in a vaginal delivery. Since increasing numbers of patients want to consider this option during their prenatal care, this is a good time to discuss your philosophy and your parameters for performing or not performing an episiotomy.

Benefits of an Episiotomy

- Straight, easily repaired enlargement of the vaginal orifice rather than a laceration
- Protection of the fetal head from the trauma of dilating the perineum
- Shortened second stage of labor
- Prevention of pelvic floor relaxation
- Reduction of third-degree mediolateral lacerations

Risks of an Episiotomy

- Extension of the episiotomy
- Unsatisfactory anatomic results (fistulas)
- Blood loss and hematomas
- Pain and edema including dyspareunia lasting three months or more
- Infection (deaths have been reported secondary to an infected episiotomy)

Rare Complications of an Episiotomy

- Lidocaine toxicity of the newborn
- The episiotomy's failure to heal

- Endometriosis in the scar
- Broken needle lost in perineal tissue

Indications for Delivery without an Episiotomy

- Expressed desire of the patient
- Normal progress in second stage of labor with no evidence of fetal distress
- Previous delivery without an episiotomy

Contraindications

- Fetal distress
- Maternal fatigue
- Forceps delivery
- Large infant
- Tight perineum

Materials

None

Preparation

After a prenatal discussion about delivery without episiotomy with the patient, instruct her in perineal massage. Patients should start the massage program 4–6 weeks before delivery.

PROCEDURE

During the second stage of labor, several maneuvers can slowly dilate the perineum and assist with delivery:

- Apply warm compresses to the perineum to lessen discomfort.
- Perform perineal massage in addition to using the compresses.
- To slow the rate of perineal dilation, encourage the patient to push while exhaling or grunting rather than with Valsalva's maneuver.
- Once the head crowns sufficiently, the pushing reflex becomes quite strong. Often, gentle pushing between contractions enhances a slow dilation rate and lets the patient feel in control.
- With crowning, try to maintain the fetal head flexion so the smallest diameter passes through the vulval ring. Use one hand to push down and back on the occiput to keep the head flexed (Figure 39-1). With your other hand, support the perineum, stretching it back and toward the ischial tuberosities, which essentially retracts the perineum over the head as it extends (Figure 39-2).

Figure 39-1

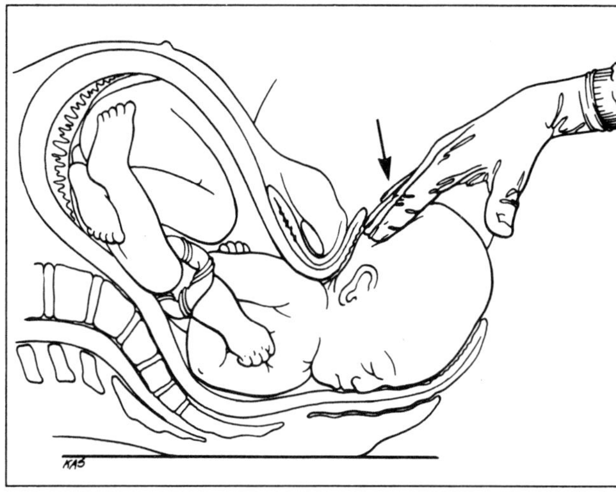

A nontraditional (standing or squatting) position may work better for the patient, allowing the perineum to retract on its own and the fetal head to stay flexed longer.

- With delivery of the shoulders, an assistant should help support the perineum, to avoid tearing at this stage. Delivering the posterior shoulder while curving the infant upward will help maintain an intact perineum.

Figure 39-2

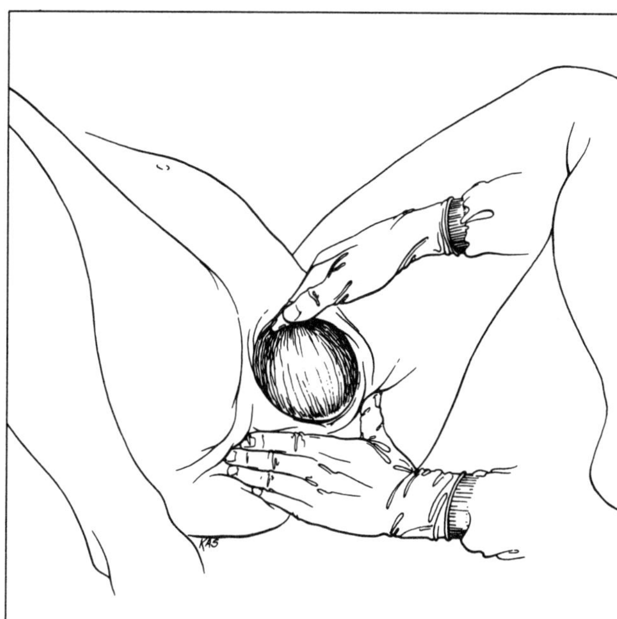

Complications of Delivery without an Episiotomy

- Perineal laceration
- Trauma to the fetal head
- Possible pelvic floor relaxation
- Women with episiotomy scars should be told there is a risk of tearing along the old scar, usually a simple-to-repair laceration
- Edema of the perineum

Follow-up Care

- Use ice packs immediately postpartum to help reduce edema
- Instruct patients in Kegel exercises, which should be started as soon as possible
- If the patient is breast-feeding, she may have symptomatic atrophic vaginitis and may require exogenous estrogen cream (Estrace, Ogen, Premarin, etc.).

Suggested Readings

Mahan CS, McKay S: Are we overmanaging second-stage labor? *Contemp OB/GYN* 1984;24(6):37-63.

McKay S, Roberts J: Second stage labor: What is normal? *J Obstet Gynecol Neonatal Nurs* 1985;14(2):101-106.

Sagov SE, Brodsky A (eds): *Home Birth: A Practitioner's Guide to Birth Outside the Hospital.* Rockville, Md, Aspen Pubs Inc, 1983.

Thacker SB, Banta HD: Benefits and risks of episiotomy: An interpretative review of the English language literature 1960-1980. *Obstet Gynecol Surv* 1983;38:322-338.

40

Minimally Invasive Endometrial Sampling

Charles E. Driscoll, MD

Minimally invasive endometrial sampling to obtain tissue in an outpatient setting is easier and better-tolerated than endometrial biopsy by curettage or suction. Done with the proper technique, the less invasive method produces very adequate specimens for examination.

Endometrial sampling may be cytologic or histologic. In cytologic as in Pap smear sampling, exfoliated cells are obtained from the endometrial cavity and smeared on a slide for fixation and microscopic examination, but this is less exact than histologic sampling for pathologic evaluation. Also, cytologic samplers such as the Endocyte are difficult to obtain in this country although they have been available for several years in Canada and Europe.

The more exact method is the histologic biopsy using an endometrial suction curet (Pipelle). This 3.1-mm-diameter, semiflexible polyethylene sampler is inserted through the cervix to the uterine fundus. When negative pressure is created in the curet lumen, rotation against the endometrial wall extracts the tissue.

Indications

In general, whenever glandular and superficial layers of the endometrial wall are needed for histologic biopsy. Common specific indications:

- Looking for endometrial carcinoma or precancerous changes (adenomatous hyperplasia) in undiagnosed uterine bleeding
- Following the course of uterine changes in response to estrogen therapy

- Endometrial dating for infertility evaluation
- Uterine tissue staging in patients with metrorrhagia

Contraindications

- Pregnancy
- Uterine or pelvic inflammatory disease
- Cervical infection such as gonorrhea or chlamydial cervicitis
- Uncooperative patient

Relative

- Cervical stenosis and inability to pass the suction curet easily

Materials

- Ibuprofen (Advil, Medipren, Motrin, etc.), 600 mg
- Sterile gloves
- Bivalve vaginal speculum
- Povidone/iodine solution (Betadine)
- Bowl for povidone/iodine solution containing cotton balls or gauze sponges
- Long ring forceps
- Sterile cervical tenaculum
- Uterine sound
- Endometrial suction curet
- 1% lidocaine HCl (Xylocaine HCl)
- Sterile scissors
- Specimen bottle containing formalin preservative

Preparation

- Explain the procedure to the patient, and obtain a written informed consent—appropriate any time you remove tissue from a body cavity.
- If desired, premedicate the patient with 600 mg of ibuprofen orally about one hour before the procedure to diminish discomfort and cramping.

PROCEDURE

1. With an assistant in attendance and the patient in lithotomy position, perform a bimanual examination to determine uterine position, and check for adnexal tenderness or signs of pelvic inflammatory disease. Then insert the bivalve speculum, inspect the cervix for signs of cervical infection or disease, and check for an open cervical os that will permit instrumentation.

2. With the speculum in place and opened to expose the cervix, cleanse the cervix and surrounding vaginal tissue with povidone/iodine solution.

3. Grasp the anterior lip of the cervix with a cervical tenaculum, and with gentle traction toward the operator, insert the uterine sound gently into the cervical os. Position the ring and little finger of your inserting hand against the perineum to block any rapid insertion movements that might cause perforation.
4. Gently push against the cervix with the uterine sound until it slides through the endocervix into the uterine cavity. Advance the sound to the fundus, withdraw it, and note the depth of insertion. Normal uterine depth is 6–7 cm.
5. Again bracing your inserting hand against the perineum, insert the tip of the suction curet into the cervical opening and gently slide it through the cervical canal, past the endocervix, and into the uterine cavity to the fundus (Figure 40-1).

Note: Stop insertion if passage seems difficult and you encounter excessive resistance. Forced passage of the curet may perforate the uterus.

6. If the procedure has been painful up to this point and the patient feels unsure about proceeding, you may inject 1% lidocaine at the 9 o'clock and 3 o'clock, 2 o'clock and 10 o'clock, and 4 o'clock and 7 o'clock positions to produce cervical block.
7. With the curet in position with its tip at the uterine fundus, have an assistant hold the cervical tenaculum while you hold the sheath steady with one hand and *rapidly* withdraw the internal plunger with your other hand (Figure 40-2). This creates negative pressure inside the curet, aspirating tissue into the open curet hole near the fundus.
8. With the plunger pulled to its full length, gently twirl or rotate the curet in your fingers as you move it from side to side. At the same

Figure 40-1

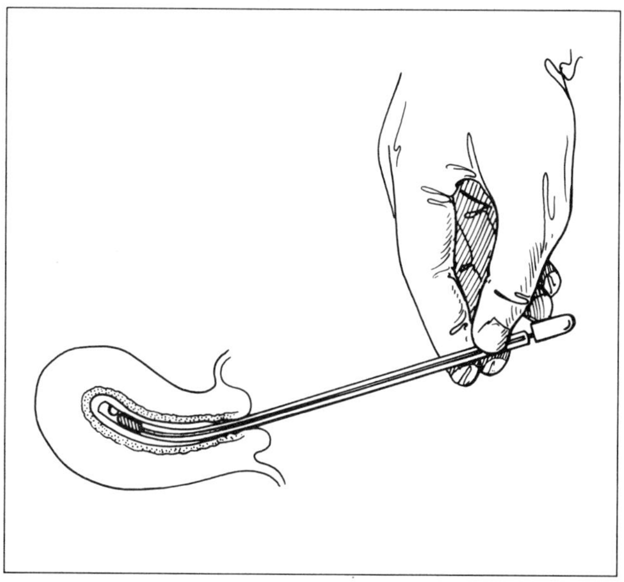

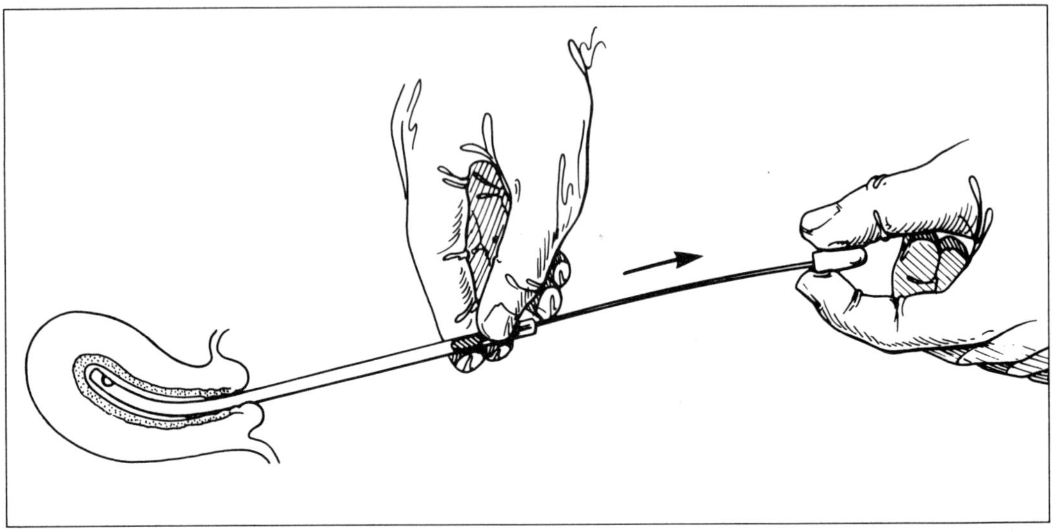

Figure 40-2

time, gently withdraw the curet toward the cervical canal, and note tissue moving into the sheath toward the plunger.

Note: Do not allow the curet hole in the tip to emerge outside the uterine cavity: If you do, all suction is lost, and further extraction of tissue is impossible.

9. Make several of these in-and-out passes keeping the curet hole just short of the internal cervical os and allowing tissue to move steadily up the inside of the sheath (Figure 40-3).

10. When the sheath is full to the plunger or when no further tissue moves after several passes, withdraw the curet with the plunger still fully retracted, and cut off the distal tip just proximal to the curet opening.

11. Grasp the plunger, and push it toward the cut-off end, expelling the sample into the formalin bottle for transport to the pathology laboratory (Figure 40-4). If one sample is inadequate, use a fresh curet, and repeat the procedure to obtain more tissue.

12. Remove the cervical tenaculum and bivalve speculum. Gently lower the patient's legs from the lithotomy position to supine recumbency.

13. Assist the patient to a sitting position after 1–2 minutes of rest.

Follow-up Care

- Bleeding and cramping are minimal; the procedure is generally quite well-tolerated.

Follow-up is indicated only to inform the patient of the pathologic analysis. No further examination or particular aftercare is required.

Figure 40-3

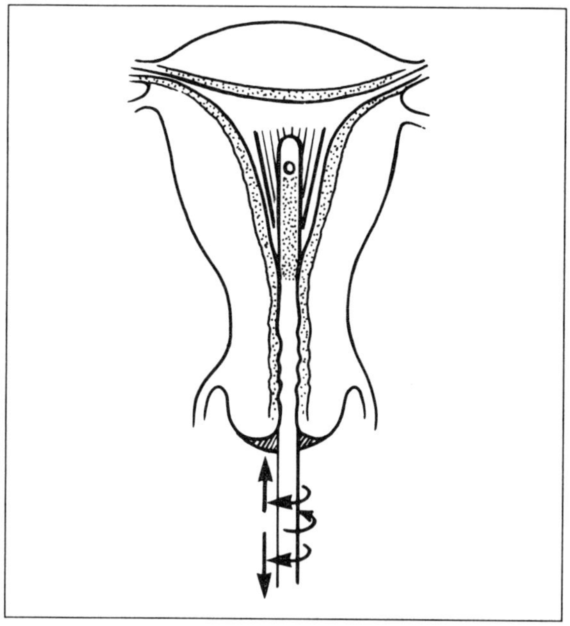

Figure 40-4

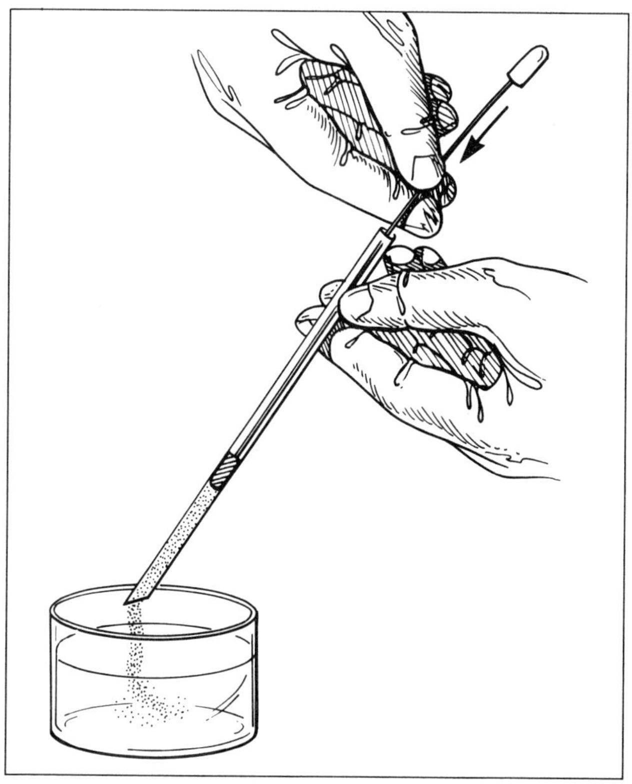

Suggested Readings

Check JH, Chase JS, Nowroozi K, et al: Clinical evaluation of the Pipelle endometrial suction curette for timed endometrial biopsies. *J Reprod Med* 1989;34:218-220.

Hill GA, Herbert CM, Parker RA, et al: Comparison of late luteal phase endometrial biopsies using the Novak curette or Pipelle endometrial suction curette. *Obstet Gynecol* 1989;73:443-445.

Honore LH, Cumming DC, Fahmy N: Significant difference in the frequency of out-of-phase endometrial biopsies depending on the use of the Novak curette or the flexible polypropylene endometrial biopsy cannula ('Pipelle'). *Gynecol Obstet Invest* 1988;26:338-340.

Kaunitz AM, Masciello A, Ostrowski M, et al: Comparison of endometrial biopsy with the endometrial Pipelle and Vabra aspirator. *J Reprod Med* 1988;33:427-431.

VII

DERMATOLOGY PROCEDURES

41

Administering Local Anesthesia

Darrell Randle, MD
Charles E. Driscoll, MD

Local anesthesia, the usual choice for office surgery, is available in three basic forms: infiltration, regional nerve block, and IV regional nerve block (Bier's block). Which type is appropriate depends on the nature of the procedure, the area to be anesthetized, the physician's experience, and the status of the patient.

The six agents commonly used in local anesthesia are lidocaine HCl (Xylocaine HCl), mepivacaine HCl (Carbocaine), bupivacaine HCl (Marcaine, Sensorcaine), cocaine HCl, procaine HCl (Novocain), and chloroprocaine HCl (Nesacaine). The first three are amide compounds and the last three, ester compounds. Little cross-reactivity exists between the two groups: A patient who is hypersensitive to an ester compound can usually be given an amide compound without difficulty. Lidocaine is the most commonly used agent because of its prompt, long lasting, intense effect. For more rapid onset, use mepivacaine; for longer duration, use bupivacaine. Cocaine, procaine, and chloroprocaine are seldom the drugs of choice.

Precautions

Toxic manifestations of anesthetics include both CNS and cardiovascular system symptoms. Common initial signs of toxicity are anxiety, restlessness, garrulousness, and tremor. Classic treatment of toxic reactions is to halt administration of the agent, give cardiovascular support, and administer diazepam (Valium), 5–10 mg IV, to control convulsions. Epinephrine, frequently given to decrease capillary oozing and prolong the action of a local anesthetic, also may produce anxiety and dysrhythmia. To avoid toxicity problems, observe these precautions:

Do not exceed the maximum dose (Table 41-1).

If the patient has a history of allergic reaction to an anesthetic agent, use an agent from the other basic group. It may be helpful to inject 0.25 mL of the suspect agent subcutaneously as a test and observe the reaction for 15 minutes.

TABLE 41-1

Maximum recommended doses of commonly used local anesthetics

Agent	Without epinephrine	With epinephrine
Lidocaine HCl (Xylocaine)	3–5 mg/kg	7 mg/kg
Mepivacaine HCl (Carbocaine)	8 mg/kg	
Bupivacaine HCl* (Marcaine, Sensorcaine)	2.5 mg/kg	3.0 mg/kg
In young, old, and very ill patients, the maximum recommended dose is roughly 25% less.		
*Not recommended for use in children under age 12.		

Do not use epinephrine with the anesthetic in fingers, toes, nose, ears, or penis. The vasoconstriction it induces may significantly compromise circulation.

Do not use epinephrine in patients who have hypertension, cardiac rhythm disturbance, or other heart disease.

If you need to use large amounts of an anesthetic, have cardiopulmonary resuscitation equipment and personnel nearby.

LOCAL INFILTRATION

Indication

Use when the area to be anesthetized is small, when it is not amenable to a regional block, or when you want to supplement a regional block.

Materials

- 1% lidocaine HCl (Xylocaine HCl) with or without epinephrine, or other anesthetic as appropriate
- 18-gauge, 1½-in. needle
- 25- or 30-gauge, 1½-in. needle
- Syringe
- Skin prep such as povidone-iodine (Betadine)

PROCEDURE

1. Prepare the injection site. Withdraw lidocaine from the vial with an 18-gauge needle to avoid dulling the fine needle used for injection.
2. Using a 25- or 30-gauge needle, slowly inject 0.1 mL of lidocaine intradermally to create a small wheal.

3. Wait 30 seconds, then very slowly inject the target area of skin, working from the anesthetized area outward. Aspirate before each bolus injection to confirm that the needle is not in a vein.
4. Wait at least three minutes after you complete injection, and test for absence of pinprick sensation before beginning the procedure.
5. In anesthetizing for wound closure, you can minimize iatrogenic pain by dripping lidocaine into the wound, waiting three minutes, then injecting the required amount through the wound edges.

REGIONAL NERVE BLOCK

Indication

Use when local infiltration would either require too much anesthetic or distort local anatomy and inhibit good closure.

Materials

- 25-gauge, 2½-in. needle (for tibial nerve block only)
- Other equipment as listed under "Local Infiltration"

PROCEDURE

1. Prepare the injection site, and withdraw lidocaine HCl (Xylocaine HCl) from the vial with an 18-gauge needle.
2. Familiarize yourself with the appropriate landmarks (see discussions of individual blocks that follow). Using a 25-gauge needle, slowly inject 0.1 mL of lidocaine intradermally to create a small wheal.
3. Wait 30 seconds before inserting the needle slowly into the target area through the wheal. The patient's report of a momentary paresthesia indicates correct placement.

Note: Persistent paresthesia indicates nerve penetration; withdraw the needle until the paresthesia clears.

4. Slowly inject the anesthetic in small boluses, withdrawing the needle almost completely and redirecting it several times to leave a fanlike distribution. Always alternate aspiration with injection to avoid intravenous administration.

DIGITAL (FINGER OR TOE) NERVE BLOCK

Indications

- Nail removal
- Closure of digital laceration
- Manipulation of phalangeal fractures or dislocations
- Digital incision and drainage

PROCEDURE

1. Raise a wheal on the dorsal aspect of the digit at the base, using lidocaine without epinephrine.
2. Slowly inject 1–2 mL of anesthetic along the lateral aspect of the digit, staying as close to the bone as possible without touching it. Advance the needle to the volar skin as you inject.
3. Withdraw and repeat on the medial side of the digit.

METACARPAL/METATARSAL NERVE BLOCK

Indications

As for digital block, when digital block could compromise blood flow to the digit or area of procedure or when a wound interferes with placing an adequate digital block

PROCEDURE

1. Using lidocaine without epinephrine, raise two small skin wheals, one on the dorsomedial and one on the dorsolateral aspect of the metacarpal near the MCP joint.[1]
2. Inject continuously as you advance the needle alongside the metacarpal until it is palpable on the volar surface of the hand (Figure 41-1). Inject a total of 2 mL of lidocaine.
3. Withdraw and repeat on the other side.

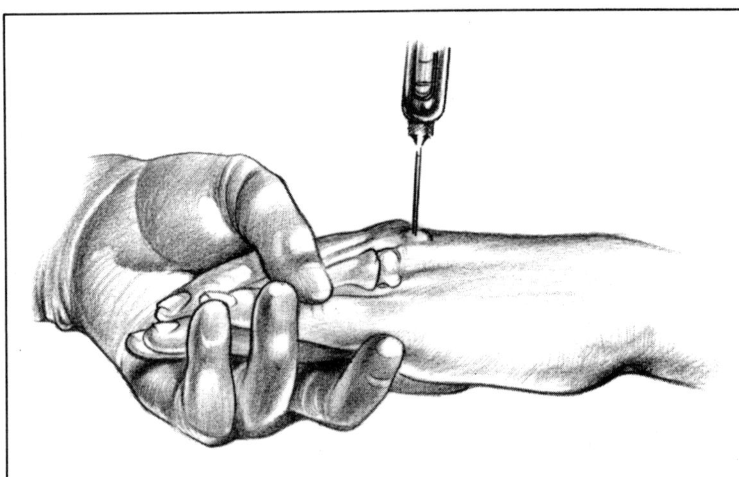

Figure 41-1 Placement of needle alongside the metacarpal for injection of lidocaine.

[1] For clarity, only metacarpal block is described; technique for metatarsal block is virtually identical.

WRIST BLOCKS

Indication

For minor procedures done in the area innervated by the ulnar, median, or radial nerve (Figure 41-2)

PROCEDURES

Ulnar nerve

1. Locate the palmar branch of the nerve by having the patient flex and ulnarly deviate his or her wrist against resistance, which should identify the flexor carpi ulnaris tendon. Palpate the ulnar artery and raise a skin wheal between the tendon and artery at the level of the ulnar styloid (Figure 41-3). The ulnar nerve lies above the flexor retinaculum.
2. Advance the needle through the wheal approximately 1 cm (3/8 in.) until you elicit paresthesia. Inject 5–10 mL of 1% lidocaine without epinephrine.
3. Block the dorsal branch of the ulnar nerve by infiltrating 5–10 mL of 1% lidocaine without epinephrine subcutaneously in a linear array of subcutaneous injections that extends from the flexor carpi ulnaris around the ulnar aspect of the wrist to the middorsal aspect.

Median nerve

1. Have the patient flex his wrist against resistance and oppose his thumb and fifth finger to make apparent the tendon of the palmaris

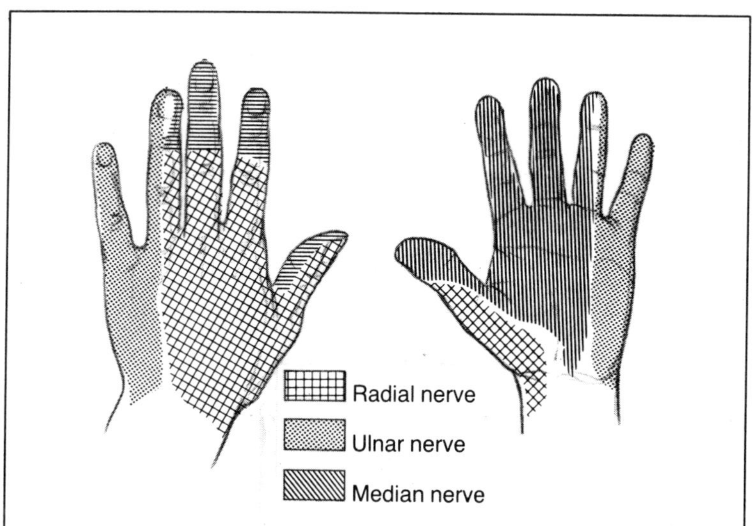

Figure 41-2 Fields anesthetized by blocks placed at three nerve innervations.

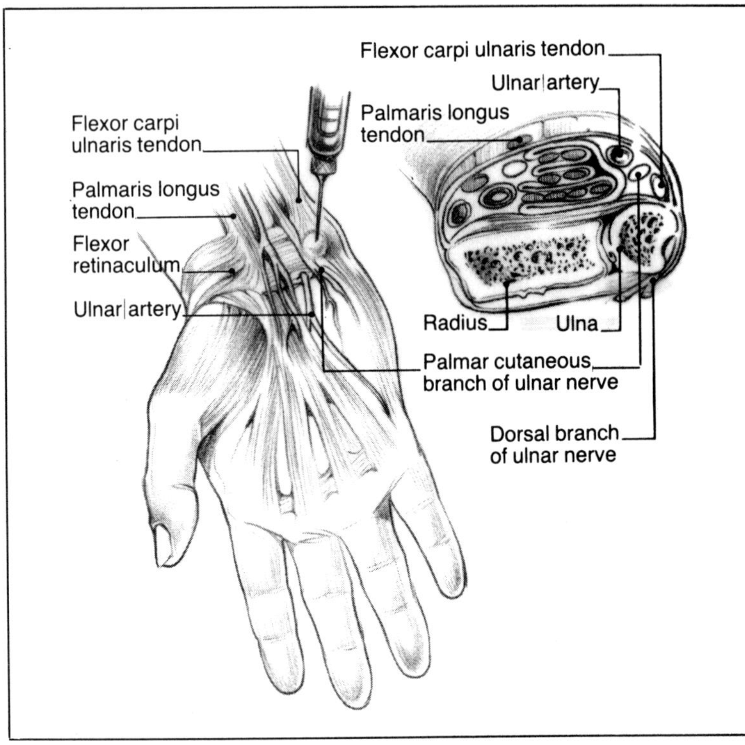

Figure 41-3 Site of needle insertion for ulnar nerve block. Determine location by palpating the ulnar artery, and raising a skin wheal midway between the artery and the flexor carpi ulnaris tendon.

longus in the volar aspect of the wrist. Raise a small wheal immediately radial to the tendon at the level of a line connecting radial and ulnar styloid processes (Figure 41-4).
2. Advance the needle 1.5–2.0 cm (½–¾ in.) through the skin wheal until paresthesia occurs, then inject 3–5 mL of 1% lidocaine without epinephrine. You may feel a faint pop as the needle passes through the flexor retinaculum; the median nerve lies 1 cm dorsal to this.

Radial nerve

1. Palpate for the radial artery and raise a skin wheal immediately lateral to it at the level of a line connecting the radial and ulnar styloid processes (Figure 41-5).
2. Inject 2 mL of 1% lidocaine without epinephrine subcutaneously through the wheal.
3. Extend infiltration laterally to the middorsal aspect of the wrist in a series of separate subcutaneous injections, for a total of 10 mL of 1% lidocaine.

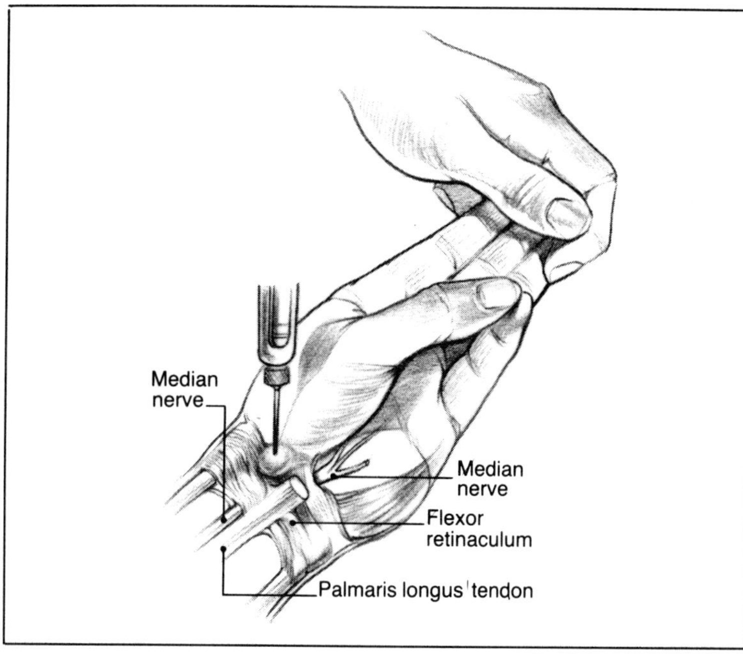

Figure 41-4 Site of needle insertion for median nerve block. Raise a small wheal immediately radial to the palmaris longus tendon.

SUPRAORBITAL NERVE BLOCK

Indication

To provide anesthesia of forehead, upper eyelid, and scalp to the lambdoid suture

PROCEDURE

1. Palpate the superior orbital rim to identify the supraorbital notch. With the patient gazing straight ahead, it should be palpable directly over the pupil. Raise a skin wheal over the notch.
2. Insert the needle through the wheal, advancing it until you elicit paresthesia. Inject 2 mL of 1% lidocaine as you apply pressure to the upper eyelid to avoid migration of the anesthetic into the lid (Figure 41-6).

INFRAORBITAL NERVE BLOCK

Indication

To provide anesthesia of the upper lip, nose, lower eyelid, and maxillary portion of the face

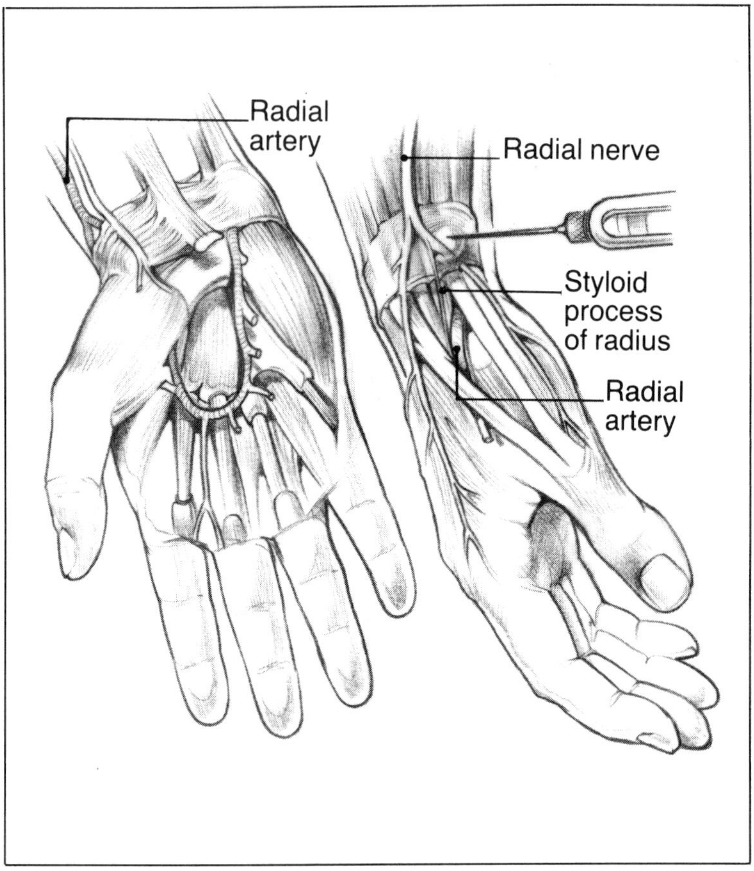

Figure 41-5 Site of needle insertion for radial nerve block. Skin wheal positioned lateral to the radial artery at the level of the radial styloid process.

PROCEDURE

1. Palpate along the inferior border of the infraorbital ridge to locate the infraorbital foramen, which should lie directly below the pupil, with the patient gazing straight ahead.
2. Placing one finger over the foramen, retract the upper lip, and raise a small wheal in the oral mucosa opposite the second maxillary bicuspid.
3. Advance the needle through the wheal until the tip is palpable at the foramen, and inject 2 mL of 1% lidocaine without epinephrine (Figure 41-7). Apply pressure over the infraorbital rim to prevent migration of the anesthetic into the lower lid.

INTERCOSTAL NERVE BLOCK

Indication

To relieve chest and abdominal pain caused by rib fractures

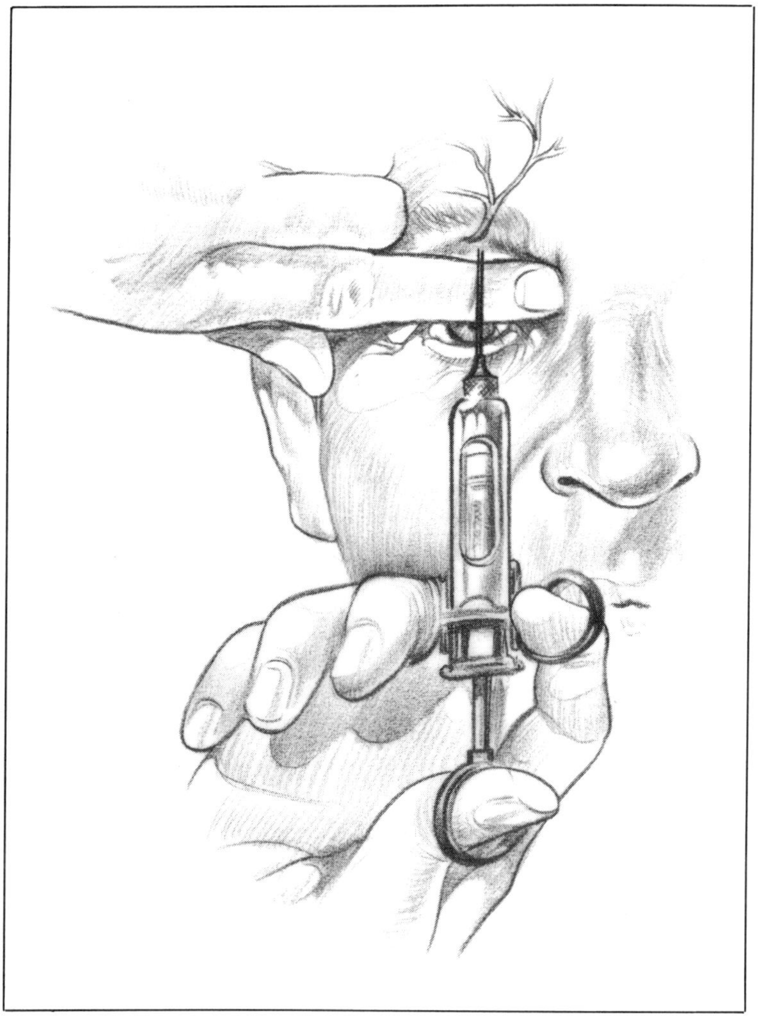

Figure 41-6 To place a supraorbital nerve block, the needle is advanced through a skin wheal raised directly over the supraorbital notch. When paresthesia occurs, begin injecting lidocaine. Note that the first finger of the nondominant hand is applying pressure to the upper eyelid. This prevents infiltration of anesthetic into the lid.

PROCEDURE

1. Have the patient sit and lean forward, arms drawn up. Identify the affected rib and the angle described by that rib and the lateral border of the sacrospinalis muscle (Figure 41-8). Place moderate cephalad-directed tension on the skin overlying this angle.
2. Raise a skin wheal over the inferior border of the rib at the apex of the angle.
3. Introduce the needle into the skin wheal until it meets bone. Withdraw slightly, tip the needle slightly caudally, and carefully advance it just under the inferior rib border for 2–3 mm (about ⅛ in.).
4. Aspirate, then inject 5 mL of 1% lidocaine with epinephrine.

Figure 41-7 For placement of an infraorbital nerve block, place one finger over the infraorbital foramen, while retracting the upper lip. Advance the needle alongside the second maxillary bicuspid until the needle tip is felt at the foramen.

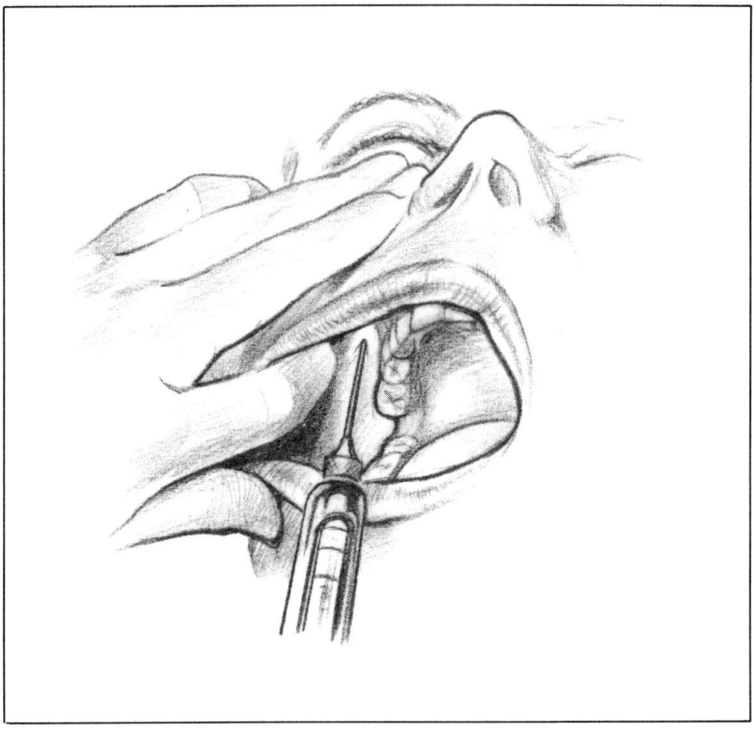

ANKLE BLOCKS

Indication

For minor procedures performed in the area innervated by the deep peroneal, superficial peroneal, sural, or tibial nerve (Figure 41-9).

PROCEDURES

Deep peroneal nerve

1. Identify the anterior tibial tendon by having the patient dorsiflex his foot against resistance. Raise a skin wheal lateral to the tendon at the level of a line connecting the superior borders of the medial and lateral malleoli (see a, Figure 41-10).
2. Insert the needle into the wheal, and advance it slightly medially. When you elicit paresthesia, inject 5 mL of 1% lidocaine without epinephrine in a fan pattern.

Superficial peroneal nerve Infiltrate 5–10 mL of 1% lidocaine in a series of separate subcutaneous injections along a line extending from the anterior tibia to the lateral malleolus at the level of the malleoli (see b, Figure 41-10).

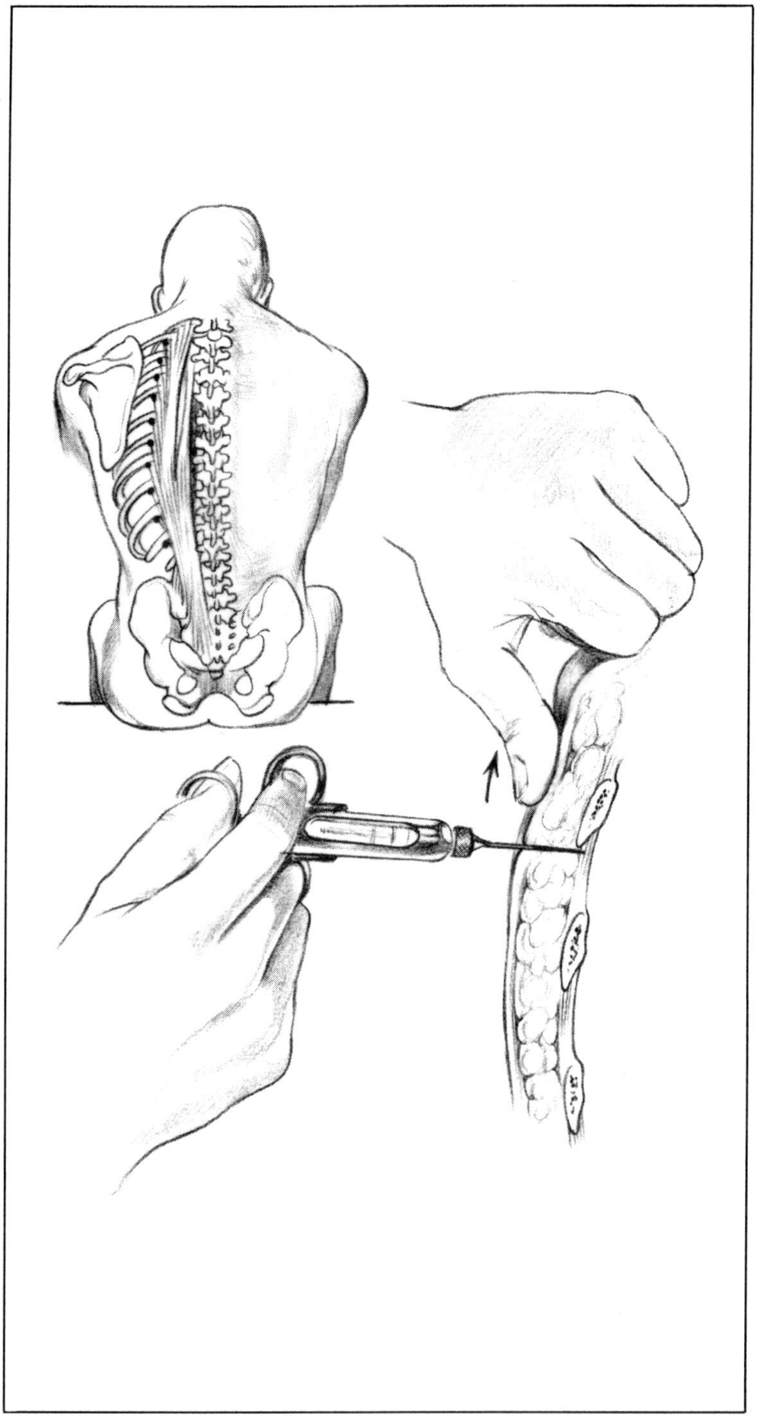

Figure 41-8 Patient is leaning forward to receive an intercostal nerve block. Arrow indicates the direction in which to apply pressure while advancing needle under the inferior border of the affected rib.

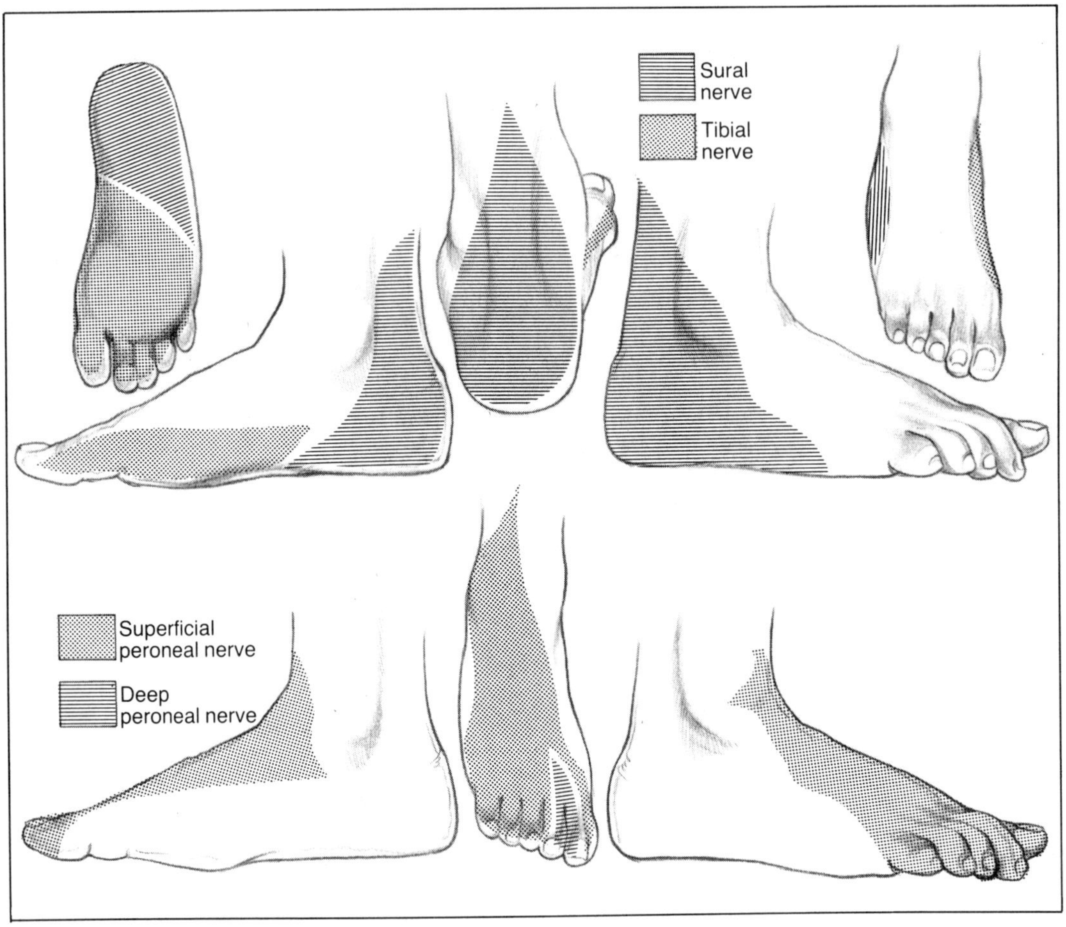

Figure 41-9 Fields anesthetized by blocks placed at different nerve innervations.

Sural nerve Infiltrate 10 mL of 1% lidocaine in a series of separate subcutaneous injections along a line extending from the lateral border of the Achilles tendon to the lateral malleolus at the level of the malleoli (see c, Figure 41-10).

Tibial nerve

1. With the patient prone, identify the Achilles tendon and posterior tibial artery by palpation.
2. Insert a 25-gauge, 2½-in. needle lateral to the artery at the level of the superior border of the medial malleolus (see d, Figure 41-10). If the artery is not palpable, insert the needle immediately lateral to the border of the Achilles tendon.
3. Advance the needle until you elicit paresthesia, then inject 5–10 mL of 1% lidocaine without epinephrine.

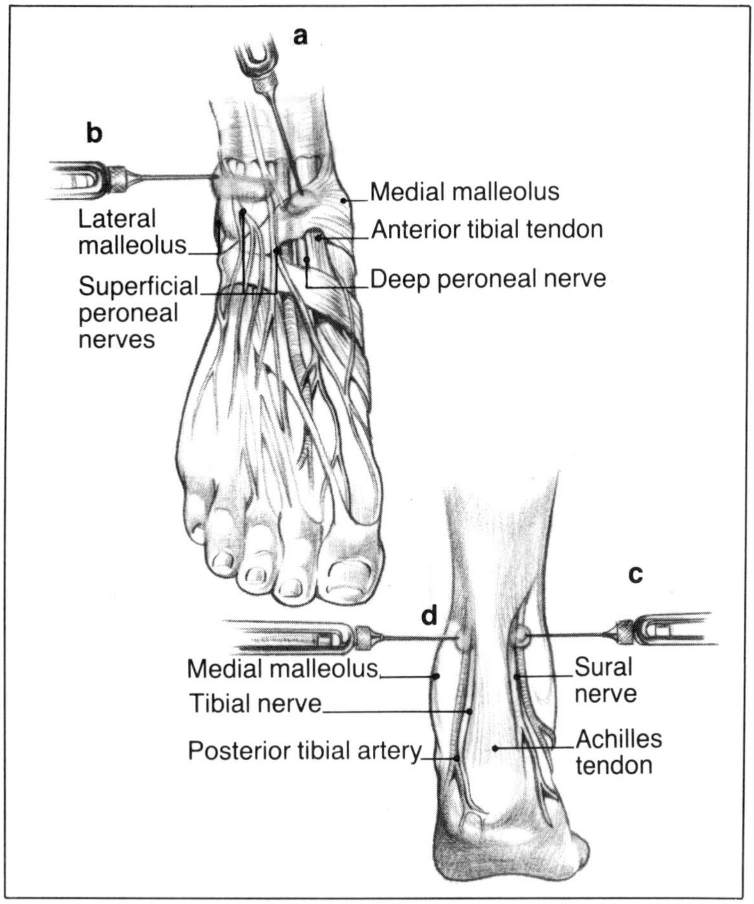

Figure 41-10 a) Deep peroneal nerve block. b) Superficial peroneal nerve block. c) Sural nerve block. d) Tibial nerve block.

4. If you do not elicit paresthesia, advance the needle to the tibia, withdraw 1 cm, and inject 10 mL of 1% lidocaine in a fan pattern.

IV REGIONAL ANESTHESIA

Indications

Reduction of long bone fractures
Extensive wound closure or debridement
Tendon repair in upper or lower extremities

Contraindication

Not to be used on patients with peripheral nervous or vascular disease

Note: Never use an anesthetic containing epinephrine for this block.

Materials

- 0.5% lidocaine HCl (Xylocaine HCl) without epinephrine
- 18-gauge, 1½-in. needle
- 22-gauge IV catheter
- Double tourniquet with inflator
- Elastic bandage
- 60-mL syringe
- IV setup
- Skin prep such as povidone-iodine (Betadine)

PROCEDURE

1. Determine the amount of anesthetic needed: 2–3 mg/kg of lidocaine for an upper extremity block, 5 mg/kg for a lower extremity block. In an average-size adult, this is about 40–60 mL of 0.5% lidocaine. Draw the desired amount of lidocaine (without epinephrine) into the syringe.
2. Establish an IV line in an uninvolved limb as a precautionary measure.
3. Preset the tourniquet pressure to twice the patient's systolic pressure and place the uninflated tourniquet on the affected limb.
4. Insert the 22-gauge cannula into a vein distal to the tourniquet in the affected limb.
5. Elevate the limb, and wrap it firmly in elastic bandage, working toward the tourniquet. When the entire limb distal to the tourniquet is compressed by the wrap, inflate the distal cuff, then the proximal cuff of the tourniquet. After inflating the proximal cuff, deflate the distal cuff, and remove the bandage.
6. Inject the anesthetic via the cannula. Remove or cap the cannula, and wait 10 minutes for adequate anesthesia to be established.
7. If the procedure lasts beyond 15 minutes, you may reinflate the distal cuff and deflate the proximal cuff to avoid tourniquet pain.

Note: Leave the tourniquet inflated for at least 30 minutes after injection of the anesthetic. Earlier deflation does not allow enough time for the anesthetic to diffuse out of the vasculature of the limb; it may release a systemic bolus of the agent.

Suggested Readings

Hill GJ II (ed): *Outpatient Surgery*, ed 2. Philadelphia, WB Saunders Co, 1980.

Posies WJ, Thomas FT (eds): *Office Surgery for the Family Physician.* Stoneham, Mass, Butterworth's, 1984.

Ramanurti CC: *Orthopaedics in Primary Care.* Baltimore, Williams & Wilkins Co, 1979.

42

Punch Biopsy of the Skin

Richard E. Munns, MD

Punch biopsy is the best way to obtain small, full-thickness skin specimens. It is much easier and more effective than the traditional scalpel method, which requires the subsequent placement of sutures. Bleeding and scarring at the punch biopsy site are minimal, suture closure is seldom necessary, and secondary infection if essentially nonexistent.

Indication

You can use the punch biopsy technique whenever you need a small, full-thickness specimen from a lesion for microscopic examination.

Materials

- Antibacterial soap and water or alcohol swabs
- Gloves
- 3 mL of 1% lidocaine HCl (Xylocaine HCl)
- 3-mL syringe
- 25-gauge, ⅝-in. needle
- Biopsy punches in 3-, 4-, 5-, and 6-mm sizes
- Skin hook
- Fine-pointed tissue forceps
- Iris scissors
- Specimen container
- Sterile gauze
- Adhesive strip
- 6.25% aluminum chloride in anhydrous ethyl alcohol 96% (Xerac AC)
- Cotton-tipped applicator
- Needle holder with small curved needle
- Suture material such as 4-0 monofilament

  Note: These suture materials are seldom necessary.

PROCEDURE

1. Cleanse the biopsy site with antibacterial soap and water or an alcohol swab. Select the precise site carefully to encompass some of the lesion and some of the surrounding normal skin.

2. Using a 3-mL syringe with a 25-gauge, ⅝-in. needle, infiltrate about 3 mL of 1% lidocaine into the subcutaneous tissue around the site. This serves to elevate the skin for biopsy as well as to provide anesthesia. The elevation protects deep tissue from injury in the unlikely case that you apply too much pressure when the punch enters the subcutaneous fat layer. Caution in applying pressure is especially important in elderly patients because of their relatively thin layer of subcutaneous fat.

3. Select the smallest size punch that will pick up an adequate specimen—usually a 3- or 4-mm punch. Be sure to confirm that the punch is sharp. With one hand, slightly stretch the skin by digital pressure at right angles to the skin lines before you introduce the punch with the other hand. Keep it stretched as you advance the

Figure 42-1 Place punch perpendicular to the skin and advance it with moderate pressure while rotating it back and forth between thumb and forefinger.

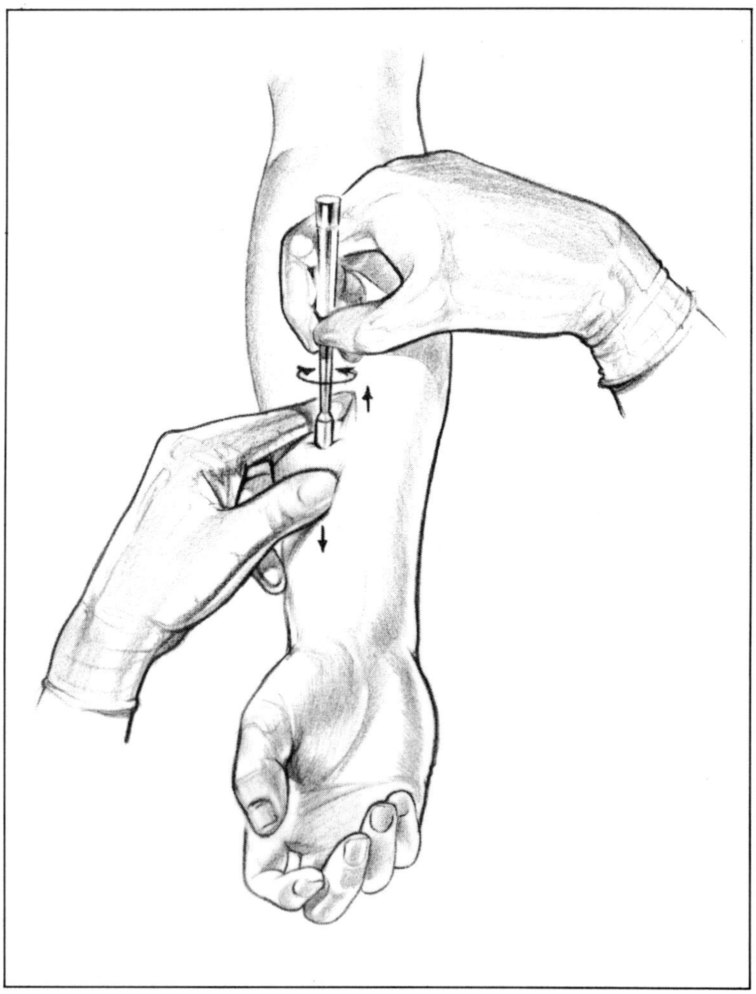

punch; this helps produce a moderately elliptic skin defect rather than a circular one and promotes quick healing.

4. Apply the punch perpendicular to the skin, advancing it with moderate pressure while rotating it back and forth between thumb and forefinger (Figure 42-1).

5. When you feel a marked decrease in resistance as the punch penetrates the dermis and enters the subcutaneous fatty layer, stop advancing the punch.

6. Remove the punch. Occasionally the specimen lifts out with the punch; if so, remove it with a small probe or skin hook. Usually the specimen remains in place. Lift the specimen up with tissue forceps, and cut the pedicle with iris scissors (Figure 42-2). Be sure the specimen contains a bit of subcutaneous fatty tissue. Place the specimen in a container for transportation to your laboratory according to the laboratory protocol.

7. Apply light pressure to the wound with sterile gauze; this nearly always stops any bleeding. An adhesive strip is usually an adequate dressing. If you've used a larger punch, you might need to cauterize with aluminum chloride solution 6.25% on a cotton-tipped applicator, or suture, but even a 6-mm punch seldom creates the need for either of these.

Complications

Punch biopsy is rarely associated with complications. If bleeding is not controlled by pressure, a well-placed suture will solve the problem.

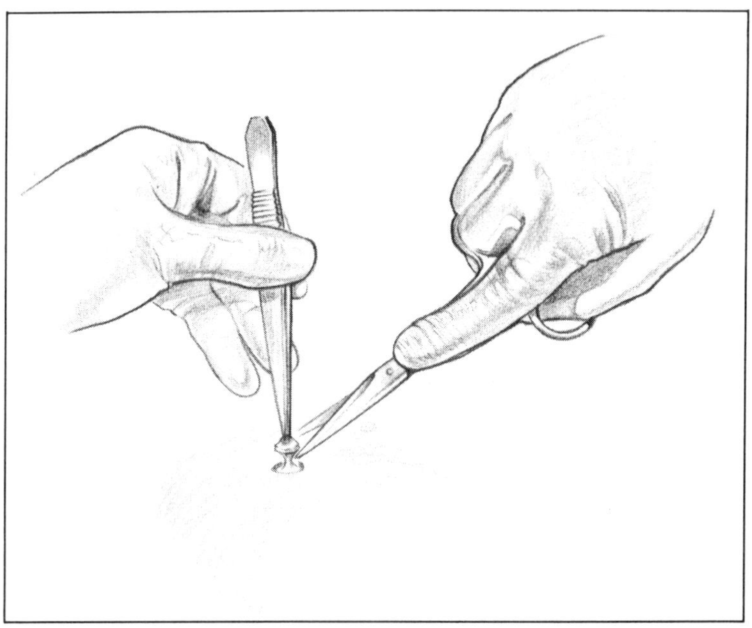

Figure 42-2 Lift specimen with tissue forceps and clip pedicle with iris scissors to free.

Using only sharp punches will permit the specimen to be cut with minimum pressure, thus avoiding injury to deep tissue when the dermis is penetrated. Return visits should be scheduled as with a skin laceration so that adequate healing of the biopsy site can be documented.

Suggested Readings

Driscoll CE, Bope ER, Smith CW, et al: *Handbook of Family Practice*. Chicago, Year Book Medical Pubs Inc, 1986.

Epstein E: *Skin Surgery*, ed 4. Springfield, Illinois, Charles C. Thomas, 1977.

Fitzpatrick TB, Polano MK, Suurmond D: *Color Atlas and Synopsis of Clinical Dermatology*. New York, McGraw-Hill Book Co, 1983.

Schultz BC, McKinney P: *Office Practice of Skin Surgery*. Philadelphia, WB Saunders Co, 1985.

43

Removing a Skin Cyst

Gerald J. McGowan, MD

Most skin cysts do not require removal. But when they become inflamed, infected, or otherwise unsightly and bothersome to the patient, they are easily remedied. Excision is not difficult, scarring is minimal, and the postoperative course is usually uneventful. You can easily excise a sebaceous or epidermoid cyst—and other simple cutaneous tumors such as small lipomas, sclerosing hemangiomas, and pyogenic granulomas—in the office or similar ambulatory setting.

You may want to arrange surgical consultation if the patient has a cyst embedded in the outer table of the skull. Similarly, you may want to arrange consultation for a patient who has any large cutaneous tumor or any tumor that is growing in a precarious site.

Indications

Consider removing skin cysts that are

- Inflamed or infected
- Unsightly and seriously bothersome to the patient

Materials

- Gloves
- Drape
- Povidone-iodine solution (Betadine)
- 10 mL 1% lidocaine HCl (Xylocaine HCl) with 1:100,000 epinephrine
- 10-mL syringe with 25-gauge, 1-in. needle
- Small Kelly clamp, straight or curved
- Small Metzenbaum scissors (optional)
- Small Allis clamp
- Sterile pads and dressing (according to cyst size)
- Small suture tray (scalpel, medium scissors, 3-0 plain catgut and 4-0 or 5-0 nylon suture)

PROCEDURE

1. If the cyst is inflamed or infected, consider incision and drainage or a course of antibiotics for 5 to 10 days and hot packs, letting the inflammation subside before you attempt to excise it.
2. Scrub the cyst and surrounding area with povidone-iodine solution. Using sterile technique, drape around the cyst. Inject 1% lidocaine with epinephrine around the cyst, not only to provide local anesthesia but also to dissect the capsule of the cyst from surrounding tissue.
3. Make an elliptic incision over the cyst in the direction of skin lines. Maximum width of the ellipse should be about 3 mm (1⁄8 in.). In length, the ellipse should extend beyond the edge of the cyst.
4. Incise the ellipse of skin through the dermis, separating both ends from the subcutaneous tissue as flaps (Figure 43-1).
5. Identify the cyst at both ends of the ellipse and carefully start to dissect it. With a small Kelly clamp or a small Metzenbaum scissors or both, spread the tissue at both ends of the ellipse (Figure 43-2). Work toward the center, spreading the tissue progressively, and cautiously separate the cyst from the surrounding tissue.
6. With careful blunt and sharp dissection, continue down and around the cyst, grasping the ellipse of skin with an Allis clamp if you need traction (Figure 43-3). When you identify the underside, remove the cyst with the ellipse intact.
7. Close the dead space with 3-0 plain catgut sutures in one or two layers. This also approximates the skin edges. If the ellipse is wide or the skin fails to come together well, undermine the dermis; you can then easily approximate the mobilized skin. For final closure, use interrupted 4-0 or 5-0 nylon sutures to minimize scarring.
8. Apply light pressure with a sterile dressing. The wound will be tender, but patients seldom require pain medication. Complications are rare. After suture removal in 4–7 days, further visits are usually unnecessary, depending on the cyst location.

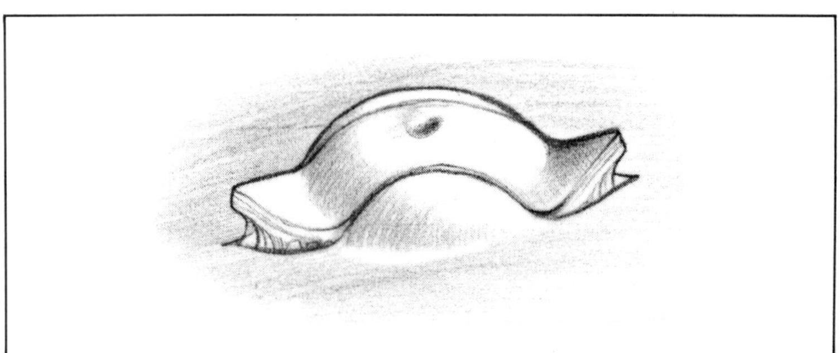

Figure 43-1 Make an elliptic incision over the cyst in the direction of the skin lines. Incise the ellipse through the dermis, separating both ends from the subcutaneous tissue.

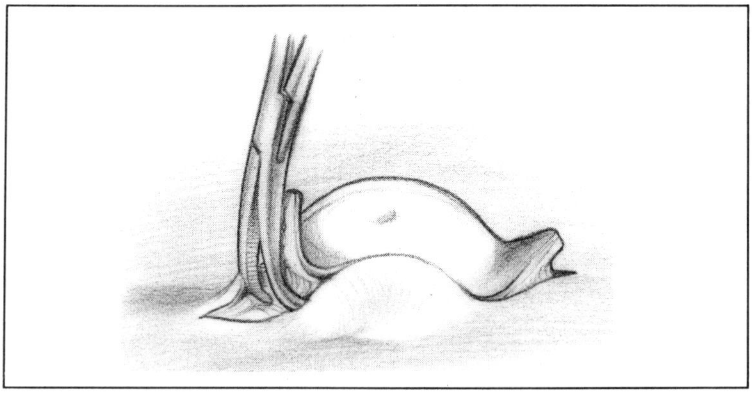

Figure 43-2 Spread the tissue at both ends of the ellipse with a Kelly clamp. Work slowly toward the center, carefully spreading tissue as you go.

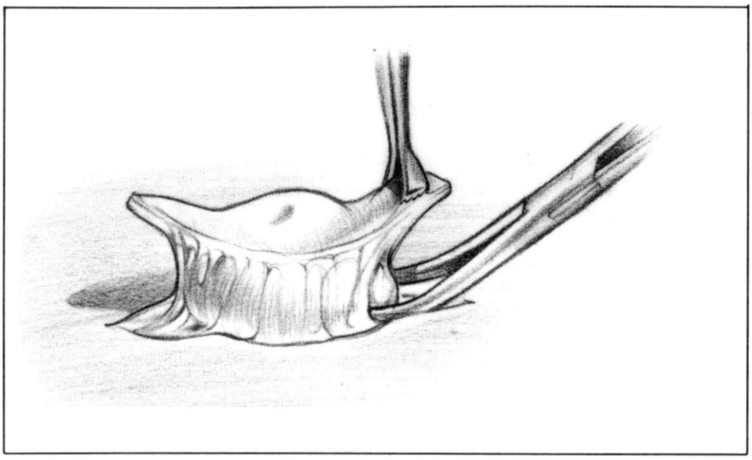

Figure 43-3 Use an Allis clamp to provide traction to the skin ellipse. When the underside is visible, remove the cyst with the skin intact.

Suggested Readings

Davis L: *Christopher's Textbook of Surgery,* ed 8. Philadelphia, WB Saunders Co, 1964, pp 192-193.

Schultz BC, McKinney P: *Office Practice of Skin Surgery.* Philadelphia, WB Saunders Co, 1985.

Thorek P: *Surgical Diagnosis,* ed 2. Philadelphia, JB Lippincott Co, 1965, pp 3, 107.

44

Cryotherapy for Skin Lesions

Charles E. Driscoll, MD
Lawrence W. Steinkraus, MD

An easy, effective procedure for destructive treatment of cutaneous lesions, cryotherapy achieves excellent cosmetic results with minimal complications. It seldom causes scarring, but hypopigmentation sometimes occurs, especially in blacks. Deeper, wider lesions such as malignancies carry some potential for permanent defects.

Different conditions require different depths of freeze, freeze-zone areas, and numbers of freeze-thaw cycles for best effect:

- Flat warts require very light freezing, often without blister formation.
- Superficial lesions in the elderly require shallow freezing because of natural thinning of the dermis. Extensive freezing, which can cause full-thickness destruction, may result in scarring and chronic ulceration.
- Periungual lesions require light, contained freezing to avoid excessive blister formation, subungual hemorrhages, and nail-bed destruction.
- Large, thick lesions may require treatment spread over more than one session.

Even with a conservative approach, cryotherapy may not achieve total effect because of discomfort and possible scarring.

Indications

- Destruction of benign cutaneous lesions including verrucae, condylomata, benign lentigines, seborrheic keratoses, hypertrophic sebaceous glands, the papules of molluscum contagiosum, epithelial nevi, and the lesions of xanthelasma
- Destruction of precancerous skin lesions—actinic keratoses, leukoplakia, and cutaneous horns
- Destruction of malignant lesions. If you suspect a tenacious type of skin cancer such as a basal cell carcinoma, obtain a biopsy before cryotherapy. This will allow cytopathologic identification and examination of the specimen's borders to help determine later on whether you have removed the entire lesion.

Contraindications

Absolute

- Cryglobulinemia, cryofibrinogenemia, or cold agglutination
- A cold-sensitivity disorder such as cold anaphylaxis

Note: It is important not to use cryotherapy to treat morphea or sclerosing basal cell carcinoma.

Relative

- Autoimmune disorders, which necessitate special caution when employing cryosurgery
- Raynaud's disease, when lesions are on an extremity or on the nose, penis, or ears
- Lesions that occupy very thin epithelium immediately over subcutaneous structures that can be injured, such as the eyelid over the tarsal plate or thin skin over the nail bed in an infant or an elderly patient
- Sun-damaged skin, irradiated skin, and skin of patients who are on a regimen of chronic corticosteroid therapy. Expect a more severe destructive action and use very conservative freezing methods.

Choices of Technique

Cryotherapy can be done with a cotton-tipped applicator dipped in liquid nitrogen, a liquid-nitrogen spray apparatus, or a cryoprobe cooled by nitrous oxide (Table 44-1).

Materials

Cotton-ball wick method

- Source of liquid nitrogen in storage unit
- A 1-qt stainless-steel-lined vacuum bottle with a venting hole in the lid

  Note: Do not secure the lid tightly.
- Cotton-tipped wooden applicator sticks
- Cotton balls

Nitrogen spray method

- Liquid-nitrogen spray unit (Figure 44-1)
- Source of liquid nitrogen in storage unit
- Spray probe tips of various sizes
- Neoprene cones
- Petrolatum

Cryoprobe method

- Cryoprobe surgical gun with silver tips of various sizes (Figure 44-2)
- Tanks of nitrous oxide with pressure gauge and regulator
- Lubricating jelly

TABLE 44-1

Cryotherapy techniques compared

Method	Rate of complications	Freeze depth	Cost	Ease of use	Accuracy/ adaptability	Specific indications	Comments
Cotton-ball wick	Low	1.5 mm	+	+++	+	Benign, relatively superficial lesions, such as seborrheic or actinic keratoses	Relatively messy; needs source and storage container for liquid nitrogen
Spray	Low-moderate	≤10 mm, roughly ¼ of freeze diameter	++	+	++	Larger or deeper lesions	Needs source and storage container for liquid nitrogen; risk of spraying adjacent structures; problems with clogging and freeze-up
Cryo-probe	Low-moderate	Roughly ½ of freeze diameter	+++	++	+++	Useful for nearly all types of mucosal and cutaneous lesions, such as hemorrhoids, cervical lesions, skin tags	Good for intraoral lesions; neat; requires bulky equipment; more working parts and more chance of breakdowns

Key: +, lowest; +++, highest

Figure 44-1

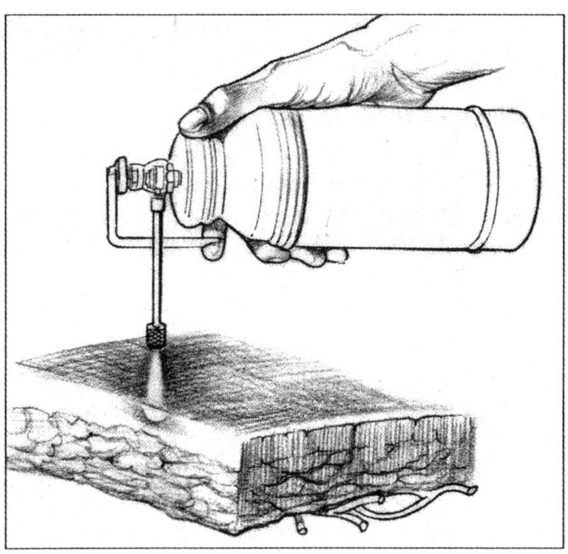

Figure 44-2

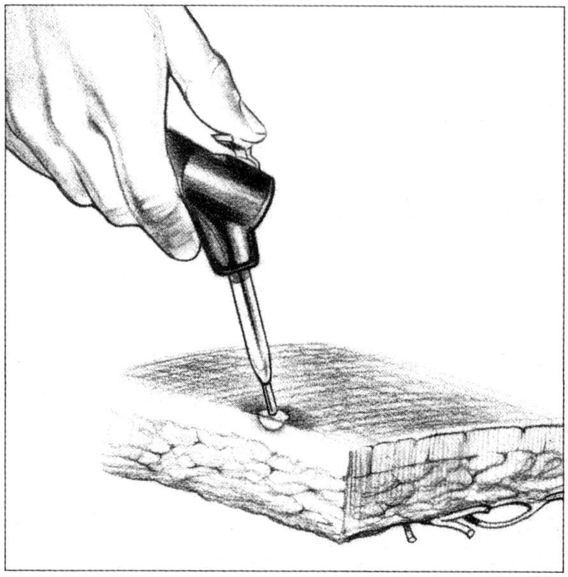

Preparation

To allay anxiety, explain the procedure and the anesthetic effects of cold. The patient sometimes feels an initial burning sensation, followed by some burning and throbbing, but these are usually mild.

If the targeted area is particularly sensitive to cold—the genital and periungual areas, for example—consider using local anesthesia:

- Infiltrate the immediate area with 1% or 2% lidocaine HCl (Xylocaine HCl).
- Do not use anesthetics that contain epinephrine.
- Pare down thick hyperkeratotic lesions before cryosurgery to remove any insulating effects.

PROCEDURE

COTTON-BALL WICK
(for small, shallow cutaneous lesions)

1. Place a supply of liquid nitrogen in a vacuum bottle and loosely secure the lid.
2. Reinforce the cotton-tipped applicator with extra cotton from a cotton ball, not too tightly wound, to carry the amount of refrigerant needed. Shape the tip to suit the targeted lesion, and be sure the cotton wad is not so bulky that it reduces your accuracy in limiting the freeze area.
3. Dip the applicator into the liquid nitrogen, and apply it to the lesion. Because liquid nitrogen evaporates quickly, you will probably have to repeat the application several times to freeze the tissue adequately.

Generally, you will have achieved adequate freezing when you create a freeze zone extending 2–4 mm into the normal tissue around the lesion, or when the frozen tissue takes approximately 30 seconds to thaw (for help in judging freeze depth, see Figures 44-3, 44-4, and 44-5). Pressure on the lesion accelerates freezing but is not recommended because it may increase discomfort. In addition, complications are more likely with pressure applications, especially in elderly patients and over superficial nerves and bone.

Note: Two cycles of freezing and complete thawing are usually required, so you may want to freeze large lesions in portions. Thick lesions may require a third cycle.

Figure 44-3

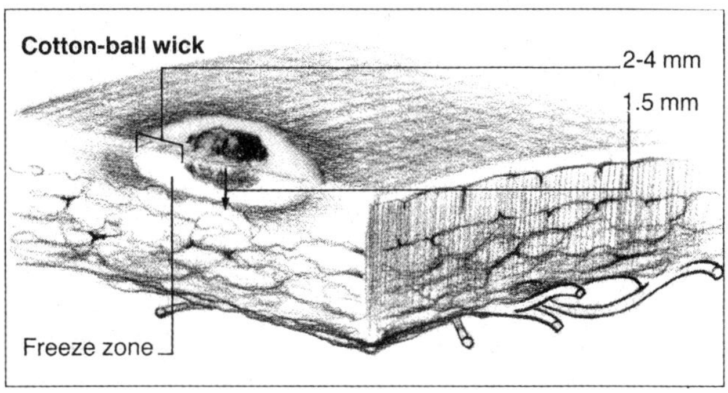

Figure 44-4

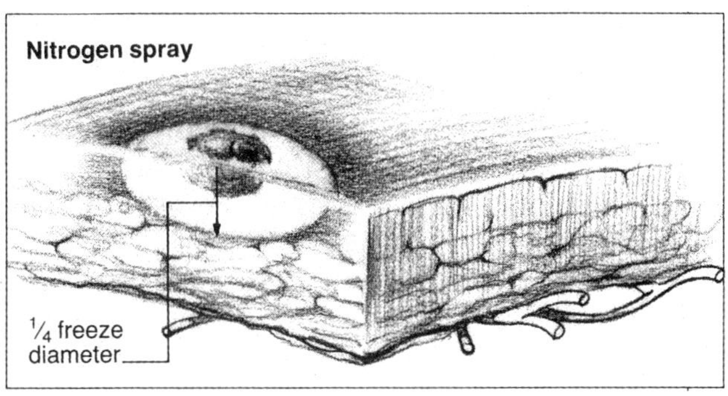

Figure 44-5

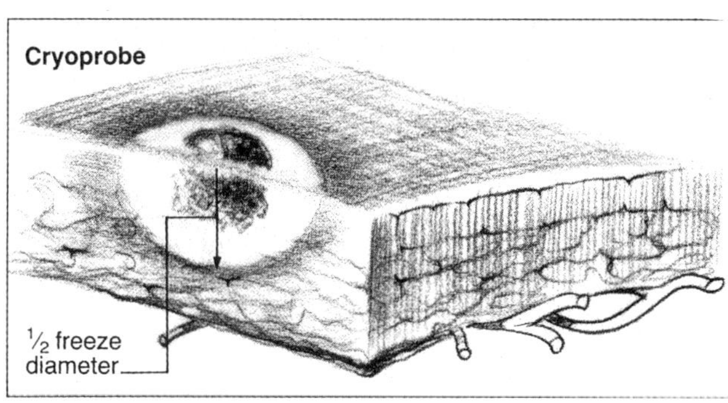

NITROGEN SPRAY
(for most cutaneous lesions)

1. Fill the spray-unit container with liquid nitrogen, and choose an appropriate tip—usually a fine, needle-type tip for better accuracy and increased concentration of refrigerant. You may choose wider tips and sprays for larger areas or for lighter freezing.
2. Spray the targeted area until you achieve a freeze zone that extends 2–4 mm into normal tissue or a 30-second thaw time. Normally, you will want to hold the spray tip 8–10 cm from the skin; closer than that causes deeper freezing. For optimal control of lateral spread, spray in short bursts rather than in one sustained spray.
3. Repeat the freeze-thaw cycle once.

Note: Neoprene cones are used occasionally to limit the area treated, with petrolatum smeared under the cone to prevent it from freezing to the skin. The freeze depth is harder to judge with the cone in place, however, and overfreezing may result.

CRYOPROBE GUN
(for mucosal and cutaneous lesions)

1. Choose a tip large enough to cover the lesion, but not so large as to injure neighboring healthy tissue. Slightly rounded or flattened tips are usually more versatile; fine-point tips are less efficient in the conduction of cold to the lesion.

Remove the protective cover from the cryogun and screw on the cryoprobe tip, checking to see that you have a firm seal.

Note: With devices that use O-ring gaskets, the gaskets will occasionally fail when you turn on the pressure, causing a loud popping noise. Warn the patient that this might happen so he or she is not unduly startled.
2. Supply the silver-tipped cryoprobe gun with nitrous oxide via a regulator valve from a pressure-monitored tank.
3. Open the regulator valve and check the pressure indicator to verify that it is reading in the green (fully pressurized) range. This indicates there is enough nitrous oxide in the tank.

Next, open the cryogun valve, and test it by pulling the trigger to allow circulation of the refrigerant. You will hear a hiss and see frost on the cryoprobe tip.

Note: Do not touch the tip to test it.
4. Apply a small amount of lubricating jelly to the area to be treated using a cotton swab. The jelly conducts the cold to the lesion and adheres the cryoprobe tip to the lesion during treatment. This fosters better cold conduction and allows you to lift the lesion away from sensitive underlying structures such as superficial nerves and bony prominences.
5. Stabilize the tip against the target area, and pull the trigger to start the flow of refrigerant.

As the tip cools, a firm frost forms and the jelly appears frozen. You now may elevate the tip slightly (1–2 mm) to avoid freezing nontarget underlying structures (Figure 44-6). The timing of this move comes with a little practice.

6. Continue the freeze until a freeze zone of 2–4 mm appears in surrounding normal skin. When you reach the desired depth and area of freeze, release the trigger, but do not remove the tip from the skin until the frost has disappeared about five seconds.

7. Allow the area to thaw, then apply a second treatment.

Follow-up Care

Warn the patient that a blister usually forms within the first few hours and that it may occasionally contain a small, insignificant hemorrhage (a "blood blister").

If you have treated a wart or other sessile lesion and the lesion lifts up to float on top of the sac in one or two days, you can remove it and the blister by cutting around the base of the blister with iris scissors. Alternatively, you can leave the blister intact and allow it to heal. Healing time is generally 2–3 weeks, with crust formation after the first 7–9 days. If you leave the blister intact, have the patient protect it with a dry dressing. Occasionally you will have to drain a blister if it becomes infected or increasingly uncomfortable. After drainage the patient can clean the area two or three times a day with hydrogen peroxide, apply a topical antibiotic if desired, and put on a clean dressing. Warn the patient to watch for signs of secondary infection, but such infections are rare.

Figure 44-6

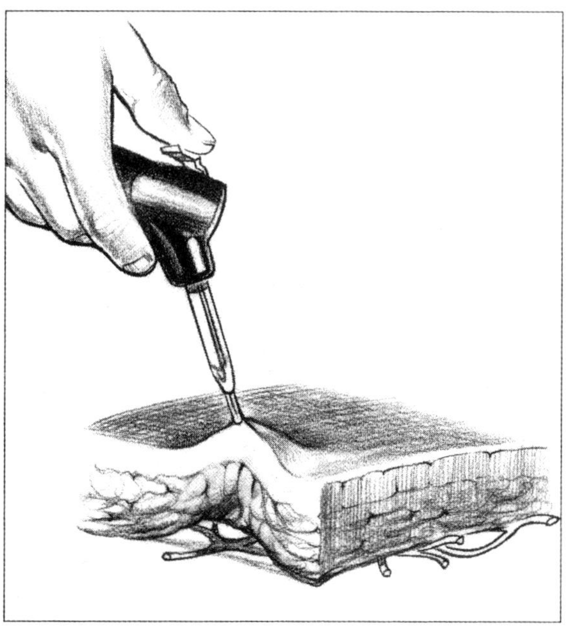

Follow up in 3–4 weeks (4–10 days with larger lesions), and recheck to make sure healing is satisfactory and to decide whether further treatments are necessary.

Suggested Readings

Elton RF: The appropriate use of liquid nitrogen. *Prim Care* 1983;10:459-478.

Elton RF: Complications of cutaneous cryosurgery. *J Am Acad Dermatol* 1983;8:513-519.

Hopkins P: Cryosurgery by the general practitioner. *Practitioner* 1983;227:1861-1873.

Torre D: Cutaneous cryosurgery: Current state of the art. *J Dermatol Surg Oncol* 1985;11:292-293.

45

Repair of Simple Lacerations

Ann Stein, MD
Paul S. Williamson, MD

Most traumatic lacerations are minor. If the wound is superficial, with no vessel, tendon, joint, or nerve involvement, you can repair it as a simple laceration on an outpatient basis. A good assistant is invaluable in most laceration repairs.

Indication

Simple laceration up to full thickness (through the epidermis and dermis but not into subdermal structures)

Note: Lacerations with linear, sharp, visible margins, such as those caused by sharp metal or glass, are generally easiest to repair. Stellate, beveled, or flap-shaped lacerations, sometimes contaminated with foreign material, are more difficult but still usually treated on an outpatient basis. Contaminated wounds needing extensive cleaning and debridement and crushed wound areas such as those resulting from wringer-type injuries often have extensive devitalized tissue and should be repaired only after demarcation with debridement.

Contraindications

The following are beyond the scope of this procedure:

- Lacerations that involve deep structures such as muscle, bone, fascia, nerves, parotid duct, or lacrimal apparatus; through-and-through lacerations of the eyelid, lip, or cheek; and lacerations requiring a large flap or graft. Superficial muscle and fascial injuries may require a layered closure. Some of these problems are better dealt with in the operating room.
- Wounds more than 8–12 hours old (or up to 24 hours old if clean) and bite wounds. These should be allowed to heal secondarily and be revised as needed later, often after debridement. Wounds to the face may be closed up to 48 hours later if clean. Dog bites may be closed if they are irrigated well and there is no extensive crush injury or necrotic tissue.
- High-pressure injection injuries. These often appear minor but can be extensive under the surface. Primary closure is not indicated.

- Thermal injuries, including electrical and chemical wounds. Gunshot wounds often have extensive thermal injury and should be widely debrided but not closed.
- Wounds with extensive edema, ecchymosis, and soft tissue injury. These may require open treatment with secondary closure to avoid compartment syndromes.
- Significant facial lacerations. Plastic surgery may be needed.

Materials

- Antibacterial skin prep, such as povidone-iodine (Betadine) or chlorhexidine gluconate (Hibiclens), in a 1-oz medicine cup
- About 12 sterile 4 × 4-in. gauze sponges
- Sterile gloves
- Skin drapes
- 1% lidocaine HCl (Xylocaine HCl) with and without epinephrine
- 5-mL, sterile, disposable syringe with a 1-in., 18-gauge needle to draw up the anesthetic and a 1½-in., 25- or 27-gauge needle to infiltrate the anesthetic
- 30–50 mL irrigation syringe with a blunt 18-gauge needle
- Warm saline
- Good operative light
- Needle holder
- Suture scissors
- Pick-up forceps with teeth (thumb)
- Pick-up forceps without teeth (for subcutaneous tissue)
- Skin hooks (optional)
- Two mosquito hemostats, one straight, one curved
- No. 15 scalpel blade with a No. 4 handle if needed for debridement
- Small pair of curved scissors for undermining (optional)
- Suture in various sizes, usually 4-0 nylon monofilament (6-0 nylon monofilament for the face) or another nonabsorbable suture such as polypropylene (Prolene, Surgilene); synthetic absorbable suture such as polyglactic acid (Vicryl) or polyglycolic acid (Dexon) for subcuticular or mucosal stitches (usually 4-0)

Preparation

In your record of the patient's pertinent medical history, include allergies (especially allergies to local anesthetics, topical antibiotics, tape and other materials used in the repair), any bleeding disorders, and tetanus immunization status. Record the time of the injury, location of the incident, the patient's own description of the mechanism of injury, and any first-aid treatment given. On initial examination, record the location and size of the laceration, estimated depth, sensory changes, structures involved, and the amount of bleeding. A small diagram may be helpful for this.

Remove any clothing that obstructs the wound; remove the patient's watch and any rings if near the wound.

Stop the bleeding with direct pressure, or use a blood pressure cuff as a temporary tourniquet if the bleeding is in an extremity. If pressure does not produce hemostasis, you may need to explore the wound for the bleeding source. Electrocautery is sometimes used to stop small bleeders. Suturing the wound is often sufficient hemostasis. Particularly with scalp wounds, large sutures placed deep in the tissue may be the only way to control the multiple small vessels involved in the laceration.

Scrub the skin surrounding the wound with antibacterial skin prep or soak it for five minutes in a sterile pan of warm soap solution. Clean the wound itself with saline irrigation using the 10–50 mL syringe with 18-gauge blunt needle, expelling the saline fast enough to produce sufficient cleaning pressure. Debride necrotic, dirty, or ragged edges mechanically if necessary. Be cautious with debridement on the face. This well-vascularized area will often heal better with ragged edges that when carefully matched will leave a less visible scar.

Note: Do not apply antiseptic within an open wound; it will impair the immune response and inhibit initial cellular repair. And do not shave the hair around the wound; this may increase the rate of infection. If the wound is above an eye, remember that eyebrows once shaved may not regrow normally. Hair can be smoothed back with water or antibiotic ointment to keep it out of the wound during repair.

PROCEDURE

1. Examine the wound under sterile conditions for depth and involved structures. If called for, assess tendon function and ductal structures before repair. Record pinprick sensation distal to the wound before local anesthesia. For fingers, document a two-point discrimination test. Search for and remove any foreign bodies in the wound. Record your search for foreign bodies whether or not you find any. Use X-ray or xeroradiography if necessary to rule out foreign bodies such as glass or associated orthopedic fracture.

2. Administer local anesthesia, aspirating before injection to make sure the needle is not in a vein. Inject approximately 1 mL of 1% lidocaine for every 2 cm (¾ in.) of laceration, to a maximum of 4 mg/kg for repair of multiple lacerations, or 28 mL for a 70-kg (154-lb) person. Infiltrate all dermal tissue within about 1 cm (⅜ in.) of the wound edge. If the wound is clean, inject through the open wound surface; if contaminated, inject through the surrounding scrubbed skin surface. Inject slowly in the subdermal space to minimize pain, then allow five minutes for diffusion and anesthetic effect before suturing. Digital blocks may be very useful for fingers and toes, especially if the nail area is involved.

Note: Lidocaine with epinephrine will prevent some vasodilation and rebleeding caused by local infiltration, but epinephrine is contraindicated in fingers, toes, penis, nose, and earlobes. Epinephrine should also be avoided in contaminated wounds as it slows the body's response to infection.

3. Excise obviously necrotic tissue and any jagged wound edges, being conservative around vital tissues and in areas where the skin is tight. Where necessary, undermine the dermis to mobilize the skin edges and permit approximating them without tension. Square off oblique cuts to leave perpendicular skin edges for approximating (Figure 45-1). Try to preserve landmarks and leave square wound edges that can be approximated by appropriately matched layers. In hair-bearing areas, excise tissue in the direction of the hair follicles to avoid buried hairs that will regrow (Figure 45-2). Eliminate dead space in subcutaneous adipose tissue by approximating it with a few absorbable synthetic sutures to leave the smallest scar possible (Figure 45-3). Reestablish hemostasis with pressure or absorbable-suture ligature of small veins. If the wound is now clean, linear, and no more than skin deep, proceed with suturing.

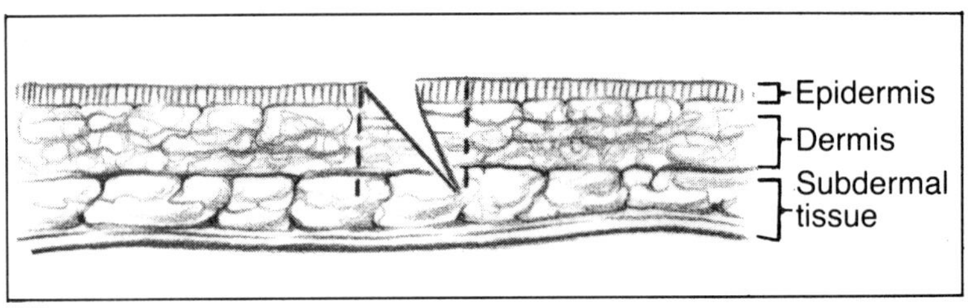

Figure 45-1 Dotted lines illustrate squaring-off of an oblique laceration perpendicular to the skin edges.

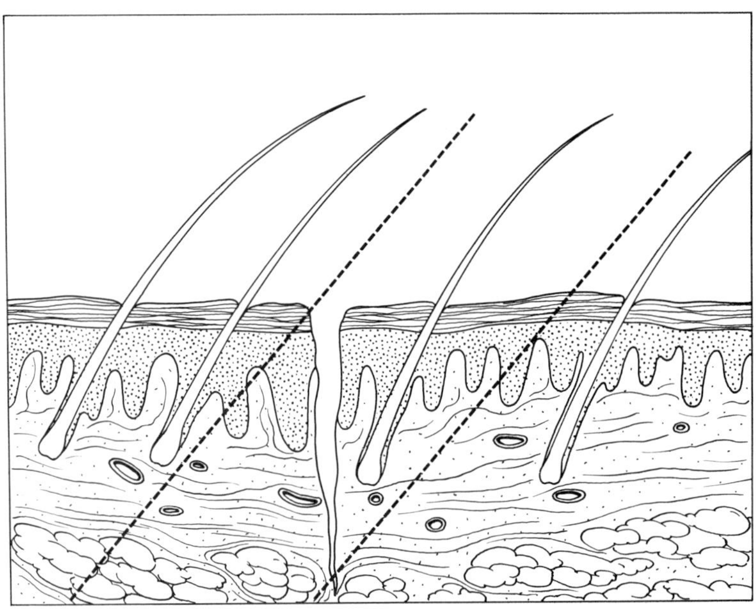

Figure 45-2 Excise tissue in the direction of the hair follicles.

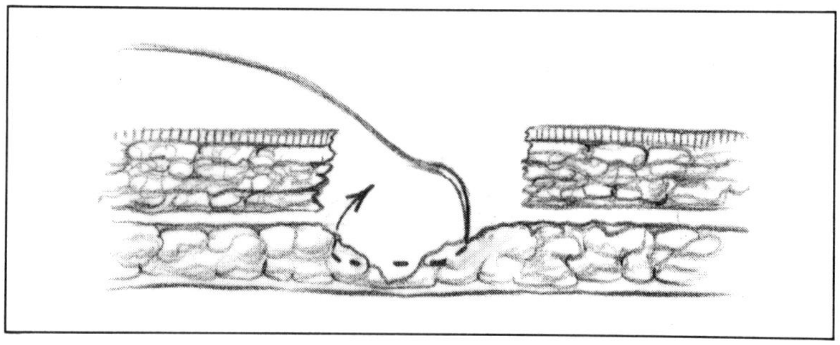

Figure 45-3 Eliminate dead space in subcutaneous adipose tissue by approximating it with a few absorbable sutures. Reestablish hemostasis with pressure.

4. Choose the smallest monofilament suture that will hold the wound well, usually 3-0 on the back, 4-0 or 5-0 on the extremities, and 6-0 on the face. For facial lacerations, consider whether subcuticular or running closure would be better than interrupted sutures. For interrupted sutures, plan the first suture to realign landmarks such as the vermilion border, skin wrinkles, or hair lines. For a V-shaped or flap laceration, place the first stitch at the vertex to realign tissue structures (Figure 45-4). For a T-shaped laceration, use the first stitch to approximate both flaps with the area where they were originally attached (Figure 45-5). Stabilize one edge of the wound with a skin hook or pick-up forceps with teeth lightly held to avoid crushing tissue.
5. Hold the suture needle perpendicular to the skin surface, as far from the wound edge as the skin is thick (Figure 45-6), and rotate your wrist to twist, not push, the needle through the skin. Hemostasis at this point is essential, since a clot interposed between skin edges will delay healing and encourage infection. Use electrocoagulation if necessary, with the proper precautions.
6. If the gap between the wound edges is small, continue moving the needle up through the opposing skin edge, exiting about one skin thickness from the wound edge.

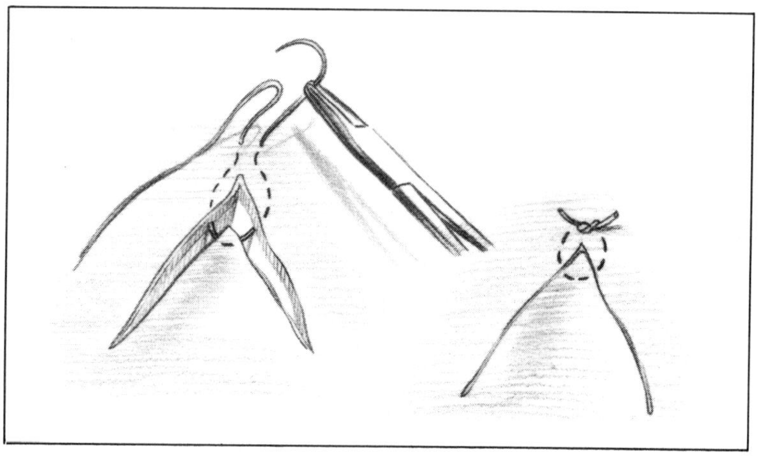

Figure 45-4 Plan the first suture to realign landmarks. For a V-shaped or flap laceration, place the first stitch at the vertex.

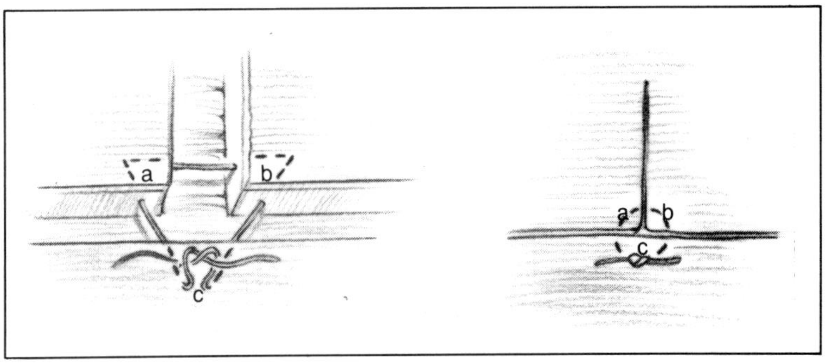

Figure 45-5 For a T-shaped laceration, use the first stitch to approximate both flaps with the area they were originally attached to.

7. With some 2 cm of suture remaining on the side of the wound where the suture needle entered, instrument-tie the suture with just enough tension to approximate but not strangulate the skin edges. Try to leave wound edges slightly everted. Mattress sutures may be required to evert adequately.

8. Place subsequent sutures as far apart as possible (0.5–1.0 cm [3⁄16–3⁄8 in.]) while allowing no gaping at the wound edges. Space between sutures should be approximately equal to the width of the stitch. Handle "dog-ears" by removing a small triangular area of skin at the end of the laceration with the dog-ear or by extending the length of the laceration (Figure 45-7).

9. Dress the wound with sterile gauze and tape.

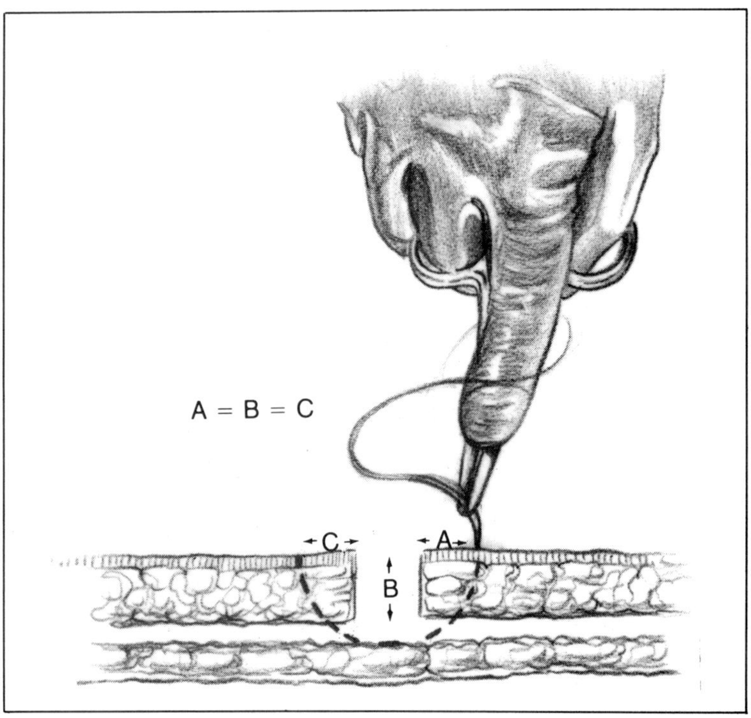

Figure 45-6 Hold the suture needle perpendicular to the skin surface, as far from the wound edge as the skin is thick, and twist the needle through the layers. Do not push the needle.

Figure 45-7 A dog-ear or pucker of excess skin may be unavoidable as you close (a). It may be removed by using a skin hook to lift the edge of the wound, incising along the side of that portion of skin (b), and pulling a triangle of skin over the suture line (c), which is then incised along the suture line to remove the excess and closed (d).

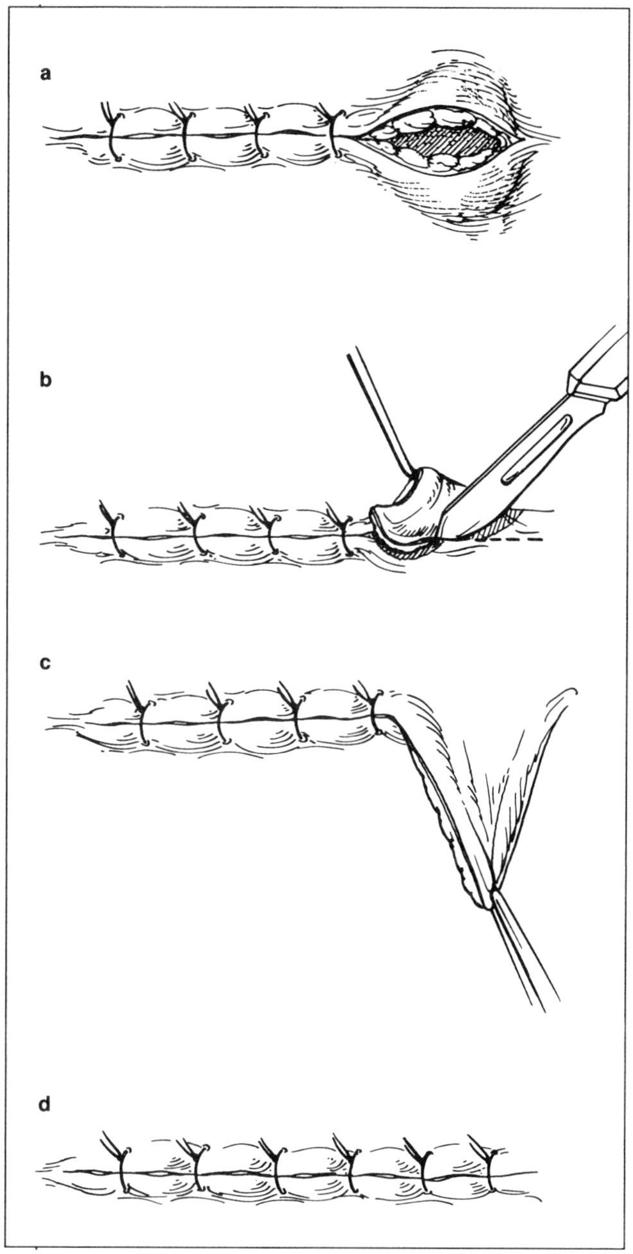

Follow-up Care

1. Instruct the patient to leave the initial dressing in place for 24 hours and, if it bleeds through, to pack it over the top with more gauze and tape, then see you immediately for reexamination. Analgesics such as aspirin or acetaminophen may be needed for discomfort as the local anesthetic wears off.

2. Have the patient change the dressing two to three times daily and wash the wound with hydrogen peroxide, then lightly coat the wound with an antibiotic ointment for the first three days. Starting with day 4, the wound may be washed with soap and water, but eschar should be kept covered with gauze until the sutures are removed. The bandages should be changed as necessary to keep them dry. The wound infection rate for so-called clean wounds is approximately 5%. In addition, lacerations across a joint may need to be immobilized with a small splint.
3. If the initial wound was contaminated with bacteria, reexamine it in 24–48 hours. Instruct the patient with a contaminated wound to return immediately if he or she develops fever, if the wound becomes red or swollen, or if it drains pus.
4. Have the patient return for suture removal in a specified number of days, generally 3–5 days for lacerations of the face, 5–7 days for the scalp, 7–10 days for the extremities and abdomen, and 10–14 days for the foot or back. Remember that a patient taking corticosteroid drugs may take two or three times as long to heal.
5. Note the condition of the wound at suture removal time. To remove a suture, elevate the knot with a hemostat, clip the suture on one side of the knot, and pull toward, rather than away from, the healing wound line to avoid tearing the wound open. If indicated, redress the wound with a dry gauze bandage for one day. For persons who are prone to scarring, areas where tension and motion will stretch a wound, or facial lacerations where cosmetic appearance is important, adhesive strips should be applied and left in place several days for reinforcement.

Suggested Readings

Bonadio WA, Wagner V: Efficacy of the topical anesthetic for repair of pediatric lacerations. *Am J Dis Child* 1988;142:203-205.

Calabro JJ, Hoidal CR, Susini LM: Extensor tendon repair in the emergency department. *J Emerg Med* 1986;4:217-225.

Howell JM, Morgan JA: Scalp laceration repair without prior hair removal. *Am J Emerg Med* 1988;6:7-10.

Maimaris C, Quinton DN: Dog-bite lacerations: A controlled trial of primary wound closure. *Arch Emerg Med* 1988;5:156-161.

Phillips LG, Heggers JP: Layered closure of lacerations. *Postgrad Med* 1988;83:142-148.

Steele MT, Sainsbury CR, Robinson WA, et al: Prophylactic penicillin for intraoral wounds. *Ann Emerg Med* 1989;18:847-852.

Stuzin JM, Engrav LH, Buehler PK: Emergency treatment of facial lacerations. *Postgrad Med* 1982;71(3):81-94.

Zukin DD, Simon RR (eds): *Emergency Wound Care: Principles and Practice.* Rockville, Md, Aspen Publishers, 1987.

46

Incision and Drainage of Cutaneous Abscesses

Ralph H. Knudson, MD

Abscesses are the end result of infections such as cellulitis, lymphadenitis, and wounds and lacerations that were contaminated. Incision and drainage provide the best and virtually only course of treatment.

Indications

Therapeutic

- When liquefactive necrosis is present in an abscess caused by bacterial infection. This may be demonstrated by palpation of fluctuance or, if the site is difficult to palpate, by needle aspiration of pus.

Diagnostic

- Culture and susceptibility testing of the abscess material occasionally helps determine a choice of antibiotic.

Contraindications

None, but areas overlying nerves or vessels, deep lesions around the eyes, perianal abscesses, and deep palmar and plantar lesions should be surgically drained with careful follow-up and parenteral antibiotic treatment.

Use of Antibiotics

Routine culturing of all abscess material from healthy patients is not considered necessary because using antibiotics to promote abscess healing after incision and drainage is questionable; many studies show no significant improvement. For the high-risk patient, the toxic patient, or the patient with a facial lesion that might be drained by the cavernous sinus, however, antibiotics are recommended. Select appropriate agents on the basis of a Gram's stain plus culture and susceptibility results.

Abscess microbiology shows mixed aerobic and anaerobic growth. *Staphylococcus aureus* is the predominant aerobic organism in cutaneous abscesses. Perineal abscesses tend to show more anaerobes and may grow *Neisseria gonorrhoeae* in vulvar bland areas. A penicillinase-resistant penicillin is generally a good choice for beginning antibiotic care.

Materials

- Sterile gloves
- Sterile drapes
- Antiseptic such as isopropyl alcohol, hexachlorophene cleanser (pHisoHex), or povidone-iodine solution (Betadine)
- Razor
- 1% lidocaine HCl (Xylocaine HCl)
- 5-mL syringe with 25-gauge needle
- 10-mL syringe with 22-gauge needle
- Blunt needle
- Ethyl chloride spray
- Scalpel with No. 11 blade
- Culture swab
- Sterile cotton-tipped swab
- Hydrogen peroxide
- ¼- or ½-in. plain strip gauze
- Sterile scissors
- Forceps
- Hemostat tape
- 4 × 4-in. gauze pads

PROCEDURE

1. Position the patient comfortably with good exposure of the site. Gently scrub the area overlying and surrounding the abscess for one minute. Vigorous scrubbing is unnecessary. Shave the site if needed for exposure. Drape the area.

2. Anesthetize the lesion:

- For a superficial lesion with obvious fluctuance, use ethyl chloride spray. The first contact of the spray on an abscess site is uncomfortable, so lead up to it by demonstrating the cooling effect on your own hand, then on the patient's hand, then on the lesion. Maintain a steady spray until a white "frost" appears, then proceed immediately to step 3.
- For a lesion that is too deep or large for a single brief incision, infiltrate the overlying dermis with 1% lidocaine. Injection is pain-

ful and adds to induration, so limit injection sites and the amount of lidocaine to the minimum necessary for anesthesia.

3. Locate fluctuance by two-finger gentle pressure, or, if necessary, use the 22-gauge needle for fine-needle aspiration of the site to demonstrate pus. Resort to fine-needle aspiration only if fluctuance is questionable, not when fluctuance is clearly not present.

Note: If you do not demonstrate fluctuance or purulence, do not proceed with incision, because it can open up tissue planes and spread infection. Instead, prescribe moist heat and elevation for 24 hours, treat any cellulitis with systemic antibiotics, and reexamine the patient. This helps reveal very early nonpalpable abscess sites and limit associated cellulitis.

4. When you achieve anesthesia, incise as follows:

- *With demonstrated fluctuance,* make a single quick incision parallel to skin lines from edge to edge across the fluctuance (Figure 46-1). Expect spontaneous drainage of some pus, occasionally mixed with blood.
- *With pus demonstrated on needle aspiration,* make a single stab incision following the needle path.

5. If no spontaneous flow occurs, try light pressure on the surrounding skin to recheck fluctuance and possibly extrude thicker purulence.

Note: Avoid this step if the site is on the face or mastoid area since it might infect the sinuses.

6. Collect a culture specimen if culture is indicated.

7. Gently probe the opened abscess with a sterile swab soaked in hydrogen peroxide to break up and clean out loculations (Figure 46-2). An abscess is seldom smoothly spherical. It is more likely to be irregular in shape, with fingerlike extensions that spread into tissue planes; it can be partially loculated by fibrous and necrotic debris.

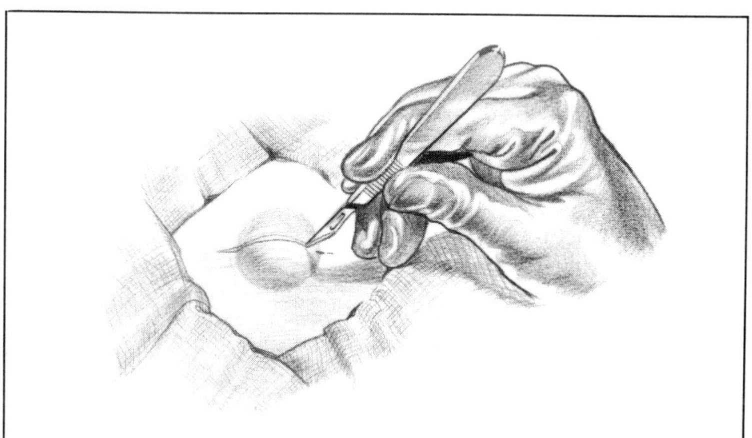

Figure 46-1 For abscesses with demonstrated fluctuance, make a single quick incision from edge to edge.

Figure 46-2 Following expression of pus, probe the cavity with a sterile cotton swab soaked in hydrogen peroxide.

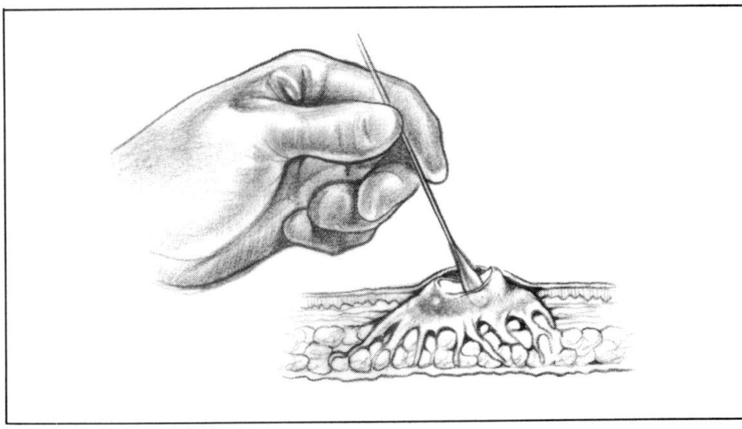

8. After probing, lavage the abscess with saline or hydrogen peroxide, using the lidocaine syringe and a blunt needle.
9. When probing and lavage no longer yield pus, examine for hemostasis. If the abscess is relatively large, packing will stop a slight oozing. In the rare case of persistent bleeding, you may resort to silver nitrate cautery or electrocautery.

Note: Do not use electrocautery in the presence of ethyl chloride, which is explosive.

10. Insert a gauze wick, or, if the abscess is relatively large, pack the abscess site with ¼- or ½-in. plain strip gauze (Figure 46-3). Cover with sterile 4 × 4-in. gauze pads, and inform the patient to expect some oozing of pus, exudate, and a little blood.

Follow-up Care

1. See the patient again in 1–2 days:

- *Facial lesion:* Reevaluate in 24 hours. If erythema is resolving and drainage is minimal, no further packing is needed. If not, replace the wick or repack loosely and continue daily follow-up examinations and repacking until both erythema and drainage are minimal.
- *Other lesions:* Replace the wick or repack in 24–48 hours, then recheck every 1–3 days, depending on patient reliability, size of lesions, and resolution of erythema, drainage, and induration.

2. Instruct the patient to use warm peroxide-and-water soaks, 2–4 times per day for 5–7 days, followed by redressing. Caution the patient not to try to reinsert packing if it falls out. Healing time varies from 7 to 21 days depending on the dimensions, depth, and location of the abscess.

Complications

Complications are few and easily managed.

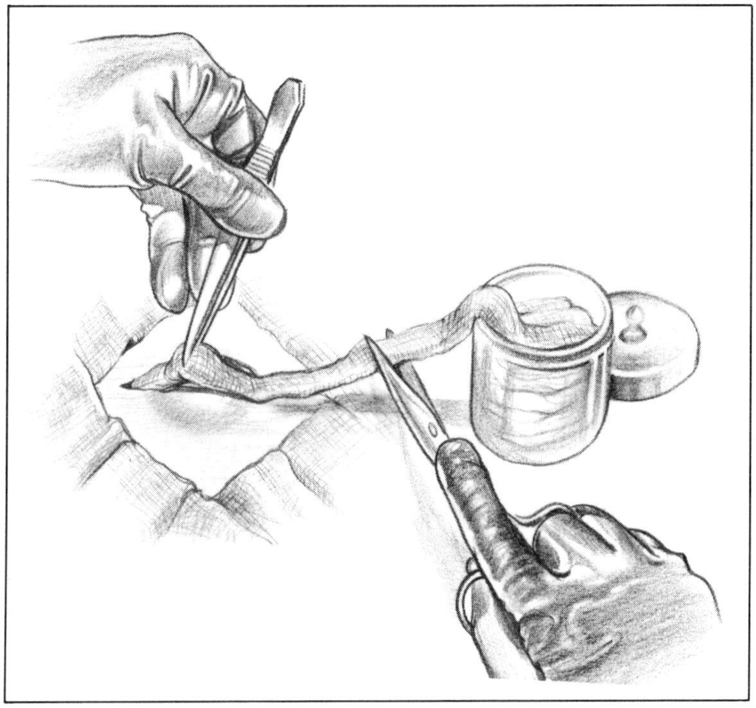

Figure 46-3 If the cavity is large, pack with ¼- or ½-in. sterile gauze strip. Then cover with sterile 4 × 4-in. gauze pads.

- Re-formation of the abscess, the most common complication, is usually due to inadequate incision, incomplete probing for loculations, inadequate lavage, or inadequate packing and soaking during aftercare. Correction usually entails reincision, using the old incision site, and aggressive drainage.
- Bleeding may occur if the abscess is in a highly vascular area or under unusual mechanical pressure or if granulation tissue is traumatized. This is nearly always corrected by packing, pressure, or cautery.
- Slow or poor healing may indicate inadequate drainage or lax aftercare.

Suggested Readings

Dodd RW, Seidenberg B: Abscess, incision and drainage, in Mayhew HE, Rodgers LA (eds): *Basic Procedures in Family Practice*. New York, John Wiley & Sons, 1984, Chap 1.

Llera JL, Levy RC: Treatment of cutaneous abscess: A double-blind clinical study. *Ann Emerg Med* 1985;14:15-19.

Meislin HW, Lerner SA, Graves MH, et al: Cutaneous abscesses—Anaerobic and aerobic bacteriology and outpatient management. *Ann Intern Med* 1977;87:145-149.

Munster AM: Infections, in Hill GJ II (ed): *Outpatient Surgery*, ed 2. Philadelphia, WB Saunders Co, 1980, pp 134-159.

47

Paronychia: Incision and Drainage

Leslie E. Weber, MD

Acute paronychia involves the nail folds of the fingers, usually as a result of minor trauma. Toenails are infrequently involved. Paronychia is nearly always bacterial, most often caused by *Staphylococcus aureus,* group A or D streptococci, or *Pseudomonas aeruginosa*. Redness, swelling, and pain surrounding the margins of the fingernail are usually the presenting complaints. Paronychia can be confused with herpetic whitlow, which is a purulent infection of the fleshy tip of the finger that needs only conservative treatment. Paronychia may also be chronic, in which case it has a somewhat different etiology and treatment. In early or mild paronychia, conservative treatment with warm saline or aluminum acetate (Domeboro) soaks may be sufficient. More often, an abscess under the nail fold causes significant pain because of tissue tension; at this stage, treatment is surgical.

Indication

Acute bacterial infection of the nail folds with redness, swelling, and pain.

Contraindications

- None, although herpetic whitlow and chronic paronychia will not respond to surgical treatment
- Periungual verrucae, which also disfigure the nail fold, call for a different treatment and should not be mistaken for infection

Materials

- 5- and 10-mL syringes
- 22- and 25-gauge needles
- 1% or 2% lidocaine HCl (Xylocaine HCl) without epinephrine
- Povidone/iodine (Betadine)

- Alcohol
- Sterile towels, gloves
- No. 11 scalpel blade and handle
- Iris scissors
- Straight mosquito forceps
- Saline solution
- ¼-in. iodoform packing strips
- Several 3 × 3-in. or 4 × 4-in. gauze pads

PROCEDURE

1. With the 5-mL syringe and 25-gauge needle, inject lidocaine HCl at the base of the involved finger for a metacarpal block. Anesthetize the dorsal and ventral digital nerve branches through small epidermal wheals on the medial and lateral aspects of the finger. Inject about 1 mL of lidocaine adjacent to each digital nerve, ventral and dorsal on each side (Figure 47-1). Aspirate before each injection.

2. Gently wash the whole finger with warm soap solution, apply povidone/iodine (Betadine) solution, and wash that off with alcohol. Drape for a sterile field.

3. Identify the point of maximum fluctuance and incise by placing the scalpel blade against the nail, the point directed into the abscess (Figure 47-2). Advance the blade approximately ¼–½ in., incising the abscess and expressing localized purulent matter. (This often provides relief from pain.) With iris scissors, excise necrotic material.

Figure 47-1

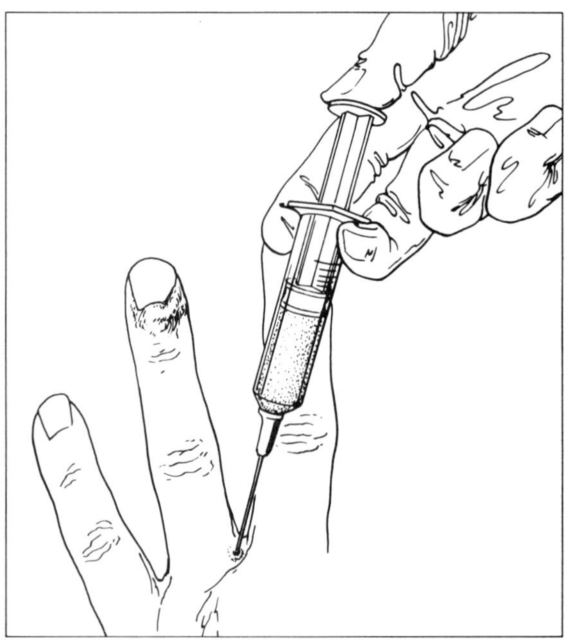

Figure 47-2

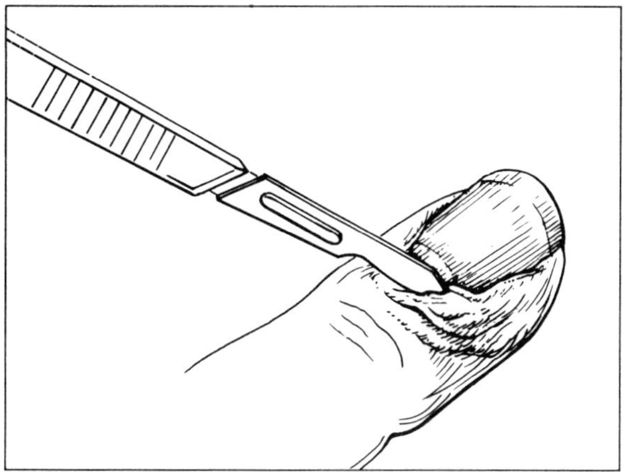

4. If the infection involves the fold at the base of the nail, subungual abscess has developed (Figure 47-3), and the base of the nail should be excised. Use blunt dissection with mosquito forceps at the base of the nail to separate and lever out the base from beneath the fold (Figure 47-4).
5. Make a transverse cut with scissors across the base of the nail and excise about ½–1 in. of nail (Figure 47-5).
6. Gently irrigate under the nail fold, using the 10-mL syringe, 22-gauge needle, and saline solution. Place iodoform packing strip under the nail fold, and cover the finger with a gauze square and occlusive dressing.
7. Surgical drainage brings about a cure in the majority of patients with paronychia, but you may want to prescribe a penicillinase-resistant antibiotic and obtain a culture of the infected material.

Follow-up Care

- Instruct the patient in routine pain control—elevation, rest, and mild analgesics. Narcotics are rarely needed since the procedure itself relieves most discomfort.
- Have the patient return in 2–3 days for removal of the packing. Afterward, instruct the patient to soak the finger for 15 minutes

Figure 47-3

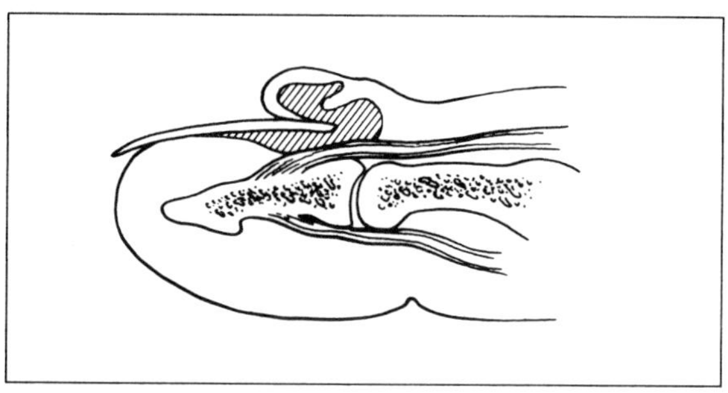

Figure 47-4

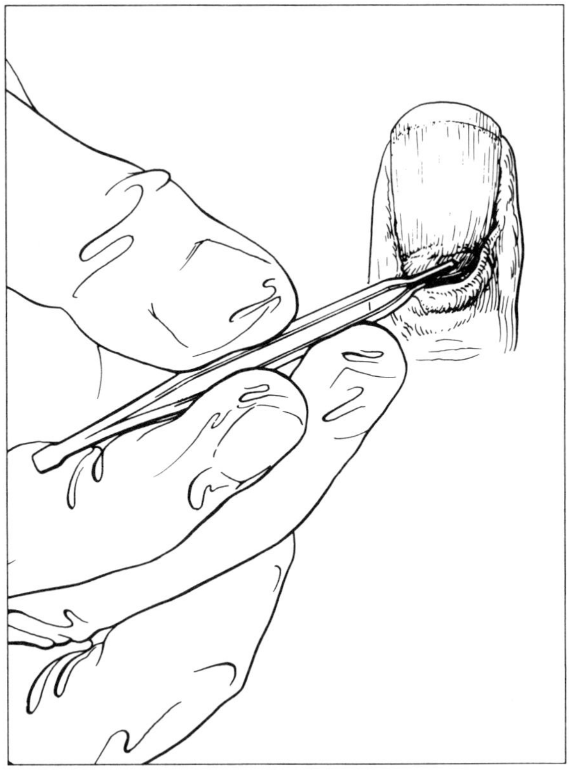

three times a day in warm water or saline solution for several days. After soaking, the patient should apply a dry dressing until healing is complete, changing as often as necessary.

Complications

- A procedure that is too extensive may damage the nail plate and cause the new nail to be disfigured.
- If the procedure is not extensive enough, infection may continue and spread along tendon sheaths or into the pulp space of the finger. Spread may result in osteomyelitis of the distal phalanx or aseptic necrosis from buildup of pressure within the pulp space.

Figure 47-5

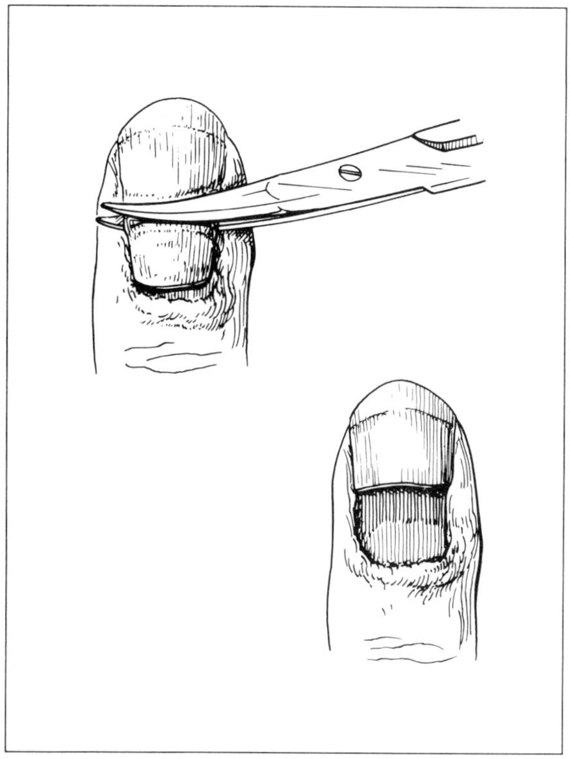

Suggested Readings

Daniel CR III: Paronychia. *Dermatol Clin* 1985;3(3):461-464.

Goroll AH, May LA, Mulley AG, et al: Dermatologic problems, in *Primary Care Medicine: Office Evaluation and Management of the Adult Patient*. Philadelphia, JB Lippincott Co, 1987, p 828.

Mercier LR (ed): *Practical Orthopedics*. Chicago, Year Book Medical Pubs, 1987, pp 88-90.

Umland BE: Paronychia, incision and drainage, in Mayhew HE, Rodgers LA (eds): *Basic Procedures in Family Practice: An Illustrated Manual.* New York, John Wiley & Sons, 1984, pp 21-24.

48

Treatment of Ingrown Toenail

Timothy Appenheimer, MD

Management approaches suggested for ingrown toenails run the gamut from conservative nonsurgical procedures to bone removal. Recurrence is a significant problem in many commonly used treatments. The following guidelines yield good results:

- For initial lesions of less than two months' duration with minimal infection and granuloma, consider using cotton wick insertion.
- For recurrent lesions, lesions of more than two months' duration, and lesions with significant infection and granuloma formation, consider partial avulsion of the nail plate with phenolization.

Note: According to several studies, simple avulsion of a strip of nail or the entire nail plate without phenolization often produces recurrence rates of 60–80%.

Either procedure can be done easily in the office and provides a satisfactory cosmetic result with an acceptable recurrence rate.

Indication

Ingrown toenail, most commonly on the tibial side of the great toe, accompanied by pain and erythema

Relative Contraindications

- Diabetes mellitus
- Peripheral vascular disease
- Bleeding abnormalities
- Pregnancy: The use of phenol is contraindicated during pregnancy because of the possibility of systemic absorption. It has not been established whether the use of injectable lidocaine HCl (Xylocaine HCl) is safe during pregnancy.

Materials

For digital block

- 4–5 mL 1% lidocaine HCl without epinephrine
- 5-mL syringe and 25-gauge, ⅞-in. needle

For cotton wick insertion
- Povidone-iodine (Betadine) or other antiseptic skin cleanser
- Sterile or clean cotton ball
- Blunt splinter forceps
- Surgical scissors
- Tincture of iodine
- Silver nitrate sticks

For partial nail plate avulsion with phenolization
- Large rubber band or small Penrose drain for use as tourniquet
- 6-in. hemostat
- Sterile surgical scissors
- Small straight (mosquito) hemostat
- Sterile cotton swabs
- Silver nitrate sticks
- Phenol (80% or 88%)
- Alcohol swabs
- Alcohol
- Antibiotic ointment
- Nonadherent dressing
- Bandage roll (Tubegauz)

PROCEDURES

For digital nerve block, cotton wick insertion, or partial nail avulsion with phenolization, have the patient supine, with knees and hips flexed to position the foot flat on the examining table.

DIGITAL NERVE BLOCK: You can use digital nerve anesthesia for both treatment methods, although in early cases of ingrown toenail application of the cotton wick may not require anesthesia.

1. Using a 5-mL syringe and 25-gauge, ⅞-in. needle, inject 0.5 mL of lidocaine beneath the skin overlying the proximal phalanx on the extensor surface of the affected side of the great toe (Figure 48-1).
2. Insert the needle to the hub in a plantar direction alongside the proximal phalanx, but do not pierce the plantar skin surface. By placing a finger on the plantar surface, you will be able to feel the approach of the needle and stop in time. As you slowly withdraw the needle, inject approximately 1–2 mL of lidocaine (Figure 48-2).
3. When the needle tip approaches the skin surface, redirect it across the extensor surface of the toe. Then reinsert the needle and inject another 1 mL of lidocaine during withdrawal (see Figure 48-2).
4. Enter the toe dorsally on the opposite side and repeat step 2.
5. Allow at least five minutes for the nerve block to take effect.

COTTON WICK INSERTION: Consider this procedure clean rather than sterile.

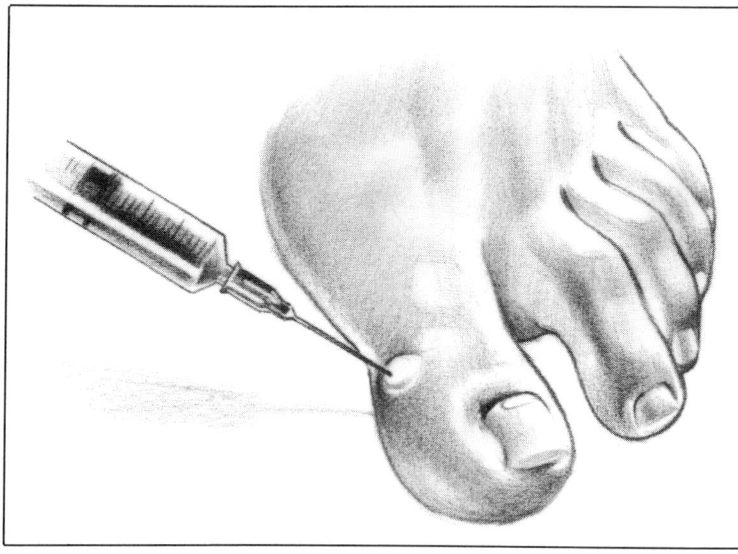

Figure 48-1 Placing the digital nerve block. Inject 0.5 mL of lidocaine HCl beneath the skin overlying the proximal phalanx on the extensor surface of the affected side of the toe.

1. Roll some cotton to a thickness of about 3 mm (⅛ in.) and an initial length of at least 2.5 cm (1 in.).
2. With splinter forceps, push the wick gently into the distal part of the lateral nail groove on the affected side, separating the nail edge from the underlying soft tissue (Figure 48-3). When you can identify the offending corner or spike of nail, remove it with the scissors.

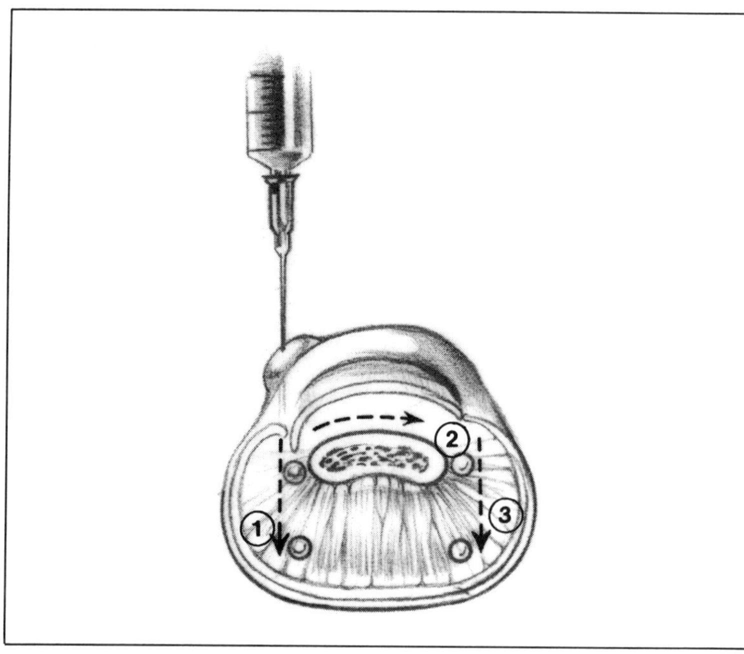

Figure 48-2 Place a finger on the plantar surface of the toe to enable you to detect the approach of the needle tip. As you feel it through the skin surface, stop advancing the needle. Withdraw the needle slowly while injecting more lidocaine. Redirect the needle in the direction of the arrows.

Figure 48-3 Push the wick into the distal portion of the lateral nail groove, separating the nail edge from the underlying tissue.

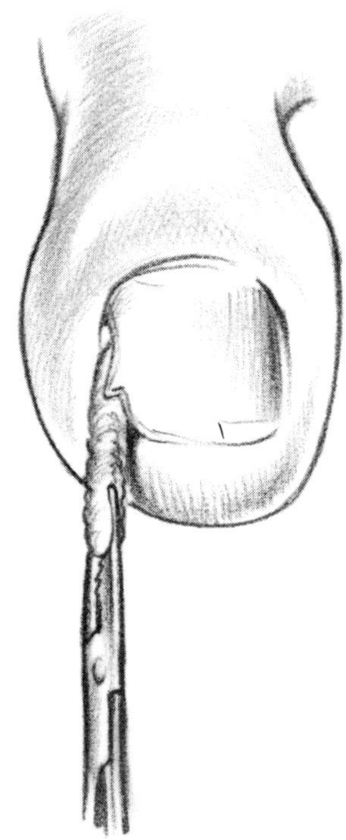

Figure 48-4 Place the small blade of the scissors in the track left by the hemostat and incise the nail to the base.

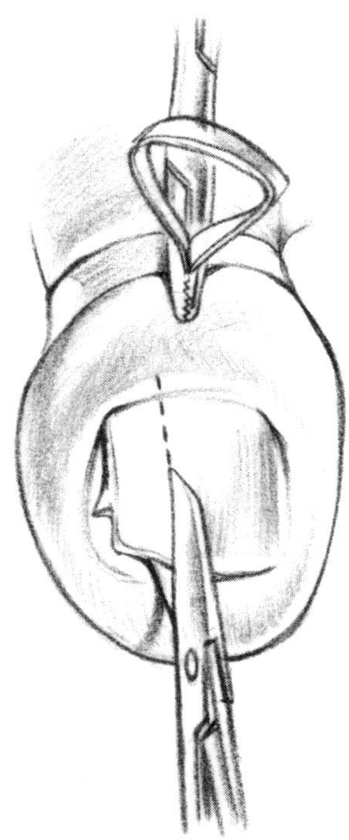

Insert the wick far enough to separate the remaining distal nail from the underlying nail groove. About 1 cm (3⁄8 in.) of the wick should remain free.

3. Apply tincture of iodine to the wick.

4. Cauterize any areas of granulation by firmly pressing a silver nitrate stick onto the tissue.

5. If you use silver nitrate, place an adhesive bandage over the granulation tissue. Instruct the patient to change it daily and to apply tincture of iodine to the wick every other day. Have him or her return weekly for replacement of the wick; at each visit, reevaluate the toe, and apply further silver nitrate if indicated. Anticipate 4–6 treatments.

PARTIAL NAIL PLATE AVULSION WITH PHENOLIZATION

1. Following nerve block, scrub the toe with antiseptic cleanser, rinse, and dry. Drape the foot if desired.

2. Place the tourniquet around the base of the toe, and secure it with the 6-in. hemostat.

3. Near the affected edge of the nail, locate the point at which the nail plate begins to curve in the plantar direction. Open the small (mosquito) hemostat, and fully insert a single blade between the nail plate and the nail bed at the point of curvature. Remove the hemostat.

4. Place the small blade of the surgical scissors in the track just opened by the small hemostat and incise the nail to the base (Figure 48-4).

5. Grasp the length of the nail portion to be removed with the small hemostat and remove it by gentle rotation toward the affected nail fold. Be sure this fragment includes the offending spike or corner of nail (Figure 48-5).

6. With cotton swabs, carefully dry the newly exposed nail bed, especially the proximal region beneath the cuticle at the germinal matrix of the nail. Phenol can effectively ablate the germinal matrix only if the matrix is completely dry.

7. Saturate a clean cotton swab with phenol, place the swab in contact with the germinal matrix beneath the cuticle, and rub. Resaturate the swab as needed to maintain contact for a couple of minutes.

8. Apply phenol to the remainder of the freshly exposed nail bed. Take care to avoid spilling the phenol, and use an alcohol swab to remove immediately any phenol that touches normal skin.

9. Cauterize any areas of granulation by firmly pressing a silver nitrate stick onto the tissue.

10. Remove the tourniquet, and elevate the patient's foot for 15 minutes to aid hemostasis. Apply antibiotic ointment, and place a nonadherent dressing on the wound. Cover this with Tubegauz.

Figure 48-5 Remove the piece by lifting it with a small hemostat and rotating it toward the affected nail fold.

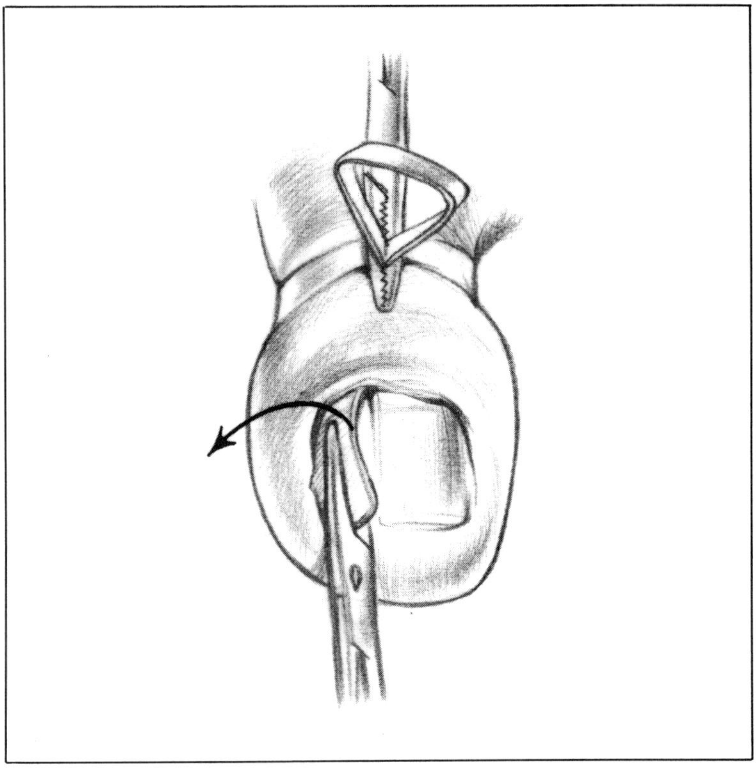

11. Have the patient return in two days so you can remove the dressing and reexamine the toe. At that visit, instruct him to cleanse the toe with soap and water, to redress it daily using a less bulky dressing, and to return in five days for reassessment. The patient can continue to care for the toe at home until healing is complete, applying a dressing during waking hours only. He can wear a shoe when dressing size and comfort allow.

Prevention

Advise the patient to wear shoes with an ample toe box. If the patient is a woman, advise her to avoid high-heeled shoes. When the nonablated nail regrows, the patient should take care to trim it straight across without rounding the corners. Cutting a V-shaped notch in the center of the distal border of the nail (Figure 48-6) may reduce the odds of recurrence.

Suggested Readings

Cameron PF: Ingrowing toenails: An evaluation of two treatments. *Br Med J* 1981;283:821-822.

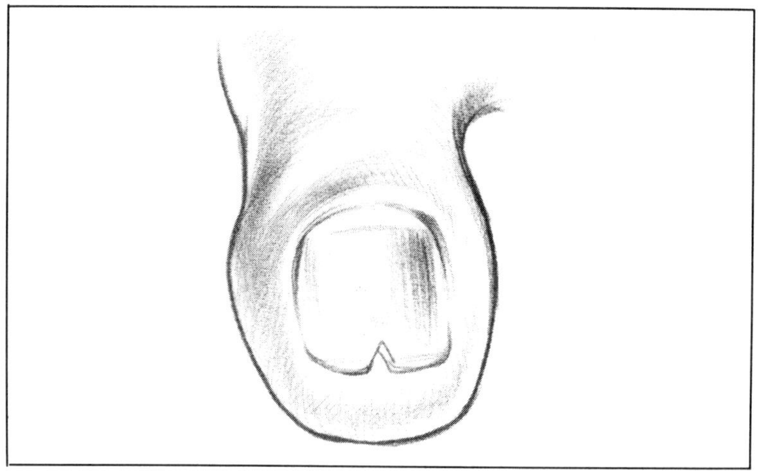

Figure 48-6 Notching the center of the nail with a V may reduce the odds of an ingrown nail recurring.

Fishman H: Practical therapy for ingrown toenails. *Cutis* 1983;32:159-160.

Rinaldi R, Sabia M, Gross J: The treatment and prevention of infection in phenol alcohol matricectomies. *J Am Podiatry Assoc* 1982;72:453-475.

49

Removing a Ring from a Swollen Finger

Charles D. Huss, MD
Robert M. Webster, MD

When you are faced with removing a ring from a swollen finger because of threatened neurovascular compromise and lubrication is not enough, you can reach for a ring cutter; but this approach has the obvious disadvantage of damaging the ring. The wrapping method described here, which preserves the ring, is successful for all but the most grossly swollen fingers. The few failures usually occur in patients who have not removed the ring for years and have bony changes in the finger, such as arthritic malformations. The proximal interphalangeal joint usually has the largest diameter and is the site of most resistance, but you can adapt the method to soft tissue swelling at any level of the digit.

With the method described here, no anesthesia is necessary because the approach physiologically forces the tissue fluids out of the finger instead of causing edema and attendant pain in the distal part of the finger.

Indication

Acute swelling of a finger on which a ring is worn, when this may result in neurovascular compromise of the finger.

Contraindications

None

Material

- Size 4 silk suture or plain cotton twine, preferably on a spool

PROCEDURE

1. Have the patient lying down, elbow on or above the table and finger maximally elevated to reduce any pain and vascular engorgement.

2. Move the ring to its loosest position on the proximal phalanx, usually near the proximal end. Insert the size 4 silk suture or string under the ring, creating an S loop (Figure 49-1).
3. Starting at a point distal to the distal interphalangeal joint, wrap the finger with moderate tension.
4. When you reach the ring, cut the string, leaving about 3 inches free. Insert the free end through the distal loop of the S, and pull this loop under the ring (Figure 49-2). The free end of the wrapping string will come through with the loop and is then ready to pull to unwrap the finger (Figure 49-3). In fact, the ring will frequently slip over the

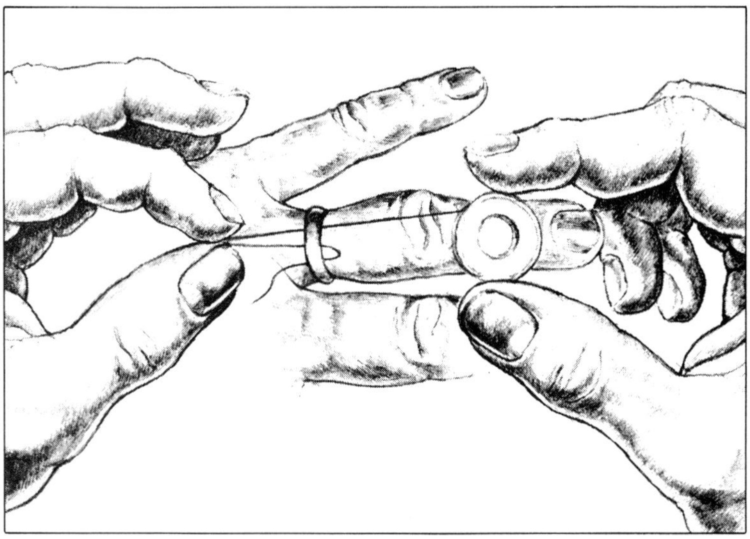

Figure 49-1 Insert string (plain cotton twine is excellent) or size 4 silk suture under the ring, creating an S loop.

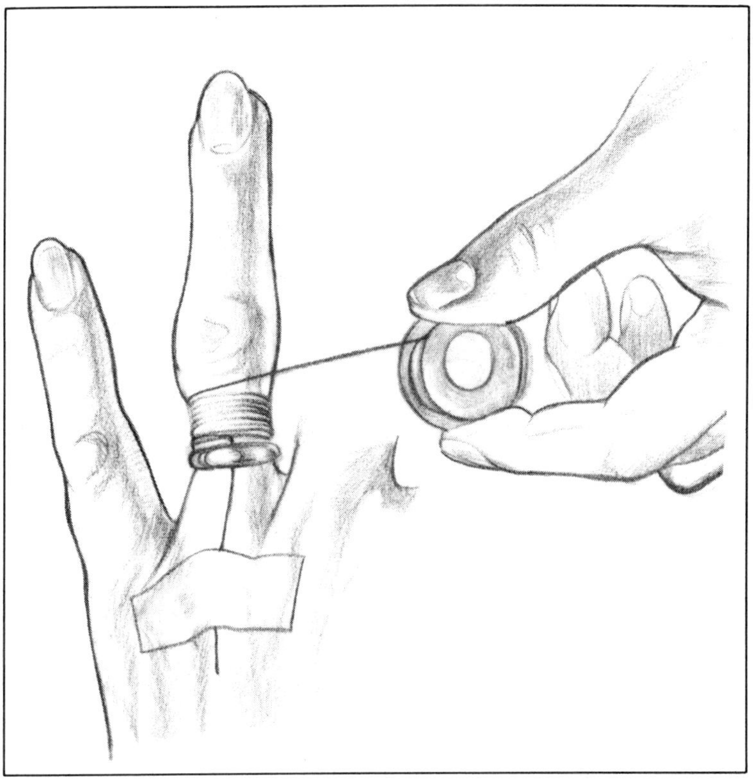

Figure 49-2 Taking the thread directly off the spool, wrap the finger distally starting at the distal edge of the ring to make a smooth single layer.

binding even without unwrapping. If the ring does not move along easily, try coating the wrapping with lubricating jelly.

5. If the finger is severely swollen, a second wrapping may be necessary.

Suggested Readings

Flatt AE: *The Care of Minor Hand Injuries,* ed 4. St. Louis, CV Mosby Co, 1979.

Roberts JR, Hedges JR: *Clinical Procedures in Emergency Medicine.* Philadelphia, WB Saunders Co, 1985.

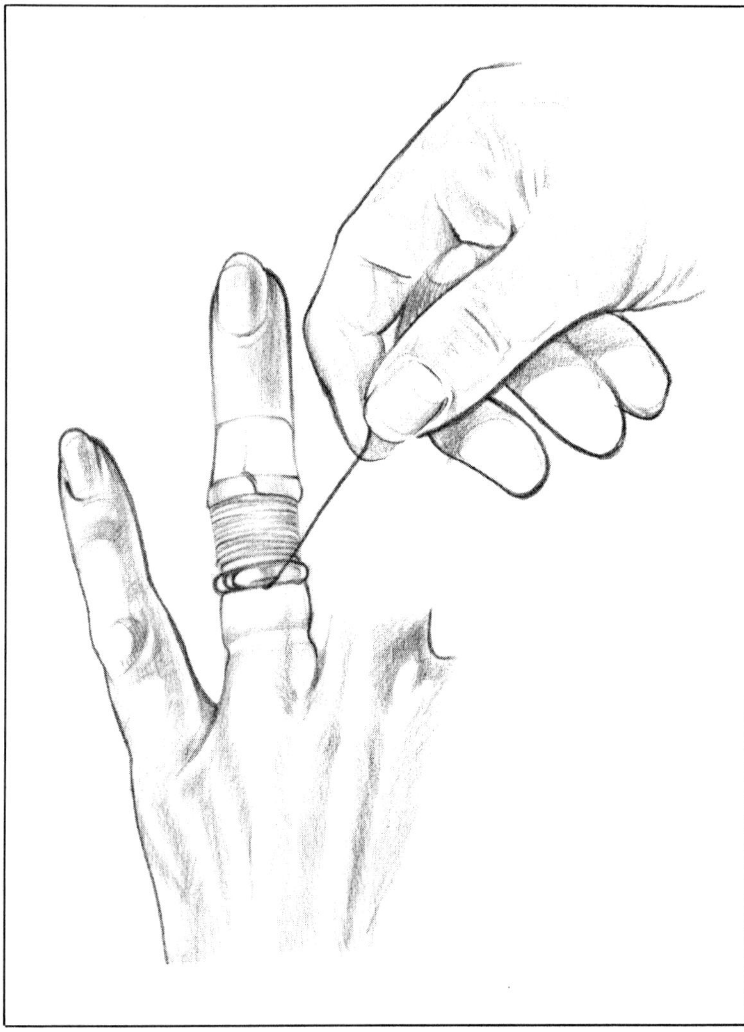

Figure 49-3 When you reach the area of greatest swelling, tape the distal end of the thread to the finger and untape the proximal end. Begin to pull on the proximal end while maintaining tension along the long axis of the finger. As you unwind the thread, keep the ring sliding distally. If the ring is not moving along easily, try coating the layer of thread with some lubricating jelly.

50

Removing Fishhooks

Leslie E. Weber, MD

With rare exceptions, fishhooks embedded in the body can be removed easily and with little pain. While the problem can be urgent, it is seldom an emergency. If the fishhook penetrates the eye, throat, or a joint cavity, refer the patient promptly to a center for appropriate treatment. In almost all other cases, you can remove the hook. The simple string technique is effective in most cases; three alternate techniques can be used in special cases.

Indication

Embedded fishhook

Contraindications

Do not use these techniques if the fishhook penetrates the eye, throat, or a joint cavity.

Note: In eye penetration, you may medicate for pain—or sedate a particularly anxious patient—then apply an eye shield to immobilize the hook, and transfer the patient for appropriate care. Sedation or pain medication may also be necessary for throat and joint penetration before transferring the patient.

Materials

- 36 in. of strong string or twine
- 1% lidocaine HCl (Xylocaine HCl) without epinephrine
- 2-mL syringe with 25-gauge needle
- No. 11 scalpel blade with handle
- Needle holder
- Wire-cutting pliers
- 22-gauge needle

PROCEDURES

The string technique, which is described first, is recommended. Resort to one of the three alternates if the string technique does not work, if more than one barb of a treble hook is embedded, or if the hook is too small or too large for string removal.

1. Stabilize the affected body part, and expose the penetration area.

2. Loop the string or twine at midpoint, over the curve of the shank of the hook near the point of entry.

3. With thumb and index finger of your nondominant hand, stabilize the shank; grasp the eye of the hook so the shank is parallel to the skin surface and the hook is perpendicular.

4. Gently depress the hook by pressure with thumb and finger to disengage the barb. Maintain the hook in this position with gentle downward pressure.

5. Hold the string in your dominant hand, make several turns around the index finger, and apply gentle traction until the string is taut.

6. With a snap of the wrist, jerk the string quickly (Figure 50-1). In most cases this disengages the hook almost painlessly, and analgesia is unnecessary.

ALTERNATE METHOD 1

1. Clean the skin, and inject lidocaine along the shaft of the hook where it enters the skin. Raise a second wheal of lidocaine in the skin overlying the point of the hook (Figure 50-2).

2. With analgesia in effect, make a small incision over the point of the hook with a No. 11 blade.

Figure 50-1

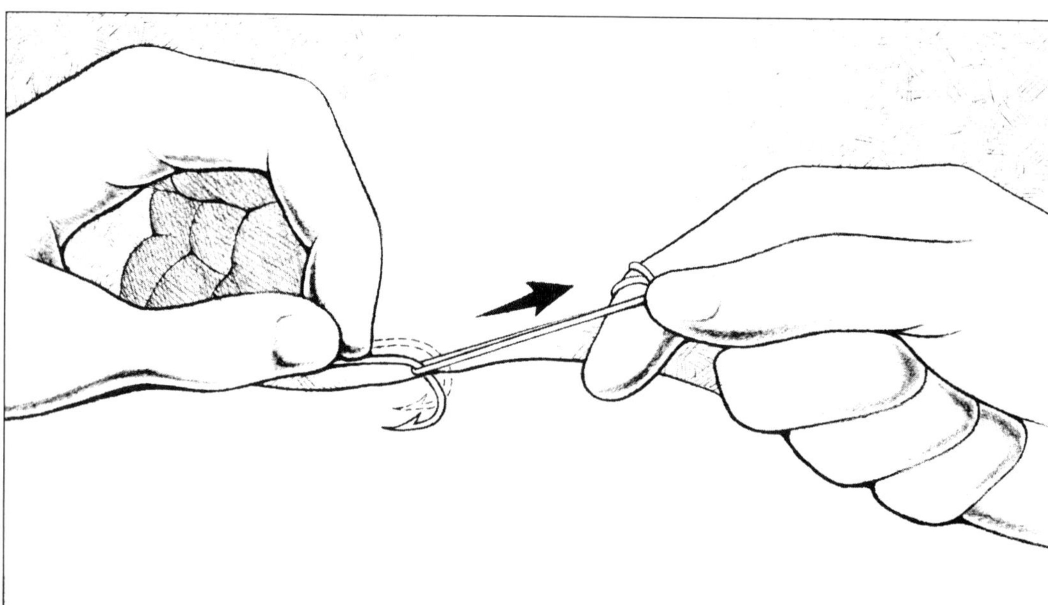

Figure 50-2

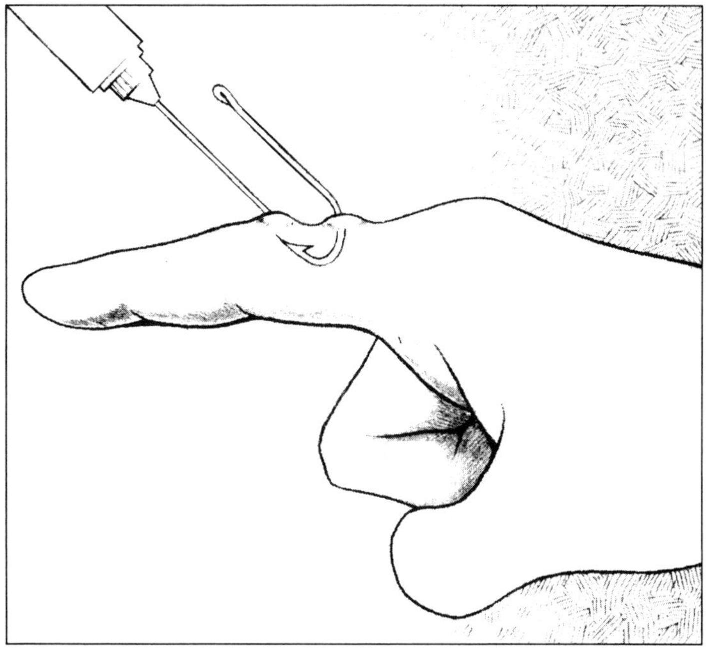

3. Grasp the shank of the hook with a needle holder, and turn the hook to bring the point through the skin incision, exposing the barb (Figure 50-3).

Figure 50-3

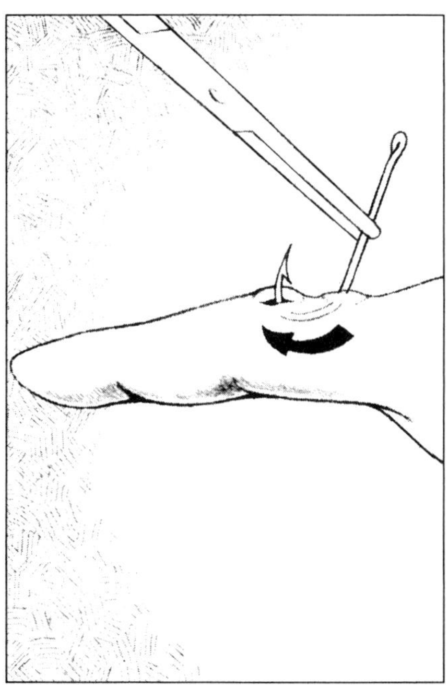

4. With wire-cutting pliers, cut the barb off, and back the hook out of the wound.

ALTERNATE METHOD 2

1. Clean the skin, and inject lidocaine along the track of the hook.
2. Slide the point of a No. 11 blade, cutting surface up, along the side of the hook (Figure 50-4).
3. This enlarges the track, and you can back the hook out with little difficulty.

Note: This technique is useful when the hook is large or when the tissues are hard to immobilize, such as an earlobe.

ALTERNATE METHOD 3

1. Clean the skin, and inject lidocaine as in the preceding method.
2. Insert a 22-gauge needle along the side of the hook, and cap the barb (Figure 50-5).
3. With the barb capped, back the hook out.

Note: This procedure is not as easy as the others because the barb may be turned.

Additional Care

- Tetanus prophylactic treatment is indicated, either toxoid or immune globulin depending on the patient's primary immunization status.
- Antibiotics are rarely needed. If the hook has been embedded for an extended time and you see evidence of acute infection, treatment with penicillin is indicated.

Complications

Secondary infections are a rare complication.

Figure 50-4

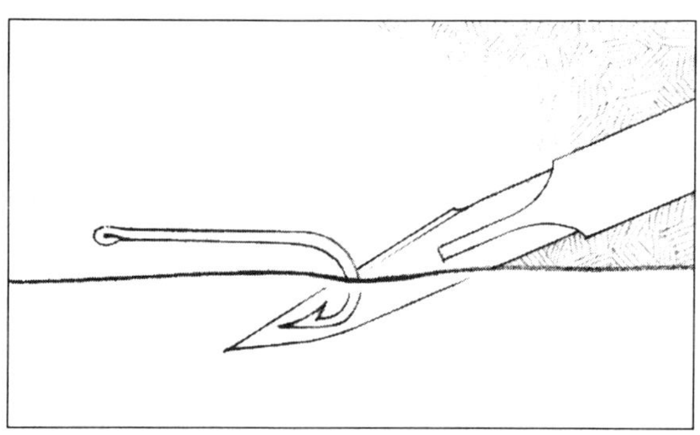

Figure 50-5

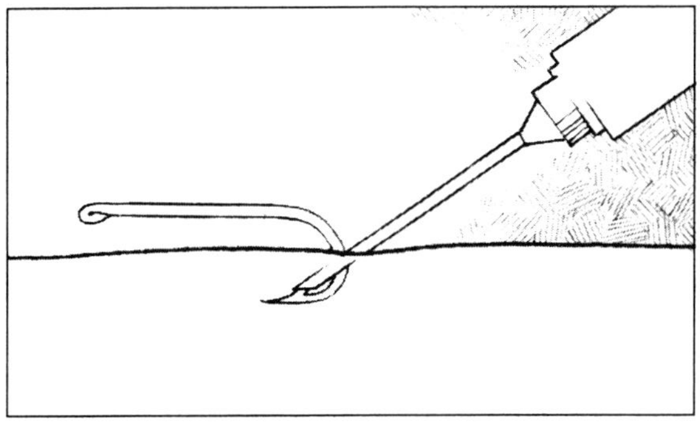

Suggested Readings

Brauer EW, Leider M: How to unhook persons hooked on fishhooks. *J Dermatol Surg Oncol* 1980;6:668-669.

Emerson EB: Fishhooks. *New York State Journal of Medicine* 1966;66:2414-2416.

Hulme J: How to remove fish-hooks. *Nursing Mirror* 1977;145:23.

51

Electrocoagulation

Leslie E. Weber, MD

Up to 15% of primary care patients have skin conditions. While many of them are simple and most are treated medically, some require surgery. Electrocoagulation techniques are particularly well-suited to an office setting since they require minimal preparation and can be performed quickly and safely with little concern for complications. Electrocoagulation is the application of very high frequency, high voltage electrical current in one of two ways. In electrodesiccation, the electrode is applied directly to the lesion and destroys it by dehydration and coagulation (Figure 51-1). Electrofulguration applies an electrical spark to the skin with no actual contact between electrode and lesion, causing superficial carbonization and light electrodesiccation (Figure 51-2). In practice, electrodesiccation is used most often; electrofulguration is used occasionally.

Selecting the Technique

Scalpel excision and punch biopsy are appropriate if you need a lesion specimen for laboratory examination or if the lesion extends into deep dermis and subcutaneous tissues. Other lesions may require wide excision of tissue for adequate treatment. Many small skin lesions in epidermis or superficial dermis can be quickly and easily removed with monoterminal electrocoagulation, however. Electrodesiccation is appropriate treatment for verrucae, xanthelasmas, fibroepithelial tags, cherry angiomas, condylomas, and other superficial lesions. Actinic keratoses and intradermal nevi can be removed by curettage or shaving, followed by electrofulguration for hemostasis. Since these lesions are superficial, you can achieve complete removal with minimal scarring. Pedunculated lesions are easily excised at their bases, with bleeding controlled by electric current.

Basal cell carcinomas confirmed by biopsy can also be treated in the office. Use curettage to remove all malignant issue and electrofulguration for hemostasis.

Contraindications and Cautions

- Do not use electrocoagulation to remove malignant melanomas, squamous cell carcinomas, or congenital giant nevi. The last are

Figure 51-1

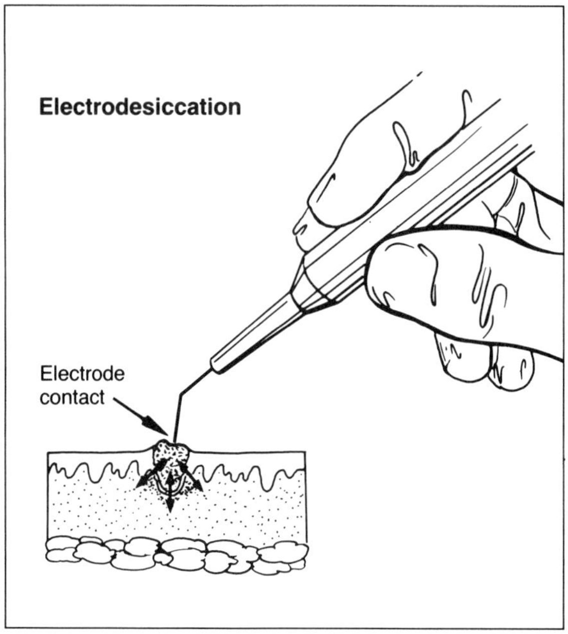

benign but have a predilection for becoming malignant. Compound and junctional nevi and other benign defects extending into the deep dermis are better treated by excision; electrodesiccation may leave undesirable scars.

Figure 51-2

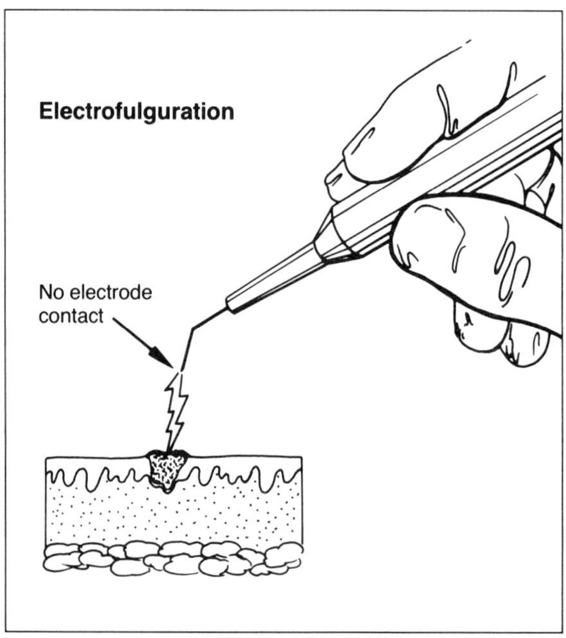

- Do not use electrocoagulation to remove lesions near the nail fold as it might damage the nail root and possibly cause abnormal nail growth.
- Be sure that alcohol or other flammable material used to prepare the skin has dried thoroughly before starting the procedure because electric current can ignite these materials.
- Generally, you do not need a ground with monoterminal electrocoagulation, but maintain contact with the patient, keeping your hand firmly on a hair-free skin surface during treatment, to assure that neither you nor the patient receives an electric shock.
- Do not turn the control to high when you use electrofulguration for hemostasis. Although brisk bleeding may tempt you to do this, avoid it because it can cause excessive tissue damage.

The Electrocoagulation Unit

Several small, portable electrocoagulation units are available, and the techniques described here are equally applicable to any of them.[1]

The Hyfrecator,[2] which is used for this discussion, weighs about 5 lb and may be mounted on a wall or on a small stand and moved from room to room. A 0-100 dial on the face panel variably controls the power delivered to the electrode, and two jack receptacles on the panel deliver low- and high-range levels of power. A cord with handle into which you insert the electrode can be plugged into the low- or high-range receptacle as desired. Several electrodes are available for specific purposes. You may choose short or long, straight or angled, and extremely fine tips for epilation or broad thick tips for coagulating bleeding vessels. The unit is controlled by an on-off foot switch.

Materials

- Electrocoagulation unit
- 1% lidocaine HCl (Xylocaine HCl) with or without epinephrine
- Marking pen
- 3-mL syringe
- 30-gauge ½-in. needle
- No. 3 oval curet
- Sterile gauze
- 35% aluminum chloride in 50% alcohol (styptic solution)
- Cotton-tipped applicators
- No. 10 or No. 15 scalpel blade and handle or thin double-edge razor blade

---

[1]Widely used electrosurgical machines include Bovie (several models), the Burton Electricator, and the Hyfrecator.

[2]Manufactured by Birtcher Corporation, El Monte, Calif.

PROCEDURE

1. Minimal skin preparation is required. Briefly prepare the skin and anesthetize with 0.5–1.0 mL lidocaine HCl injected immediately under the lesion. For some small superficial lesions, anesthesia may not be needed with a low instrument setting; let the patient decide. If the lesion is not pigmented, you may color it with a marking pen since infiltration may obscure the borders. If the lesion is fairly large, a field block may be indicated (Figure 51-3). Be sure to wait until anesthesia is effective.

2. Use a fine electrode for most lesions. Start with the unit dial at a low setting—20 or less—and the cord plugged into the low-range jack receptacle. Place the needle on the center of the lesion, nearly perpendicular to the skin. Place your hand firmly on the patient to establish a ground.

3. To lessen the risk of injuring normal tissue, momentarily depress the foot switch, and note the amount of current being delivered. Evaluate tissue destruction, and adjust the setting until the desired amount of power is being delivered. This may involve plugging the cord into the high-level jack receptacle. Experience will help you select the appropriate setting.

4. Turn the current on and off in short bursts. Holding the needle in contact with skin too long will cause a noticeable heat buildup, and this is uncomfortable for the patient. Treat small lesions by coagulating in a widening circle (Figure 51-4a). If the lesion is large and elevated, such as a verruca, needle the base of the lesion at its margins around its circumference.

Figure 51-3

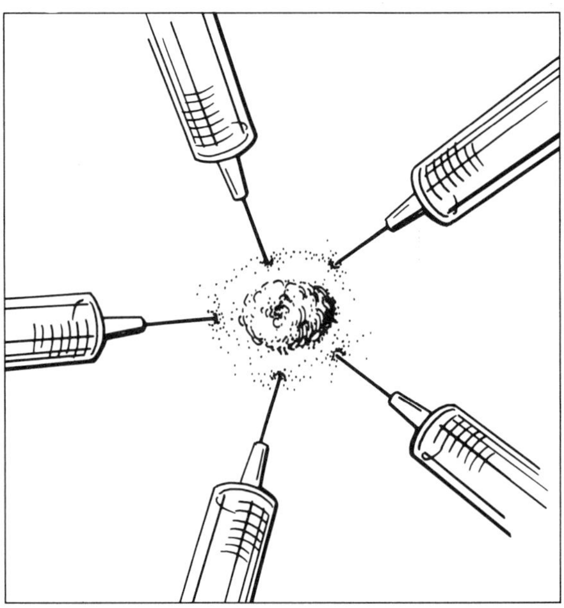

Figure 51-4

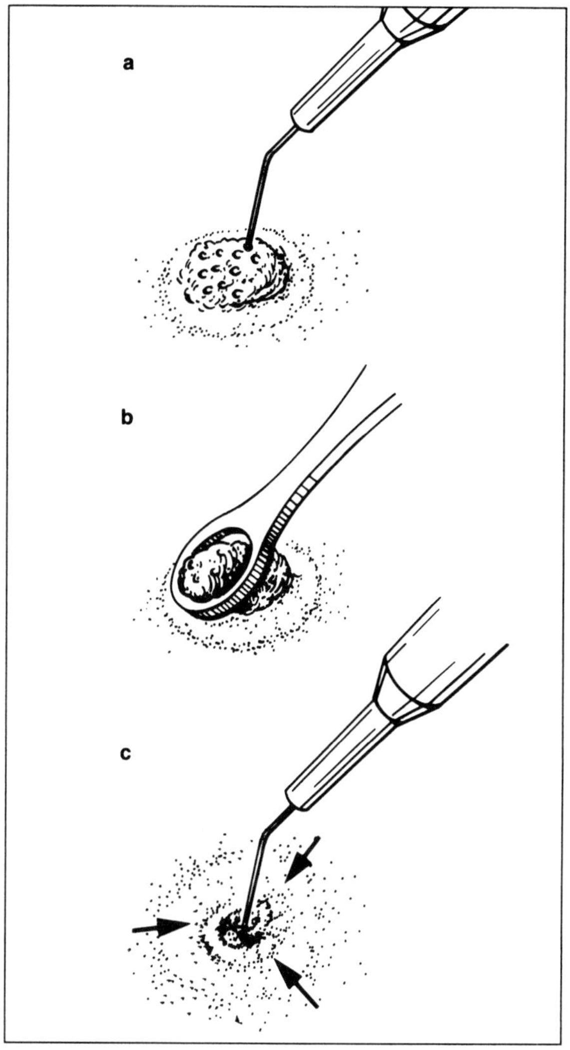

5. As the heat separates epidermis from dermis, use a curet or gauze to separate the lesion from its base with a slight downward pressure (Figure 51-4b).

6. After you expose the base, you may curet away the underlying abnormal tissue and repeat as necessary. Touch bleeding points lightly with the needle to stop blood flow (Figure 51-4c). You may also apply a styptic solution with a cotton-tipped applicator.

7. For basal cell carcinomas, you may use electric current to control bleeding. First, curet until abnormal tissue is no longer seen, then use electrofulguration. Try to control bleeding with pressure for a moment, then apply short bursts of spark at a lower setting. Blot quickly before each burst, and move over the surface until bleeding has stopped.

Figure 51-5

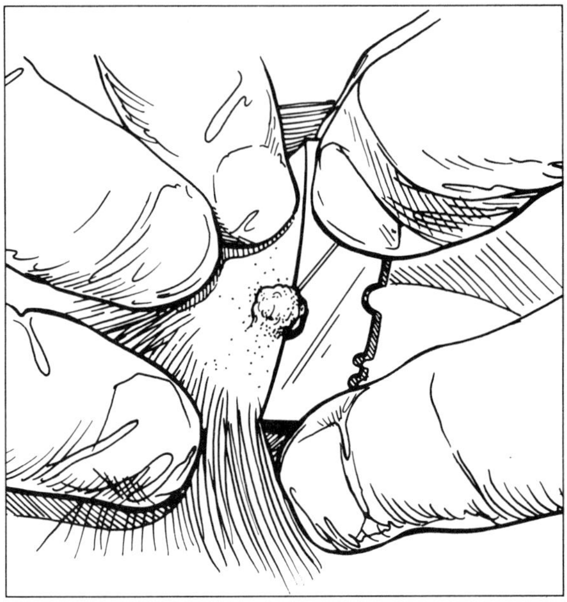

8. Benign skin lesions are easily removed by shaving. With scalpel or razor blade, excise the lesion tangentially at or slightly below skin level (Figure 51-5). Use electrofulguration if needed to control bleeding at the base of the lesion.

Note: Experience will help you judge the depth of destruction. As depth increases, bleeding will increase. After you remove a surface crust, you will note a slight depression in the skin. It is important not to destroy too much tissue under the lesion.

Follow-up Care

Electrocoagulated lesions do not usually require a dressing although some patients may want a small covering for aesthetic reasons or for protection if the lesion is located where irritation may occur. This can usually be removed in several hours. The treated area may look charred. Reassure the patient that this is not abnormal and that the discoloration will disappear over the next several days. Large lesions, especially verrucae, should be examined in 1–2 weeks to assess healing and the need for further treatment.

Complications

- Complications are few and minimal. If a lesion is inadequately electrofulgurated, bleeding may occur later.
- The base of large lesions may look ulcerated, but this usually heals without problems over a period of days to weeks.
- Deeper-than-usual lesions treated overenthusiastically might show excess scarring. Try to eliminate this possibility by screening carefully beforehand to select such lesions for scalpel excision.

Note: The electric currents used in these procedures are localized and present no danger to those who wear cardiac pacemakers.

Suggested Readings

Pearce JA: *Electrosurgery.* New York, John Wiley & Sons, Inc, 1986.

Schultz BC, McKinney P: *Office Practice of Skin Surgery.* Philadelphia, WB Saunders Company, 1985.

Sebben JE: *Cutaneous Electrosurgery.* Chicago, Year Book Medical Pubs, Inc, 1988.

52

Wood's Light Examination

Nancy L. Cwach, MD
Charles E. Driscoll, MD

Wood's light (black light) is valuable in clinical practice because fluorescence emitted from components of hair, skin, and urine may provide early clues and sometimes be diagnostic (Table 52-1). It is especially helpful in diagnosing microbial diseases and pigmentary disorders and is also used in photopatch testing and treatment of such diseases as alopecia areata and palmar psoriasis.

A Wood's light produces an invisible long-wave UV radiation from a mercury vapor source. The essential component is the Wood's filter (a nickel-chromium oxide silica glass filter) that transmits radiation only in the band between 320 and 420 nm. Porphyrins produce fluorescence that becomes visible when light rays of about 365 nm (3,650 Angstrom units) strike the affected area.

Recommended Applications

FUNGAL INFECTIONS

- Wood's light examination helps detect certain varieties of dermatophytosis of the hair shaft and may help distinguish tinea capitis from other inflammatory alopecias of the scalp. Hairs infected with anthropophilic *Microsporum audouinii* and zoophilic *Microsporum canis* fluoresce with a bright yellow-green color since both produce the chemical pteridine when the fungus invades the hair. It is the hair, not the scale or skin, that fluoresces in a dermatophyte infection. Of the *Trichophyton* genus, *T. tonsurans* and *T. verrucosum* do not fluoresce; and the rare *T. schoenleinii* produces a pale green fluorescence of the hair. Generally, tinea infections caused by fungi from animal or human sources fluoresce whereas those acquired from soil do not.
- Tinea versicolor, caused by a lipophilic yeast organism, is the only fungal infection of the skin that is fluorescent. Actively infected areas fluoresce golden yellow or coppery-orange and are often more extensive than visual examination suggests. The budding

TABLE 52-1

Dermatologic guide to Wood's light examination

Condition	Fluorescent color
Erythrasma	Coral-red or pink*
Pigmentary alterations	
Albinism	Cold, bright white
Depigmentation	Cold, bright white; blue-white
Hyperpigmentation	Purple-brown
Hypopigmentation	Pale white
Leprosy	Blue-white
Tuberous sclerosis	Ash-leaf-shaped spot
Vitiligo	Cold, bright white; blue-white
Porphyria cutanea tarda (urine)	Pink to pink-orange
Pseudomonas aeruginosa infections	Aqua-green to blue (rarely yellow-green)
Tinea capitis	
Microsporum audouinii	Bright yellow-green
Microsporum canis	Bright yellow-green
Trichophyton schoenleinii	Pale green
Tinea versicolor	Golden yellow

*Patients who bathe shortly before Wood's light examination may show little or no fluorescence.

Adapted with permission from Eaglstein WH, Pariser DM: *Office Techniques for Diagnosing Skin Disease.* Chicago, Year Book Medical Publishers, Inc, 1978.

forms of yeast are found down in the hair follicle, which makes diagnosis with potassium hydroxide (KOH) more difficult. Affected skin may be darker or lighter than surrounding areas; relative depigmentation occurs because the infected skin does not tan in sunlight. A Wood's light examination will distinguish this condition from depigmented skin lesions such as vitiligo.

BACTERIAL INFECTIONS

- Erythrasma, a superficial skin infection caused by the gram-positive bacillus *Corynebacterium minutissimum,* frequently occurs as irregular pale brown patches with minimal scale in the intertriginous areas and interdigital spaces. It may be confused with tinea cruris and tinea pedis with which it may coexist. Erythrasma can be differentiated from a tinea infection by the brilliant coral-red fluorescence from the porphyrins produced by *C. minutis-*

simum. The water-soluble porphyrins may not be present if the area has been washed recently. Erythrasma is easily treated with erythromycin; without treatment, the infection tends to persist indefinitely.

- *Pseudomonas aeruginosa* infections form fluorescein, which fluoresces blue-green to blue and is detectable before obvious signs of infection. The Wood's light is used to screen patients for pseudomonal infections in burn centers before the infection can be detected by cultures or visual inspection. Bluish fluorescence may be found in otitis externa, intertrigo pedis, or secondary pseudomonal infection of the scrotum.

PORPHYRIA The most common porphyria with cutaneous manifestations is porphyria cutanea tarda. The urine of someone with this disease will fluoresce pinkish-red to orange-red under Wood's light, which makes a presumptive diagnosis. The color will intensify with the addition of dilute hydrochloric acid (add 1.0 mL of 5.0% hydrochloric acid to urine).

PIGMENTARY ALTERATIONS

- Wood's light accentuates pigment in the epidermis, increasing the contrast between normal and hyperpigmented skin, but it does not enhance pigment in the dermis. Wood's light examination thus helps distinguish epidermal from dermal melanin hyperpigmentation by defining the extent and level of pigmentary change. For example, circumscribed hypermelanosis such as freckles or melasma (chloasma) will be more apparent and look purple-brown under Wood's light; dermal melanin such as a mongolian sacral spot and some instances of postinflammatory hyperpigmentation look relatively unchanged under Wood's light compared with ambient light.
- Wood's light helps to estimate lightness of lesions compared with normal skin color in both fair-skinned and dark-skinned persons. It can distinguish hypomelanoses as in tuberous sclerosis, tinea versicolor, pityriasis alba, and postinflammatory hypopigmentation from totally amelanotic or depigmented areas as in vitiligo, albinism, or piebaldism. Hypomelanotic regions appear pale white with decreased intensity, and previously unnoticed lesions may become apparent under Wood's light. Amelanotic areas have a true white to blue-white fluorescence. The greater the pigment loss, the more intense the whiteness under the light.
- Wood's light is a useful screen in nurseries for tuberous sclerosis. Small, ash-leaf-shaped, white macules 2–3 cm long, are present at birth and are the first manifestation of this autosomal dominant condition with serious CNS effects and other organ involvement.

DRUG DETECTION The teeth of people who took tetracycline in childhood while the deciduous teeth were forming will fluoresce yellow. The skin of patients applying topical tetracycline will also fluoresce, as will nails and bones of adults taking the antibiotic.

SCABIES In the diagnosis of scabies, it may be difficult to find the burrow or mite. Topical tetracycline painted on the area, allowed to dry for three minutes, then washed and dried will point up the burrows under Wood's light.

Materials

Essential

- A Wood's light (traditionally, a medium-pressure mercury vapor light with a nickel-chromium oxide silica glass filter). Newer models are low-pressure, UVA-emitting fluorescent lights with a UVA-transmitting, visible-light-absorbing glass envelope; they are smaller than traditional lights.

Optional

- Glass microscope slides with cover slips
- No. 10 and No. 15 scalpel blades
- 10–20% KOH solution
- Sterile scissors
- Sterile collection tube
- Suitable fungal culture such as Sabouraud's or Mycosel media or dermatophyte test medium (DTM)

PROCEDURE

1. Instruct the patient to avoid bathing or shampooing for 24 hours before the examination because porphyrins wash off with soap and water.
2. Let the Wood's light warm up for several minutes for maximum intensity, seat the patient, turn off the room lights, and wait for your eyes to adjust to the darkness.
3. Hold the Wood's light 4–5 inches from the area you are examining, and avoid shining the light directly at the cornea if using the short-wavelength lamp.
4. If necessary, confirm a clinical diagnosis by sending specimens of skin or hair for microscopic examination and culture. Scrape the skin lightly with a scalpel blade to collect superficial cells and scale on a glass slide. Cover with a coverslip, and analyze with KOH solution, or send it to the laboratory for culture. For hair, clip with scissors, place in a sterile vial, and send to the laboratory.

Sources of Error

- Not all cases of tinea capitis fluoresce since not all species produce porphyrins. Thus a negative Wood's light examination does not rule out tinea capitis.

- Washing before the examination may cause false-negative results.
- *Microsporum* infection of glabrous skin does not fluoresce. It is the infected hair, not the skin, that fluoresces.
- Do not confuse the bright fluorescence of fungus-infected hairs with the white, dull yellow, or purplish fluorescence that comes from such sources as lint particles, sulfur-laden scales, serum exudate, or ointments containing petrolatum. In addition, deodorants, soaps, makeups, and tetracycline in sweat may fluoresce blue or purple.
- Watch for errors from an insufficiently darkened room or inadequate light source.
- Keep in mind that distinction between epidermal and dermal pigmentation with the Wood's light is more useful for lighter skinned persons (skin types 1 to 4) than for brown- or black-skinned persons (skin types 5 and 6).

Suggested Readings

Eaglstein WH, Pariser DM: *Office Techniques for Diagnosing Skin Disease.* Chicago, Year Book Medical Pubs, Inc, 1978.

Fitzpatrick TB, Freedberg IM: *Dermatology in General Medicine*, ed 3. New York, McGraw-Hill Bk Co, 1987.

Flowers FP, Krusinski PA: *Dermatology in Ambulatory and Emergency Medicine.* Chicago, Year Book Medical Pubs, Inc, 1984.

Habif T: *Clinical Dermatology: A Color Guide to Diagnosis and Therapy*. St. Louis, CV Mosby Co, 1985.

Hurvitz S: *Clinical Pediatric Dermatology*. Philadelphia, WB Saunders Co, 1981.

Moschella SL, Hurley HJ: *Dermatology*, ed 2. Philadelphia, WB Saunders Co, 1985.

Murtagh J: Wood's light examination. *Aust Fam Physician* 1985;14:525.

VIII

EAR, NOSE, THROAT PROCEDURES

53

Laryngoscopy

Charles E. Driscoll, MD

You can make laryngoscopy work for you routinely. All you need are the right tools, the right technique, and practice.

Visual examination of the nasopharynx, especially the larynx, is both universally recommended and almost universally ignored in primary care practice. One reason physicians tend to avoid the procedure is that the traditional method, using headlamp and angled visualizing mirrors, is difficult to learn. Two relatively new techniques—indirect viewing with a laryngeal telescope and direct viewing with a flexible fiberoptic nasopharyngolaryngoscope—enable you to view the larynx more easily in children as well as adults.

Most primary care physicians who try the fiberoptic instrument find they succeed in viewing the larynx on the first try in 9 out of 10 patients, even in uncooperative children or semicomatose patients. Primary care physicians usually have best results with the flexible fiberoptic scope, next best with the laryngeal telescope, and worst with mirrors. Cost may influence your choice of technique: A flexible nasopharyngolaryngoscope can cost more than $3,500–6,900, while a laryngeal telescope may cost $500, and the cost of laryngeal mirrors is negligible by comparison. If you can become skillful in any of the methods by using it routinely, you'll not only gain obvious advantages in examining symptomatic patients, but also be more able to spot the early lesions or other pathology present in 10–15% of asymptomatic patients.

Indications

- Routine use in physical examinations
- Persistent hoarseness
- Pain in the throat or neck with stridor
- Recurrent pneumonia, bronchitis, or sinusitis
- Dysphagia
- A foreign body in the throat
- Persistent nasal drainage
- Unilateral serous otitis media
- Cervical lymphadenopathy
- Earache with normal examination results

PROCEDURE

USING THE FLEXIBLE NASOPHARYNGOLARYNGOSCOPE

Materials

- Comfortable chair for the patient and stool for the physician
- 5% cocaine solution or tetracaine HCl (Pontocaine) and an adrenalin solution
- Flexible fiberoptic nasopharyngolaryngoscope with light source (Figure 53-1)

1. Direct your viewing during laryngoscopy by means of the landmarks of the nasal chamber and nasopharynx (Figure 53-2).
2. Anesthetize and decongest the patient's nose by spraying with 5% cocaine solution or tetracaine in an atomizer or by inserting cotton-tipped applicators soaked in either of these anesthetics, gradually advancing them to the rear of the nasal cavity. Have adrenalin ready in case a rare allergic reaction to the solution occurs. Alternatively, one may use 0.5–1.0% neosinephrine and 4% lidocaine topical spray in a dose less than 4.5 mg/kg (in general, less than 300 mg) if the patient has cocaine allergy.
3. Have the patient breathe through his or her mouth. Introduce the scope through a naris, and slide it along the floor of the nose.

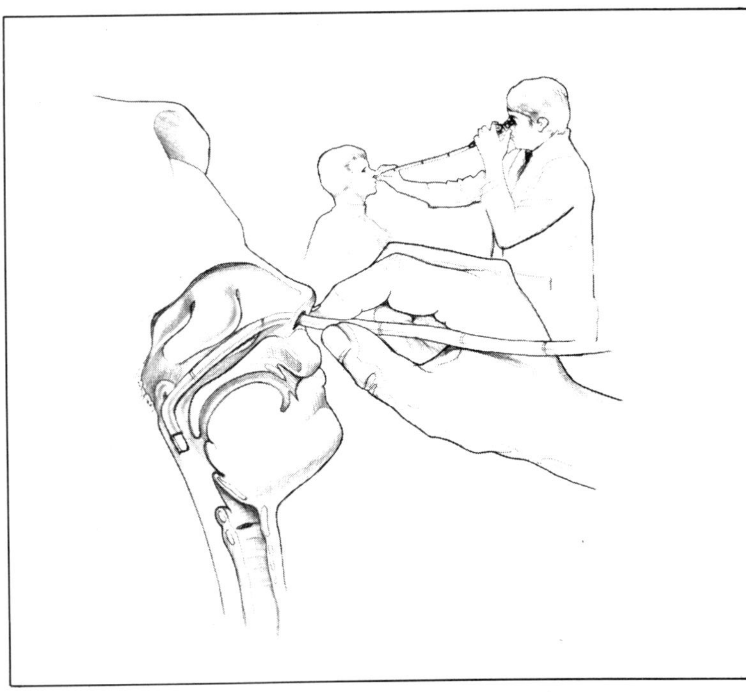

Figure 53-1 Flexible fiberoptic nasopharyngolaryngoscope.

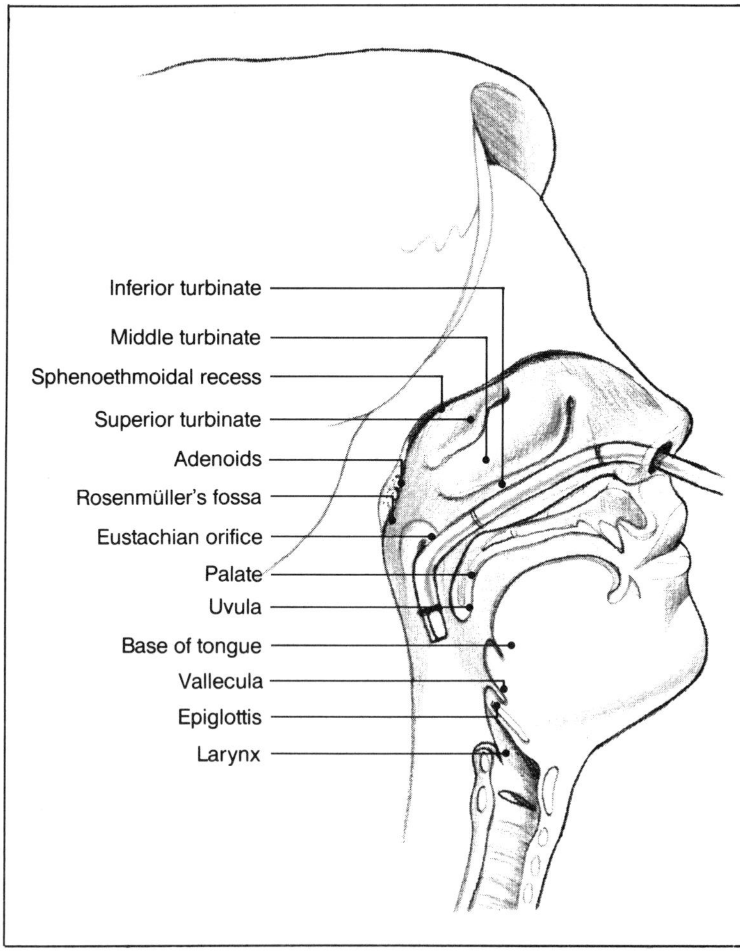

Figure 53-2 As you advance the scope through the nose, check the accuracy of your progress by looking for these landmarks.

When you reach the end of the septum, note the ipsilateral eustachian tube orifice (Figure 53-3).

4. Rotate the instrument 90 degrees, and angle the tip of the tube to inspect the contralateral eustachian tube orifice.

5. Rotate the scope back to its upright position, and have the patient breathe through his nose. This causes the soft palate to fall away from the posterior pharyngeal wall. Angle the scope 90 degrees downward to view the larynx (Figure 53-4), and advance the scope to the epiglottis, exercising care not to transcend the glottis. If mucus accumulation occludes the lens, have the patient swallow, sniff, or blow air through his nose.

6. At this position, being careful to avoid the vocal cords with the scope, take time to visualize the larynx. Have the patient phonate so you can view the laryngeal mechanism in action (see Figures 53-5, 53-6, and 53-7). The procedure is comfortable for the patient, and the

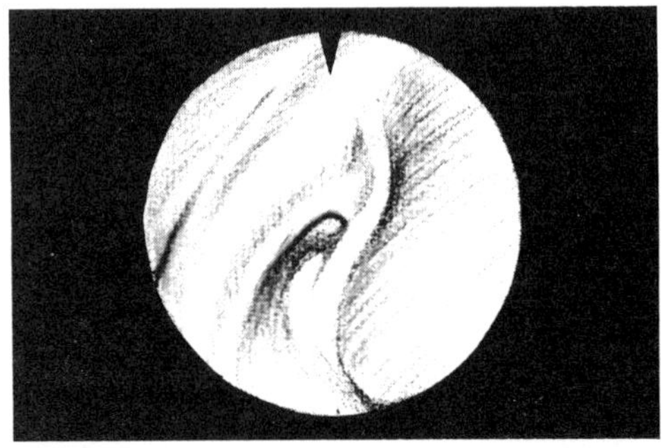

Figure 53-3 Appearance of the ipsilateral eustachian tube orifice at the end of the septum.

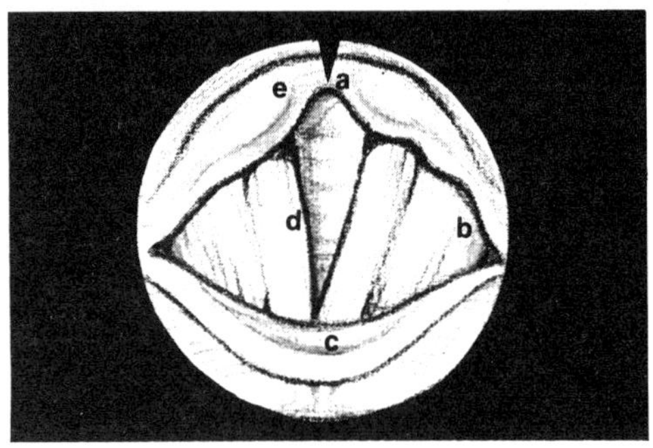

Figure 53-4 Appearance of the larynx. a) Interarytenoid fold, b) vestibular fold, c) epiglottis, d) vocal cord, e) cuneiform tubercle.

scope is narrow enough not to occlude the airway. You will be able to view the larynx clearly in almost every attempt.

Caution: Avoid transcending the larynx, which causes laryngospasm.

USING THE LARYNGEAL TELESCOPE

Materials

- Comfortable chair for the patient and stool for the physician
- Laryngeal telescope (Figure 53-8)
- Thumb guide for steadying the advancing scope (optional)
- 4 × 4-in. gauze pads for grasping the tongue
- Benzocaine spray (Hurricaine) (optional)

1. Grasp the patient's extended tongue with a gauze pad. If he needs distraction, have him hold his own tongue. Gagging is not common with this procedure so you seldom need anesthesia; for some patients, however, you may find benzocaine spray helpful.

Note: If you do spray with benzocaine or other topical anesthetic, tell the patient to eat nothing for the next two hours; the anesthetic prevents him from feeling heat or cold on the palate and also inhibits the gag reflex.

2. Insert the scope transorally and watch the insertion directly until the tip enters the throat. Then—and only then—look through the

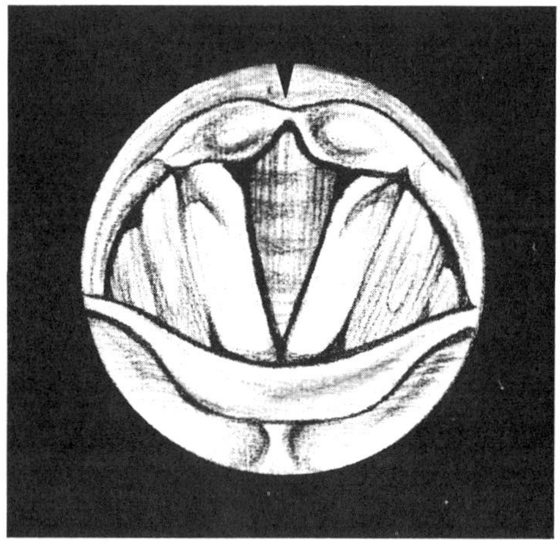

Figure 53-5 Appearance of larynx at rest.

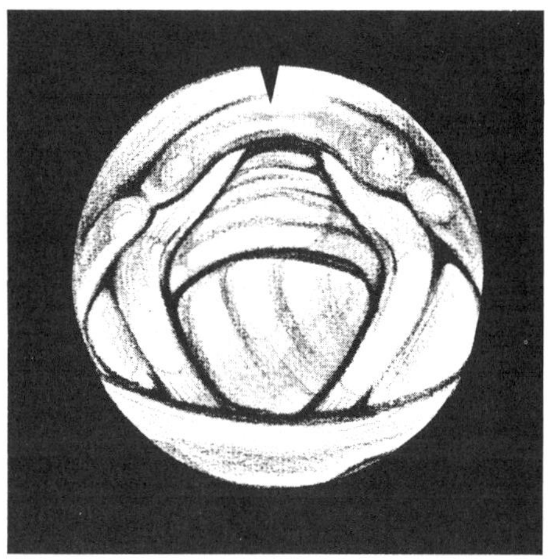

Figure 53-6 Appearance of larynx while patient is inhaling.

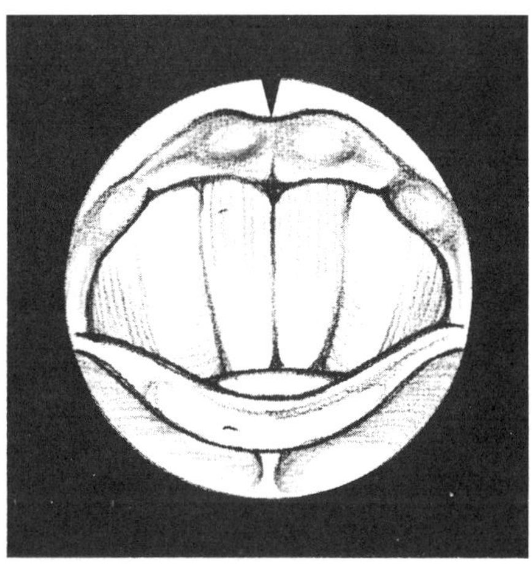

Figure 53-7 Appearance of larynx while patient is phonating.

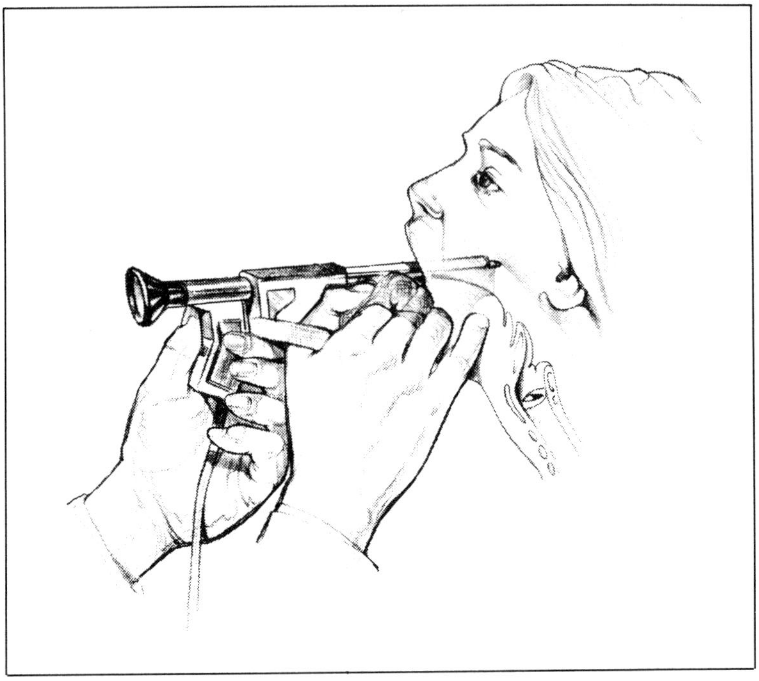

Figure 53-8 Laryngeal telescope.

eyepiece. Direct visualization of the insertion helps you avoid striking the uvula, the posterior pharyngeal wall, or the back of the tongue, all of which can cause gagging.

3. With the scope in place, ask the patient to pant like a puppy. This opens the airway for better visualization.

4. To view the nasopharynx, rotate the scope 180 degrees. Do your viewing quickly and repeat the process if necessary; patients undergoing this procedure tire quickly.

USING MIRRORS

Materials

- Comfortable chair with high back for the patient and movable stool for the physician
- 4 × 4-in. gauze pads for grasping the tongue
- Tongue blades for depressing the tongue
- Long-angled laryngeal mirror (Figure 53-9) and smaller pharyngeal mirror
- Headlamp or head mirror with illumination from behind the patient
- Benzocaine spray (Hurricaine)

1. Try the procedure without anesthesia, but don't hesitate to spray the nasopharynx with benzocaine if gagging is a problem. Sometimes having the patient supine prevents gagging.

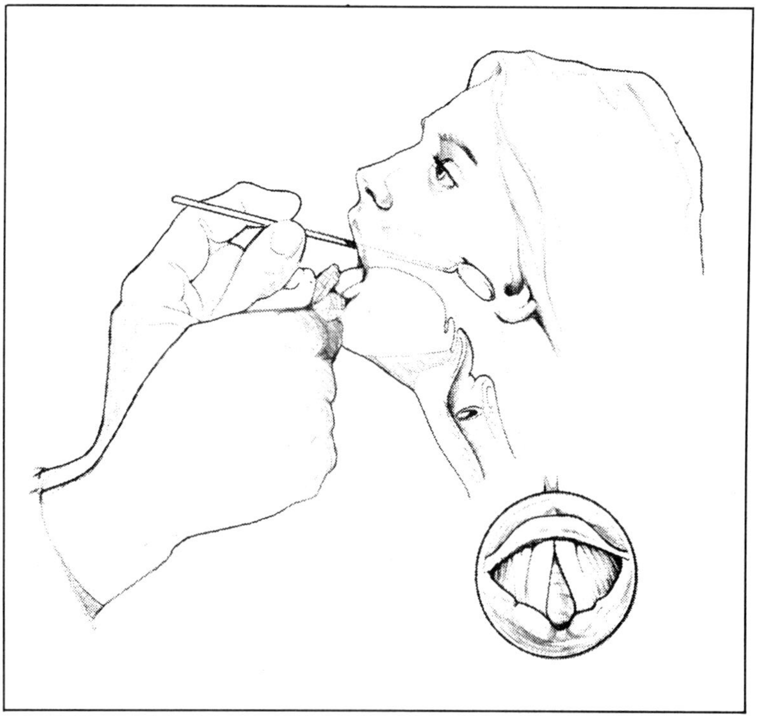

Figure 53-9 Positioning of long-angled laryngeal mirror. Insert illustrates the approximate area of visualization.

2. Use a gauze pad to grasp the patient's extended tongue. Protect the tongue from front-teeth laceration by positioning the middle finger of the hand grasping the tongue between the teeth and tongue and pulling the tongue forward.
3. Keep the tongue extended as you insert the angled mirror. If the patient begins to gag as you advance the mirror, tell him to pant like a puppy; this drops the tongue base down and elevates the uvula—also providing easier passage for the mirror to the back of the throat. Remember to lift the uvula rather than push it back.
4. With the angled mirror in position, have the patient phonate a high pitched E to relax the glottis, improve visualization of the larynx, and demonstrate movement of the cords.
5. Take a brief look, and return once or twice more if necessary, allowing the patient to rest between examinations. Many patients tire quickly during this procedure.
6. To examine the nasopharynx, use a tongue depressor to keep the tongue against the floor of the mouth. Asking the patient to breathe through his nose, insert the small pharyngeal mirror, angling it to reflect the nasopharynx. Thorough examination of the area with this technique requires considerable practice.

Note: If your mirror fogs, wipe it with hexachlorophene (pHiso-Hex) or hold it over a light bulb for heat. If you warm the mirror, test it on your cheek before reintroducing it to avoid burning the patient.

Suggested Readings

Grossan M: Indirect laryngoscopy and nasopharyngoscopy. *Ear Nose Throat J* 1978;57:430-433.

Klein HC: Why can't physicians examine the larynx? *JAMA* 1982;247:2111.

Silberman HD: Advances in the optical examination of the upper airway. *Otolaryngol Clin North Am* 1978;11:355-363.

Silberman HD: The use of the flexible nasopharyngolaryngoscope in the pediatric upper airway. *Otolaryngol Clin North Am* 1978;11:365-370.

Vanderstock L, Vermeersch H: A new flexible fiberoptic nasopharyngolaryngoscope. *Endoscopy* 1981;13:243-245.

54

Removing Impacted Cerumen from the Ear

Elizabeth A. Burns, MD
Bev L. True, PharmD

Earwax impacted in the external meatus hinders the thorough examination of the auditory canal, particularly in children. In as many as 30% of all children with signs and symptoms of acute otitis media (AOM), cerumen removal was required before the physician could make an accurate diagnosis. It is incorrect to assume that the heat generated by the middle ear infection will melt or loosen the earwax. Cerumenosis and AOM can and do coexist.

Keep in mind that the procedure usually causes reddening of the tympanic membrane, which may obscure a diagnosis of AOM. If you strongly suspect AOM at the start, remove earwax without irrigating, or check for membrane motility after removing the irrigation fluid from the canal. Tympanometry can be performed in equivocal cases.

Contraindications

- Do not irrigate or syringe the auditory canal in young children or infants if it is not absolutely necessary. Perforations are more likely to occur in this age group.
- Do not irrigate in the presence of tympanostomy tubes, a perforated tympanic membrane, a previous membrane perforation that has healed poorly, or recent surgery of the middle ear.

Note: If you have already begun the cleaning procedure with a syringe and you find a perforation that you did not know was present, administer a systemic antibiotic prophylactically.

- Avoid using a curet to remove earwax when you can't be sure that the patient's head will remain immobile. Even with good head control, the procedure incurs some risk for eardrum and auditory canal trauma. Be aware that pulling out hardened earwax can cause bleeding.

Materials

- Blunt ear curet (Buck) size 0 or wire curet (commonly called cerumen spoons)
- No. 5 and No. 7 French suction tips
- Pomeroy ear syringe or suitable substitute
- Oral hygiene appliance (Water Pik)
- Bulb syringe (can be used by the patient at home)
- Towels or plastic apron
- Ear basin
- A container of tap water at body temperature (optional additives: several tablespoons of hydrogen peroxide or 1 tsp baking soda/pint water)
- Wax softening agents (optional; see Table 54-1)
- Monsel's solution

TABLE 54-1

Agents commonly used to soften earwax

Ceruminolytics may aid removal if earwax is hard and dry although they are not necessary in all cases of impaction.

- Most ceruminolytics take 3–4 days to be effective. They are virtually useless if administered just before irrigation.
- When you prescribe a ceruminolytic, advise the patient or parent to instill the solution into the ear canal at bedtime, plug the canal with cotton, and remove the cotton in the morning. If a twice-daily regimen is required, any remaining solution should be drained by gravity before the next dose.

Brand name	Ingredients
Auro Ear Drops (OTC) Cerumenex Drops (Rx)*	6.5% Carbamide peroxide 10% Triethanolamine polypeptide oleate-condensate, 0.5% chlorobutanol, propylene glycol
Colace liquid (OTC)**, ***	Docusate sodium
Debrox Drops (OTC) Murine Ear Drops (OTC)	6.5% Carbamide peroxide glycerin
Various	Baby oil (OTC) Mineral oil (OTC) Virgin olive oil (OTC)

*This product achieves effectiveness in 15–30 minutes.
**Earwax removal is not an FDA-recognized indication for this product.
***Use liquid, not syrup, forms of docusate products.

PROCEDURE

1. If irrigation is contraindicated, proceed to step 5. Otherwise plan to use either an ear syringe or a Water Pik to flush impacted cerumen from the external meatus.

2. Be sure the water used for irrigation is at body temperature to avoid triggering the vestibular reflex and producing vertigo, nausea, and vomiting.

3. For best results, have the patient assume a sitting position, and direct the liquid toward the wall of the canal not obscured by the earwax plug (usually superiorly) to build up pressure behind the plug and push it out (Figure 54-1). To reduce the risk of trauma, take care to use the lowest possible pressure. Use an ear basin to collect the irrigating fluid.

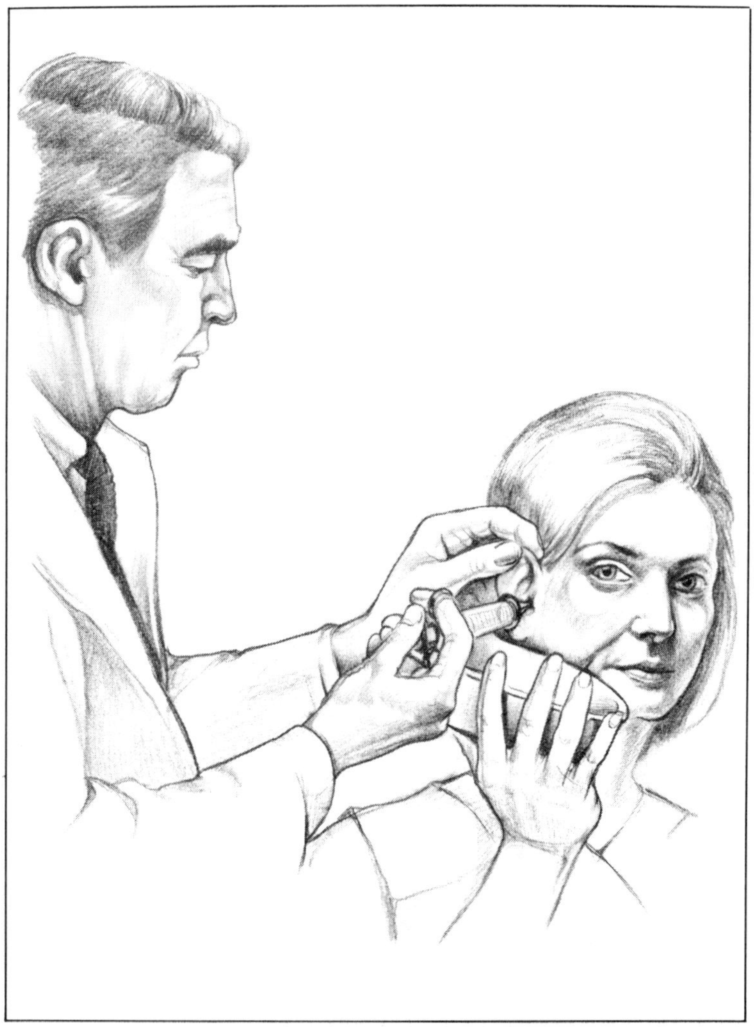

Figure 54-1 With the patient sitting, have him or her hold an ear basin under the ear to catch draining fluid. Aim body-temperature water toward the wall of the canal that is not obscured by earwax. This allows pressure to build behind the plug, which helps push it out.

4. If the wax plug dislodges, dry the canal with 70% alcohol to prevent maceration and subsequent otitis externa. If the plug does not dislodge, continue with step 5.
5. Use a blunt wire curet to remove cerumen. If the patient is a young child, have an assistant restrain him or her firmly (Figure 54-2).
6. Insert the curet alongside and just past the plug, and spoon or roll out the wax plug (Figure 54-3). Exercise extreme caution to avoid nicking or irritating the ear canal.
7. If bleeding occurs, swab the area with Monsel's solution, and administer a combination antibiotic such as hydrocortisone, neomycin sulfate, and polymyxin B sulfate (AK-Sporin H.C. Otic, Cortisporin Otic) or hydrocortisone and polymyxin B sulfate (Otobiotic Otic) prophylactically to avoid an external ear infection.

Follow-up Care

The key to a successful procedure outcome and proper follow-up care is patient education.

- Urge your patients not to use cotton-tipped swabs to remove earwax, as these devices can push the wax deeper into the auditory canal, thereby increasing the chance of impaction. Always point out the extreme hazards of putting anything into the ear, such as bobby pins, paper clips, or any other common objects people use to

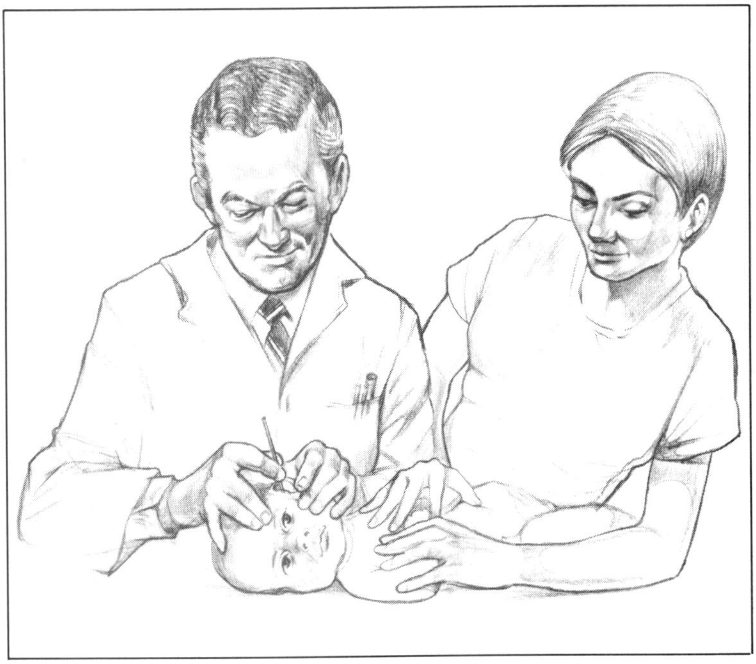

Figure 54-2 An assistant immobilizes the infant while the physician uses a curette to remove impacted earwax.

Figure 54-3 Gently slide curette past the cerumen plug and spoon or roll the plug out. Try not to nick the ear canal.

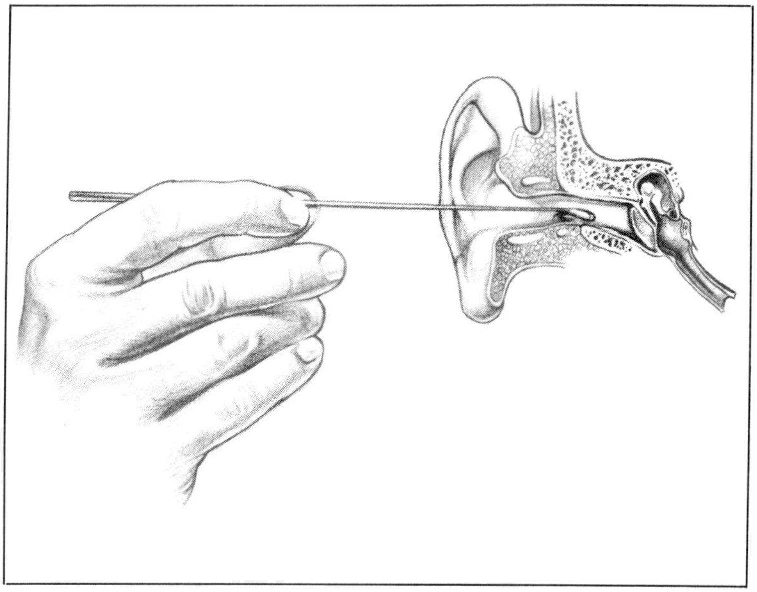

get at earwax. These objects easily traumatize the lining of the ear canal and therefore increase the risk of otitis externa.

- Let the patient know that over-the-counter wax-softening products do not remove earwax, as they may be advertised to do. These products do, however, soften the wax enough to facilitate removal by a professional. Sometimes it is helpful to instruct a patient a few days before an appointment for earwax removal to instill one of these products in the ears. Baby oil or mineral oil are also effective and have a long shelf life.
- Before your patient leaves the office, demonstrate the careful and proper use of the bulb syringe as adjunct home therapy for the patient who has a continuing earwax problem and who is capable and willing to perform the irrigation procedure himself or herself.

Suggested Readings

Bailey BJ: Removal of cerumen. *JAMA* 1984;251:1681.

Carne S: Ear syringing. *Br Med J* 1980;280:374-376.

Schwartz RH, Rodriguez WJ, McAveney W, et al: Cerumen removal: How necessary is it to diagnose acute otitis media? *Am J Dis Child* 1983;137:1064-1065.

55

Tympanometry

Charles E. Driscoll, MD

Tympanometry provides an objective measurement of tympanic membrane mobility, affirms the presence of an intact membrane, and helps confirm the integrity of the ossicular chain with results that are reproducible from test to test. The technique is sensitive to subtle changes produced by middle ear disease. Little training is required to perform satisfactory examinations with a modern tympanometer. The recommended devices are fully automatic and require little maintenance or calibration.

Tympanometry measures tympanic membrane mobility during variation of the air pressure in the sealed ear canal. Mobility is plotted graphically, with distance traveled by the membrane on the Y axis and pressure change on the X axis. Pressure is gradually decreased from a reference level of $+200$ mmH_2O through 0, to at least -200 mmH_2O. You can also measure the volume of air required to fill the ear canal. This aids in the diagnosis of tympanic membrane perforation when insufflated volume exceeds normal range. Mobility of the tympanic membrane and integrity of the ossicular chain may also be measured when you test the stapedial reflex by presenting a pure tone through the earphone probe unit.

This technique does not replace traditional pure tone audiometry, but it adds useful information on several conditions that alter the architecture or volume of the middle ear.

Indications

- To detect or follow progress of a middle ear condition such as effusion, cholesteatoma with possible perforation, or a retracted tympanic membrane with adhesions
- To detect negative middle ear perforation
- To detect tympanic membrane perforation
- To detect ossicular chain disruptions
- To check ventilation tubes for patency
- To screen children who may need audiometry

Contraindications

Tympanometry has no absolute contraindications. Otitis externa with purulent exudate that can cross-infect patients through contaminated equipment is a relative contraindication.

Materials

- Otoscope with ear specula of various sizes
- Cerumen spoon
- Automatic tympanometer composed of an ear probe unit for delivery of air and a pure tone pulse to the middle ear and a recording unit with self-contained manometer and a strip chart recorder to provide hard copy of test results
- Soft rubber ear pieces of various sizes for the ear probe unit

PROCEDURE

1. Emphasize the need for the patient to sit quietly and to look straight ahead while you perform the test, without talking, swallowing, moving the jaw, or moving away from the ear probe (thus breaking the hermetic seal). For accurate diagnosis in a patient unable to cooperate, such as a young child, you will need repeated measurements taken during quiet periods.
2. After inspecting the external ear, grasp the helix between your thumb and forefinger, and move it in several directions to evaluate pain.
3. Using an otoscope, examine the ear canal to be sure it is free of cerumen or exudate (as in otitis externa). If cerumen occludes the canal, remove it with a cerumen spoon or by irrigation until you can see a portion of the tympanic membrane. Do not use irrigation if perforation is expected.
4. Inspect the tympanic membrane surface for architecture, perforation, and visible positive or negative signs of middle ear disease.
5. Turn on the automatic recording device so that it will be triggered when you apply the probe to the ear. You may also trigger it manually if you prefer.
6. Select a soft rubber tip for the ear probe. The tip that fits properly occludes the opening of the external ear, producing a hermetic seal against the soft tissues of the ear, without being able to advance past the opening into the ear canal (Figure 55-1).
7. Grasp the helix of the ear firmly as before. Pull up and outward in older children and adults, down and outward in young children, to straighten the ear canal while the probe is sealed (Figure 55-2). Remind the patient not to move. When the probe is properly positioned, the automatic recording device will be triggered.
8. Leave the ear probe sealed to the external ear canal until the tympanometer signals the conclusion of the test (3–8 seconds). The signal is a light or tone on most units. Concentrate on positioning the ear probe in the ear while the test is in progress; do not move and look at the tracing until the test is completed.
9. Repeat the procedure in the opposite ear. If you obtain any tracings of doubtful validity, repeat the test.

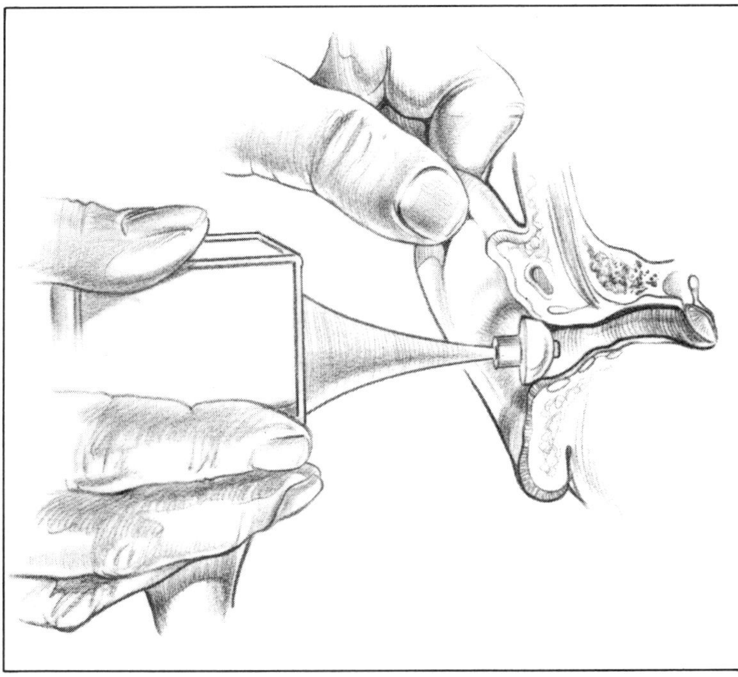

Figure 55-1 The rubber tip of the ear probe is the correct size if it creates a hermetic seal against the soft tissues of the ear, completely occluding the opening without advancing into the ear canal.

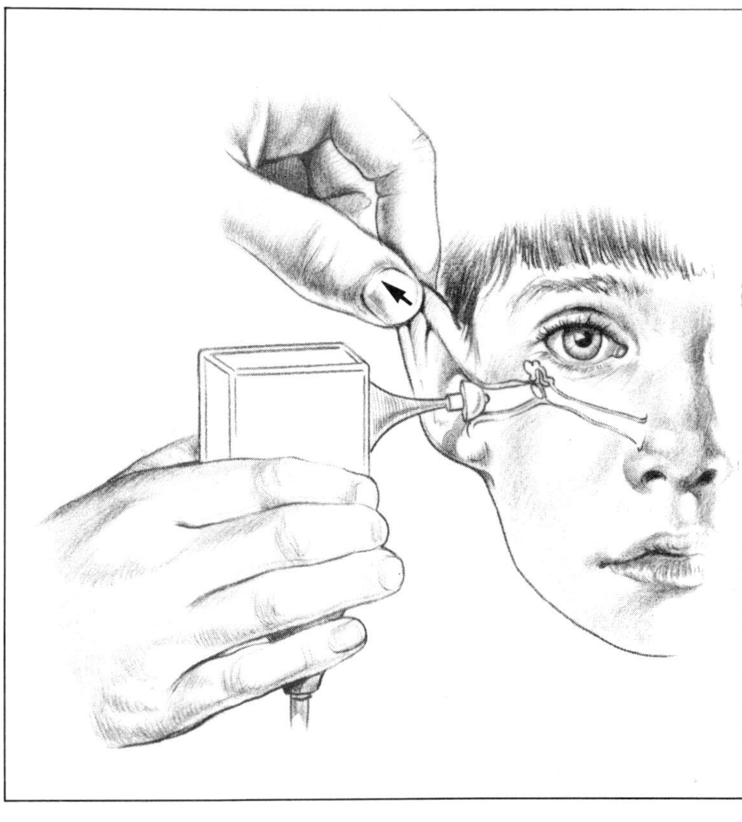

Figure 55-2 In an older child or adult, the arrow indicates the direction to pull the helix, which is up and outward.

Interpretation

Tympanogram tracings made by the method described (called the American method) usually fall into three types:

- Type A is normal with a peak of eardrum compliance at or near an air pressure of 0 mmH_2O, indicating that air pressure in the middle ear is in equilibrium with that of the atmosphere (Figure 55-3).
- Type B shows little change in compliance as the air pressure changes, suggesting fluid in the middle ear (Figure 55-4).
- Type C shows greatest compliance when air pressure in the ear canal is below atmospheric pressure, indicating low (negative) middle ear pressure (Figure 55-5).

You will occasionally obtain maximum compliance at a pressure of +10 to +50 mmH_2O. This suggests either that the patient may be developing acute otitis media or that he or she applied positive pressure through the eustachian tubes during the test.

The volume needed to insufflate the ear canal and move the tympanic membrane is generally recorded on the tracing. Normal volume for children is 0.6–1.0 mL and for adults, 0.8–2.5 mL. If you need to insufflate an abnormally high volume of air to move the tympanic membrane, increase your suspicion of a perforation.

A normal variant can occur with hypermobile tympanic membrane. In that setting, the peak is near zero, but it is so high it seems to go off the chart (Figure 55-6). You can chart the peak by changing the air pressure applied to the tympanic membrane to bring the peak down to traceable range: Turn the switch to alter the amount of air displacement from 1 mL (the usual normal) to make 5 mL the normal level, thereby accommodating a bigger swing.

Stapedial reflex testing involves presenting a pure tone to the tympanic membrane to elicit movement that registers on the tympanogram. Failure to obtain motion of the tympanic membrane on pure tone stimulus in a patient with reduced hearing may indicate disruption of the ossicular chain.

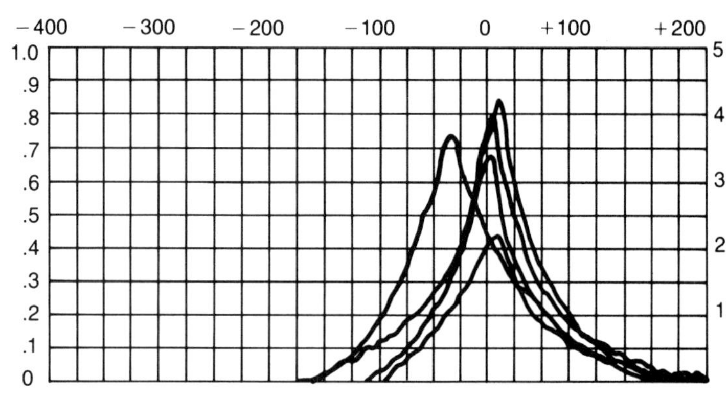

Figure 55-3 Type A tracings of the American method. Air pressure in the middle ear is in equilibrium with the atmospheric pressure.

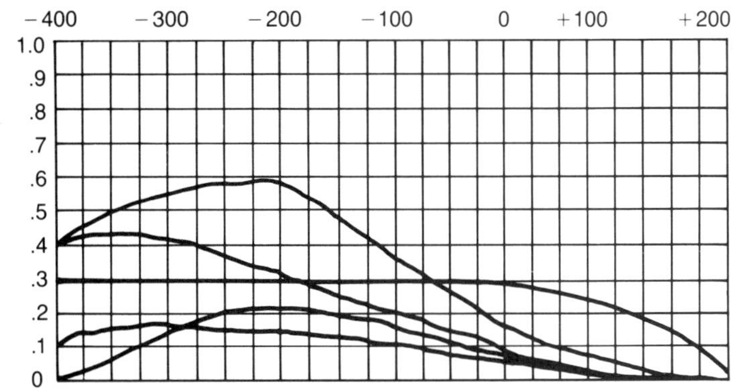

Figure 55-4 Type B tracings. Suggests presence of fluid in the middle ear.

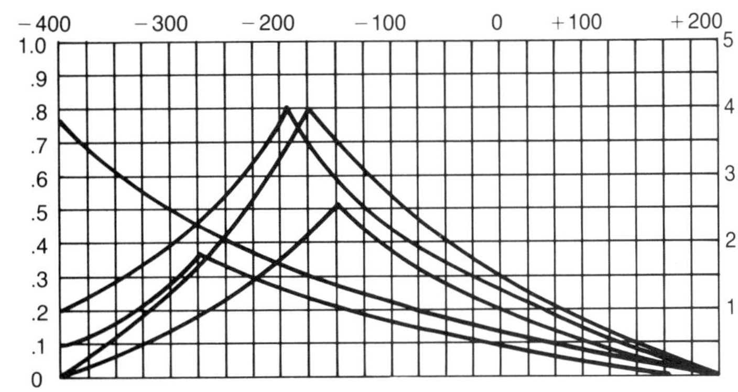

Figure 55-5 Type C tracings. Evidence of negative middle ear pressure.

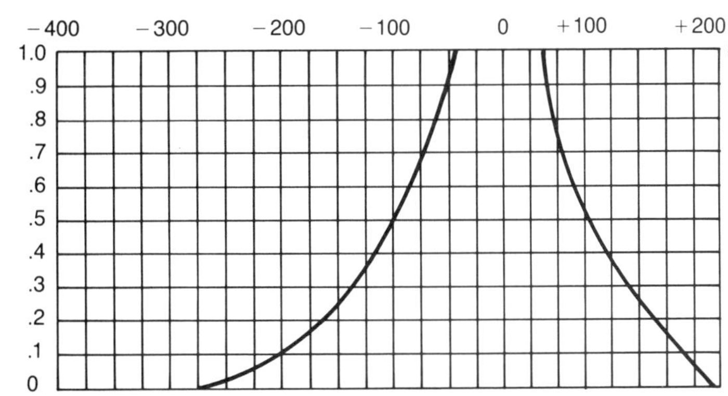

Figure 55-6 Illustrates hypermobile tympanic membrane. The peak is near zero and can be charted by adjusting the air pressure applied to the membrane to 5 mL, thereby accommodating the bigger swing, bringing the peak down to traceable range.

Suggested Readings

Harford ER: Tympanometry, in Jerger J, Northern JL (eds): *Clinical Impedance Audiometry*, ed 2. American Electromedics Corp, Acton, Mass, 1980, pp 40-64.

Stool SE: Medical relevancy of immittance measurements. *Ear Hear* 1984;5:309-313.

56

Controlling Posterior Epistaxis

Leroy R. Schlesselman, MD
Rafael Ivan Iriarte, MD

Ninety percent of nosebleeds are anterior. These usually involve Kiesselbach's plexus of the nasal septum. The other 10% are posterior and arise from the sphenopalatine or ethmoidal vessels that supply the upper recesses of the nasal chamber (Figure 56-1).

In patients younger than 40, bleeds are usually anterior and venous, most of them resulting from trauma. In those 40 and older, bleeds are often posterior, arterial, and associated with systemic disease although the precise etiology is frequently not clear. Possible causes include degenerative processes of the blood vessels, neoplasms of the nose and paranasal sinuses, infections, hypertension, and bleeding diathesis. Many cases, however, must be classified as idiopathic spontaneous epistaxis.

Anterior epistaxis usually responds to pressure, application of 4% cocaine, or cauterization with silver nitrate. Patients with posterior epistaxis, however, often require sedation, posterior nasal packing, and hospitalization.[1]

A conventional gauze nasal pack is difficult to insert and remove, is poorly tolerated by most patients, and has a high rate of complications. Several types of intranasal balloons minimize these disadvantages, but a Foley catheter serves the same purpose and is available in most primary care settings.

In addition, the catheter procedure allows for quicker insertion than the conventional packing method. It is also less painful to insert and remove, less uncomfortable in place, less likely to cause a nasal

---

[1] High posterior bleeds are rarely controlled by packing; they usually require ligation. Some authorities recommend treating a *severe* posterior bleed with arterial ligation initially.

Figure 56-1 Vessels involved in posterior epistaxis.

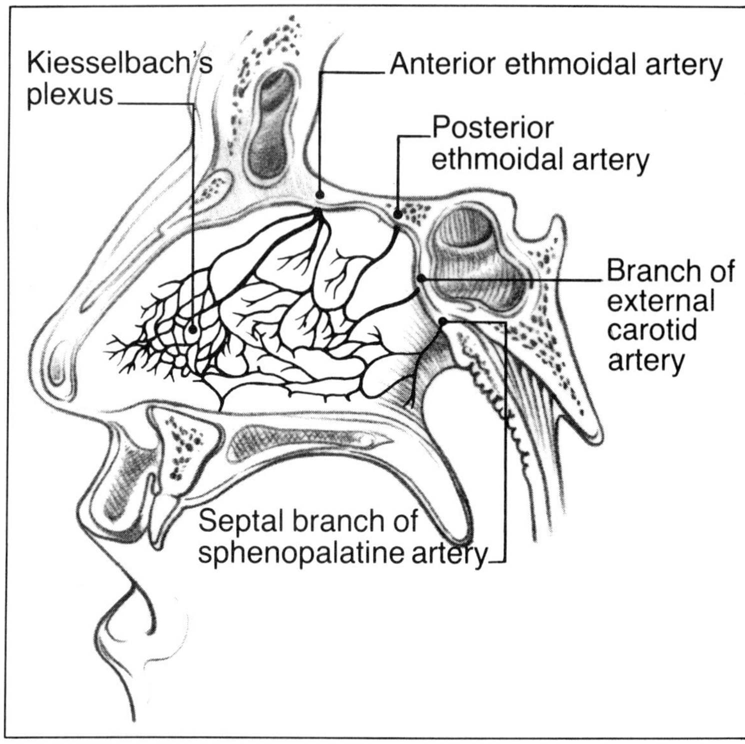

infection, and less odoriferous. And less need for sedation helps decrease the risk of hypoxia.

Indication

- Posterior epistaxis

Contraindications

- Obstruction of oral airway
- History of tumor in the nasopharynx

Materials

- 4% topical cocaine solution, with or without epinephrine (1:1000), tetracaine, or 2% lidocaine HCl with epinephrine
- Cotton swabs
- Foley catheter, No. 12 or No. 13 French, with 30-mL balloon
- 20-mL syringe
- Absorbable gelatin sponge (Gelfoam) (optional and expensive)
- Petrolatum gauze for nose packing
- Antibiotic ointment
- Umbilical clamp
- Piece of foam rubber or other padding

- Nasal speculum
- Bayonet forceps

PROCEDURE

1. Anesthetize the nasal fossa with topical cocaine solution. This is necessary to avoid vasovagal side effects from insertion.
2. Remove and discard the tip of the Foley catheter distal to the balloon. Lubricate the catheter with antibiotic ointment. Introduce the catheter into the bleeding nasal fossa past the choana.
3. With a syringe, introduce 5 mL of air or saline into the balloon, and apply gentle traction to bring the balloon into contact with the choana. Then fill the balloon with an additional 10–15 mL of air or saline (Figure 56-2). Check the soft palate for any bulging; if present, the pressure of the balloon is excessive and should be decreased.
4. Continue to apply constant moderate traction to the catheter, or have an assistant do so. Using bayonet forceps, fill the posterior and medial portions of the nasal cavity with absorbable gelatin sponge smeared with antibiotic ointment, then pack the anterior part of the nasal fossa with antibiotic-coated petrolatum gauze in a conventional ribbon-layer manner (Figure 56-3). If the gelatin sponge is unavailable, pack the entire cavity with petrolatum gauze.
5. After completing the anterior packing, fix the Foley catheter in position with an umbilical clamp, using a piece of foam or other padding between the clamp and the nose. Fasten the remaining length of

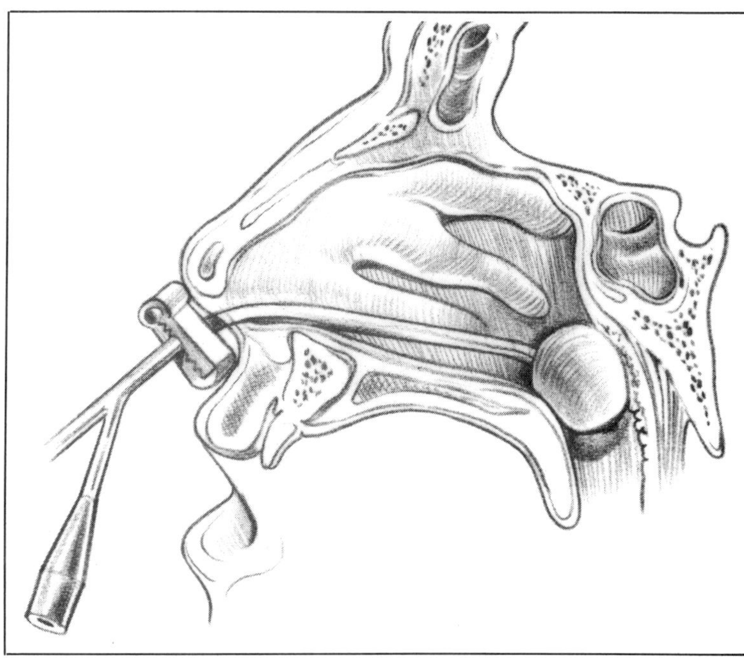

Figure 56-2 Lubricate a Foley catheter with antibiotic ointment and insert it into the bleeding nasal fossa, past the choana. With a syringe, inflate the balloon.

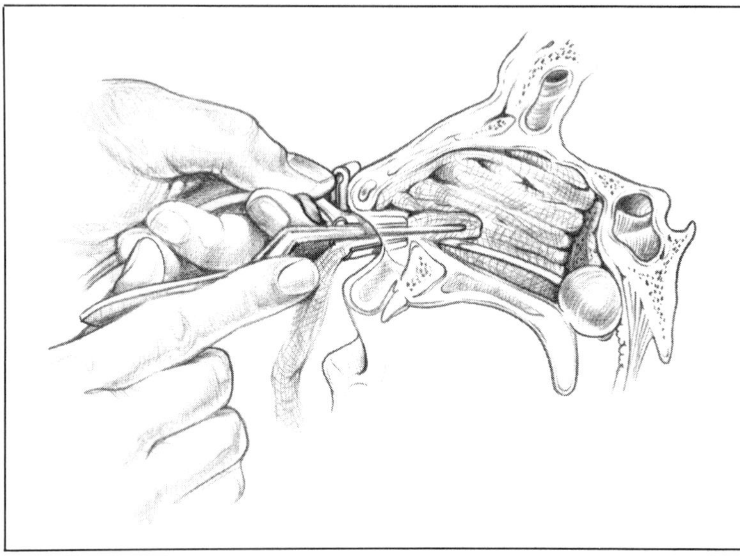

Figure 56-3 Pack the anterior portion of the nasal fossa with antibiotic-coated petrolatum gauze (if available), using bayonet forceps.

catheter around the ear with tape (Figure 56-4). Plan to keep the patient under observation for 24 hours. To prevent pressure necrosis of the skin under the clamp, have the position of the clamp adjusted every few hours.

6. When bleeding stops, deflate the balloon gradually and leave the catheter in place for 4–6 hours in case of rebleed.

7. If no rebleed occurs, remove the catheter, and leave the anterior pack in place if possible; remove the pack in 24 hours if bleeding does not recur.

Note: If this method fails to control bleeding, arterial ligation may be indicated: Consult an otolaryngologist.

8. Follow-up care should include increased humidification of the nares with normal saline nose spray several times per day.

Complications

- Acute sinusitis from blocked drainage
- Hemotympanum, middle ear effusion, or acute otitis media from blocked eustachian tube
- Hypoxia from the nasopulmonary reflex
- Balloon leakage (if air is used to inflate)
- Rupture of balloon and aspiration of saline (if liquid is used to inflate)
- Necrosis of mucous membranes from balloon pressure (rare but the risk is high if the balloon is inflated more than 24 hours)
- Pressure necrosis of skin under the umbilical clamp
- Toxic shock syndrome—controlled with antibiotic ointment and antistaphylococcal antibiotic therapy during use of the balloon and packing

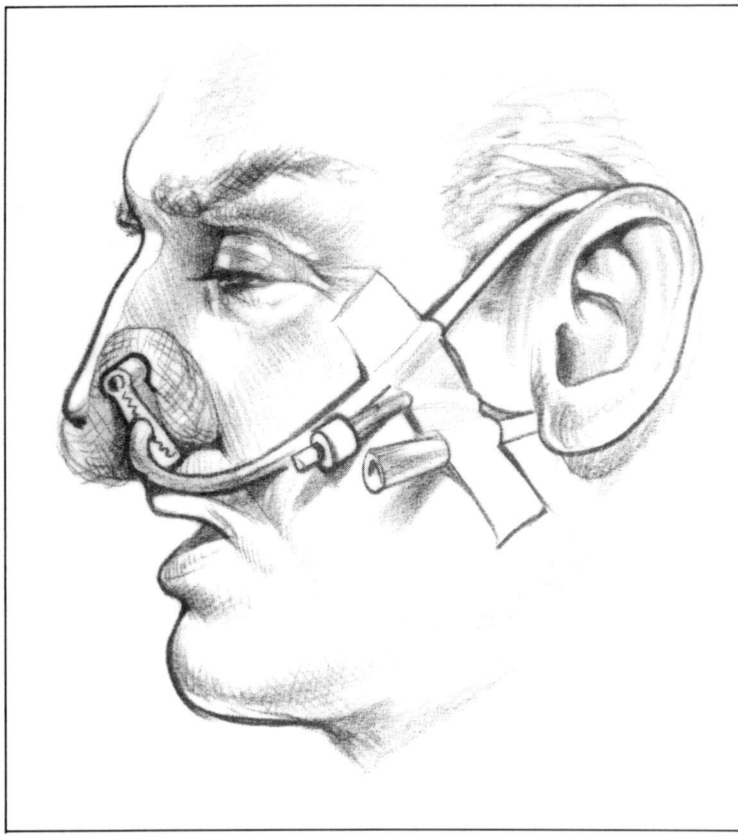

Figure 56-4 Fix the catheter in position by applying an umbilical clamp, which should be padded by a piece of foam or gauze. Hook the free end of the catheter around the ear.

Suggested Readings

Bierman SF: To air is humane. *N Engl J Med* 1983;309:243.

De La Haye, Davies H: Managing epistaxis. *Practitioner* 1983; 227:1011-1014.

Elwany S, Kamel T, Mekhamer A: Pneumatic nasal catheters: Advantages and drawbacks. *J Laryngol Otol* 1986;100:641-647.

Kirchner JA: Current concepts in otolaryngology: Epistaxis. *N Engl J Med* 1982;307:1126-1128.

Nassif AC: How I do it—head and neck and plastic surgery. A new procedure in nasal packing to stop bleeding. *Laryngoscope* 1983;93:1222-1224.

Perretta LJ, Denslow BL, Brown CG: Emergency evaluation and treatment of epistaxis. *Emerg Med Clin North Am* 1987;5:265-277.

Wang L, Vogel DH: Posterior epistaxis: Comparison of treatment. *Otolaryngol Head Neck Surg* 1981;89:1001-1006.

IX

Eye procedures

57

Removing a Foreign Body from the Eye

Phillip G. Couchman, MD

Most particles that get into the eye from the environment produce no symptoms or only mildly annoying ones and are washed away by tears. Even when symptoms are severe or prolonged, some patients may be able to remove a particle safely with your telephone instructions. Caution every call-in patient to avoid rubbing his or her eyelids. Then ask whether it was a rapidly moving object that entered the eye—a circumstance indicating immediate examination and possible referral to an ophthalmologist. But if you can rule out dangerous trauma, suggest that the patient try remedies such as the following:

- If the foreign body is visible in the lower conjunctival sac, the patient or someone else can try to remove it with the corner of a clean handkerchief or a paper tissue.
- If the patient feels the foreign body behind the upper lid, advise him or her to look down, then grasp the upper lid and lift it away from the globe. This often decreases pain and allows tears to wash away the irritant.
- If the patient is resourceful enough, encourage him to irrigate the eye once or twice with an eyecup or by simply flooding the eye and using a salt water solution (½ tsp salt dissolved in an 8-oz glass of warm water). Tell the patient to call you right away if these measures do not work.

If home remedies don't help or if telephone instructions are inappropriate to begin with, arrange an immediate appointment to evaluate the patient and then refer him or remove the foreign body, using techniques to be described here. When the patient arrives, see him promptly.

Materials

- Bright light source
- Magnifying glasses

- Snellen's chart
- Sterile cotton-tipped applicators
- Sterile eye spud or 18-gauge needle
- Sterile fluorescein sodium strips (Fluor-I-Strip, Fluorets)
- Sterile saline or water and eyedropper
- Topical anesthetic such as 0.5% proparacaine HCl (Alcaine, Ophthaine, Ophthetic, etc.)

Optional, often Useful Equipment

- Cycloplegic drops such as cyclopentolate HCl (Cyclogyl)
- Examination table
- Ophthalmoscope (20–40 diopter lens)
- Sterile eye patches and 1-in. paper tape
- Wood's light

Preparation

1. For easier examination, have the patient lie supine on the examining table.
2. Anesthetize the affected eye with 1–2 drops of the topical anesthetic. This is not mandatory, but a patient quickly relieved of much acute pain responds better to your questions and treatment. While you anesthetize the eye, review or take the history. Explain that the anesthetic will not block sensation completely but will prevent severe pain and will take effect within one minute. As soon as anesthesia is effected, proceed with the examination.

Examination

Most eye injuries resulting from foreign bodies in the cornea or conjunctiva are superficial. Unless emergency referral is indicated, continue to examine all areas even after you find one foreign body; there may be several particles in the eye.
1. Expose the eyeball by opening the lids wide, using thumb and index finger. You may want to use a bright light and magnifying glass to examine the sclera and cornea more carefully.

Introduce fluorescein dye. Avoid the multiple-dose dropper bottles; fluorescein is a fertile culture medium for *Pseudomonas.* Use fluorescein strips instead. Moisten a strip with sterile water, saline, or anesthetic solution, and place it in the lower conjunctival sac for 3–5 seconds. The dye quickly disperses throughout the conjunctiva as the patient blinks. Flush the eye with the sterile solution; denuded areas that have accepted the brilliant yellow stain will be easily identifiable. The dye may reveal mucus or tears around a foreign body in the conjunctival sac.

A Wood's light sometimes helps reveal a small foreign body in the cornea surrounded by a halo of stained tissue. It might also show a corneal scratch that feels like a foreign body to the patient. If you find a foreign body in the cornea, use Snellen's chart to check the patient's visual acuity. If the foreign body is outside the visual axis or just superficially embedded in the visual axis, use the removal technique for a particle in the cornea before proceeding with the exam.

Caution: Refer the patient immediately to an ophthalmologist if the patient is uncooperative or if you find any of the following:

- A foreign body inside the eyeball or deeply lodged in the sclera or cornea
- A penetrating wound
- Blood in the anterior chamber of the eye
- Fixed, distorted, or dilated pupils

Unless you are highly experienced or remote from an ophthalmologist, also refer if you see a fleck of steel or iron surrounded by a rust ring in the patient's visual axis. Inadequate removal of the rust ring may cause low-grade inflammation and impaired vision. Removing too much corneal tissue along with the rust may produce a distorted cornea or excess scarring.

2. Evert the upper eyelid to examine the upper conjunctiva. Have the patient look downward. Grasp the upper eyelashes between thumb and index finger, and with the tip of the other index finger or the side of the pad of a cotton-tipped applicator, press gently on the skin at the upper lateral border of the tarsal plate (Figure 57-1). Pull outward on the lashes and rotate the tarsal plate upward until it forms a right angle with the eyeball. A gentle tug upward should flip the plate into eversion, clearly exposing the conjunctival surface of the upper lid (Figure 57-2). Withdraw your finger or the applicator; the lid will

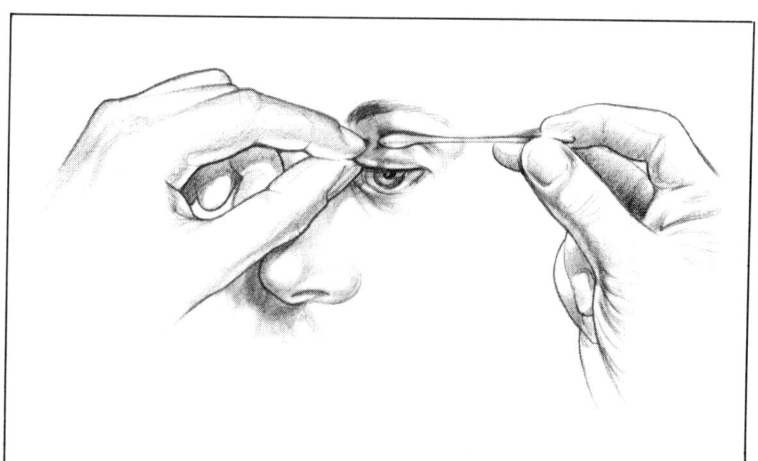

Figure 57-1 Grasp the upper eyelashes with one hand, and with the other, press gently on the skin at the upper lateral border of the tarsal plate with a cotton-tipped applicator.

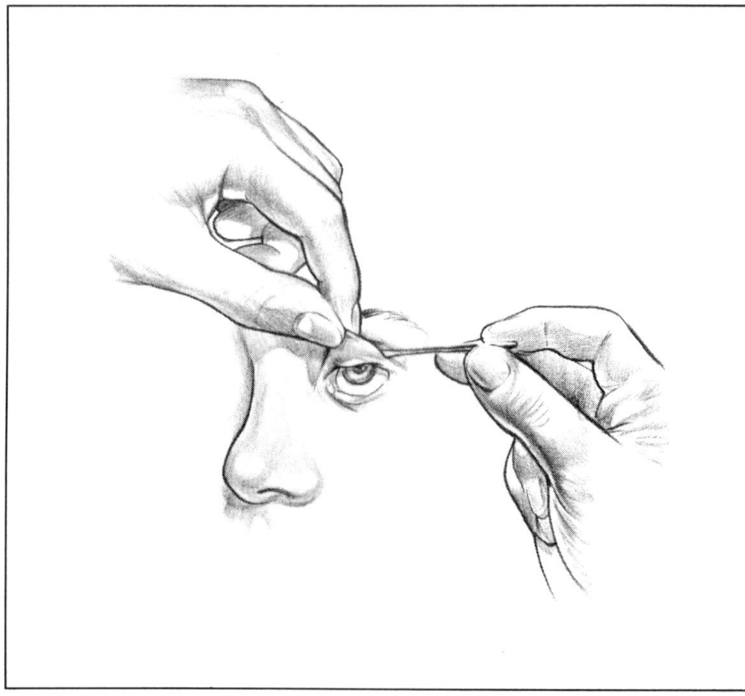

Figure 57-2 Pull outward on the lashes. A gentle tug out and up should flip the tarsal plate into eversion, exposing the conjunctival surface. The lid should stay everted on its own so you can remove the cotton-tipped applicator.

remain everted until you have the patient look upward after examination. If you find a foreign body, remove it using the removal technique for a particle in the conjunctiva and proceed with the examination.

3. Have the patient fix his gaze upward. Gently grasp the lower eyelashes between thumb and index finger and pull the lid away from the eyeball. Place the tip of your free index finger on the cheek over the inferior orbital margin and push the skin upward to help lift the lower lid further from the eyeball. If you see a foreign body, use the removal technique for a particle in the conjunctiva.

PROCEDURES

PARTICLE IN CORNEA

1. Have the patient fix his gaze on a distant object. Holding the eyelids apart with thumb and index finger, begin by wiping the cornea once with a moistened cotton swab. This occasionally dislodges the particle.

2. If this is unsuccessful, slip an eye spud or the point of an 18-gauge needle under the particle, and lift it off the cornea. When using a needle, hold it bevel up. You may have to make several attempts. Keep the instrument parallel to the surface of the cornea to avoid perforation (Figure 57-3).

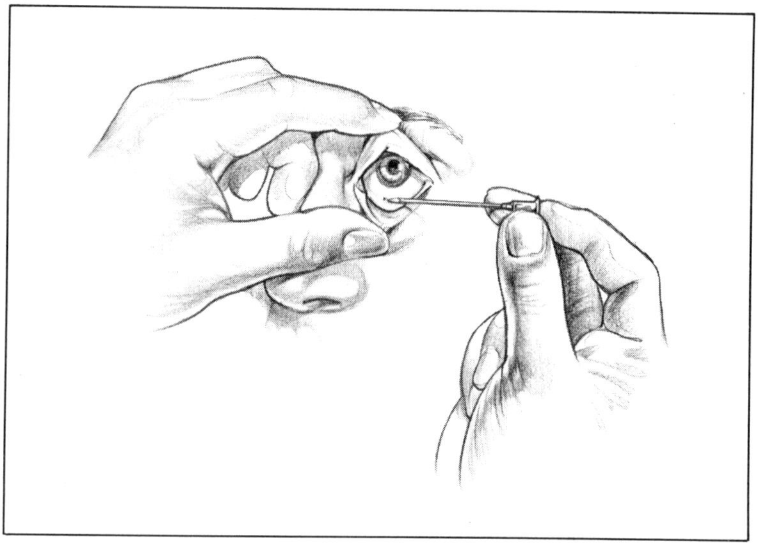

Figure 57-3 When using a needle to lift a particle off the surface of the cornea, always keep it parallel to the corneal surface to avoid perforation, with the bevelled side away from the cornea.

If rust stain is present and you are confident of your ability to remove it safely, scoop it up bit by bit with the tip of the needle or spud. Magnifying glasses (8–10 power) are useful here; an ophthalmoscope (20–40 diopter lens) can help locate any residual fragments.
3. Once you have removed the foreign body, retest the patient's vision.

PARTICLE IN CONJUNCTIVA Remove a foreign body from the conjunctiva by wiping with a moistened cotton swab. In rare cases you may need to use a spud or needle to lift a particle out.

Follow-up Care

1. After removing the foreign body, remind the patient that the anesthesia lasts about 15 minutes and that even though he may experience paresthesias while the effect is dissipating, he must avoid rubbing the eye. Antibiotic drops, cycloplegic drops, and eye patches are seldom necessary unless corneal scratching is extensive; and they are often counterproductive in that they interfere with the patient's activities. Healing usually occurs within 24 hours after the foreign body is removed.
2. If the corneal lesion is painful after treatment, have the patient apply moist compresses as needed to provide relief. He should stop as soon as the discomfort abates to avoid iatrogenic disability.
3. If the cornea has been scratched, follow up with a fluorescein stain in 1–2 days. If healing is not complete, repeat every 1–2 days until the injured area will not accept the stain, watching closely for signs of infection and referring if necessary.

Note: At some point during your follow-up care, remind patients to wear safety goggles if appropriate to help keep foreign bodies out of the eye.

Suggested Readings

Bankes JL: *Clinical Ophthalmology: A Text and Colour Atlas.* New York, Churchill Livingstone Inc, 1983, pp 45-54.

Miller D: *Ophthalmology: The Essentials.* New York, John Wiley & Sons, 1979, pp 219-268.

X

NEUROLOGY PROCEDURES

58

Lumbar Puncture in Adults

Elliot D. Schmerler, MD
Glenys O. Williams, MD

Indications

- Symptoms of meningitis, including seizures, intractable vomiting, unexplained fever, headache, stiff neck, and positive Kernig's and Brudzinski's signs
- Suspicion of leukemia or CNS malignancy
- Instillation of therapeutic agents (chemotherapy, for example)

Contraindications

- Raised intracranial pressure, especially from a space-occupying lesion. Performing a lumbar puncture in such conditions could result in a possibly fatal cerebellar pressure cone or herniation of brain substance through the tentorial falx.
- Infection of the neighboring skin.
- Blood dyscrasias and full anticoagulant treatment. Intradural and extradural bleeding may occur.
- Stiff and unyielding back from any cause.

Relative Contraindications

- Obesity makes landmarks hard to find.
- Elderly patients, even thin ones, may have a long, bone-hard supraspinous ligament that is hard to penetrate.
- Patients with severe degenerative changes in the spine and those who have trouble bending into the necessary position cause special difficulties.

Materials

- Sterile gloves and towels
- Antiseptic solution containing iodine, such as povidone-iodine (Betadine)
- 70% alcohol solution
- Gauze pads, 2 × 2 in.
- Spinal needle (22–25 gauge, 1½ in., with stylet)
- Manometer with three-way stopcock

- 0.5–1.0 mL 1% lidocaine HCl (Xylocaine HCl) and 2-mL syringe with 25-gauge needle
- Three sterile test tubes
- Adhesive strip

Preparation

1. Have the patient lie on one side. A sitting position can occasionally be used if the patient cannot lie down, but this does not allow accurate measurement of CSF pressure. The risk of herniation also increases with the patient sitting; avoid this position when intracranial pressure is elevated.
2. See that the lumbar vertebrae are flexed on each other as far as possible so that the inferior articular processes of the upper vertebrae ride up on the superior articular processes of the lower, the ligamenta flava are stretched, and the interlaminar spaces are increased, all of which expand the target area.

Flexion of the hips on the spine does not necessarily produce flexion of the lumbar vertebrae. Telling a patient "Draw your knees up to your chin" is insufficient. A better instruction is "Try to roll your head into your lap." Or you can put your fingertip on the lumbar area and say "Push out this part of your back." If the patient is lying down, an assistant can firmly flex the neck and raise the knees to meet the head.

Caution: Be careful that your assistant's head or breath does not contaminate the sterile field during the procedure.
3. Identify the site for puncture by drawing an imaginary line between the highest points of the patient's two iliac crests. This line passes just below the fourth lumbar space (Figure 58-1).
4. Provided the site for lumbar puncture is below L-2, the exact location is unimportant: At this level, the spinal cord becomes the cauda equina in adults. Distances between lumbar vertebrae may vary; choose the space where the gap is greatest.
5. Observe strict antiseptic technique. Using gauze pads, scrub the back first with antiseptic, then with alcohol. Cleanse the puncture site

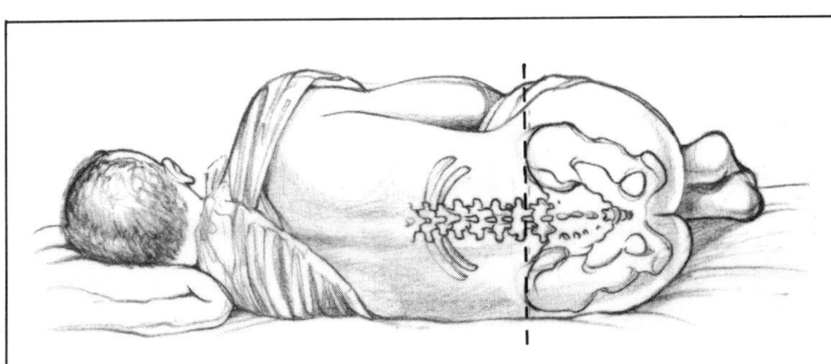

Figure 58-1 With the patient in the correct position, try to imagine a line drawn between the highest points of the patient's iliac crests. This line passes just below the fourth lumbar space. As long as the puncture is directed below L-2, the exact location is unimportant.

first, then, using concentric circles, cleanse the area surrounding the puncture site.

6. Drape the patient's back with sterile towels.

7. Using a 2-mL syringe and a 25-gauge needle, inject 0.5–1.0 mL 1% lidocaine subcutaneously at the site.

PROCEDURE

1. Line up your eye behind the hub of the needle, looking down the shaft. Keep the bevel facing cephalad. The median approach is recommended although some physicians prefer a paramedian or lateral approach.

2. Direct the needle slightly cephalad, toward the umbilicus. Advance it cautiously, either in millimeter steps or continuously, in the median plane.

3. When you have advanced the needle 1.0–1.5 cm (3/8–5/8 in.), you will feel a drop in resistance as the needle penetrates the ligamentum flavum. You will sometimes get the sensation that the needle is "popping" though the ligament.

4. Once the needle point penetrates the ligamentum flavum, remove the stylet, advance the needle a little further to puncture the dural arachnoid (dura and arachnoid are virtually homogeneous in the lumbar area). CSF should appear (Figure 58-2).

5. Check for free flow of fluid. If necessary, rotate, fractionally advance, or withdraw the needle. You may have to create negative pressure by attaching a 2-mL syringe and aspirating before CSF flows freely (Figure 58-3).

6. Once free-flowing fluid appears, attach a three-way stopcock and manometer to measure the CSF pressure. Then allow 0.5–1.0 mL CSF to drip into each of three sterile test tubes—the first for glucose and protein measurements; the second for Gram's stain, culture, and sus-

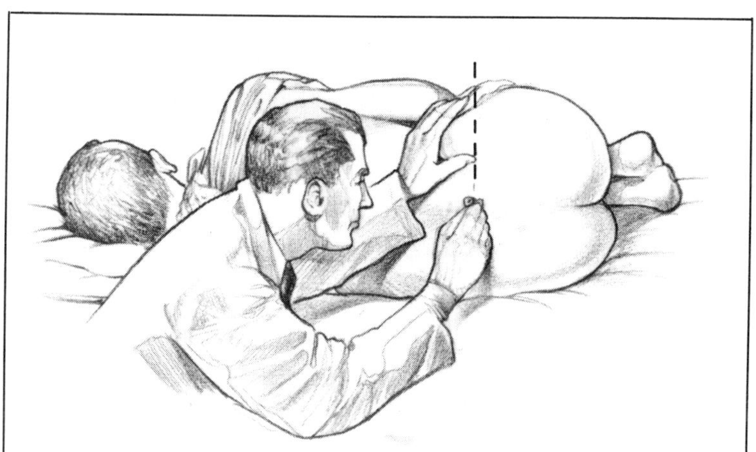

Figure 58-2 With the hub of the needle at eye level, advance it cautiously and slightly cephalad toward the umbilicus.

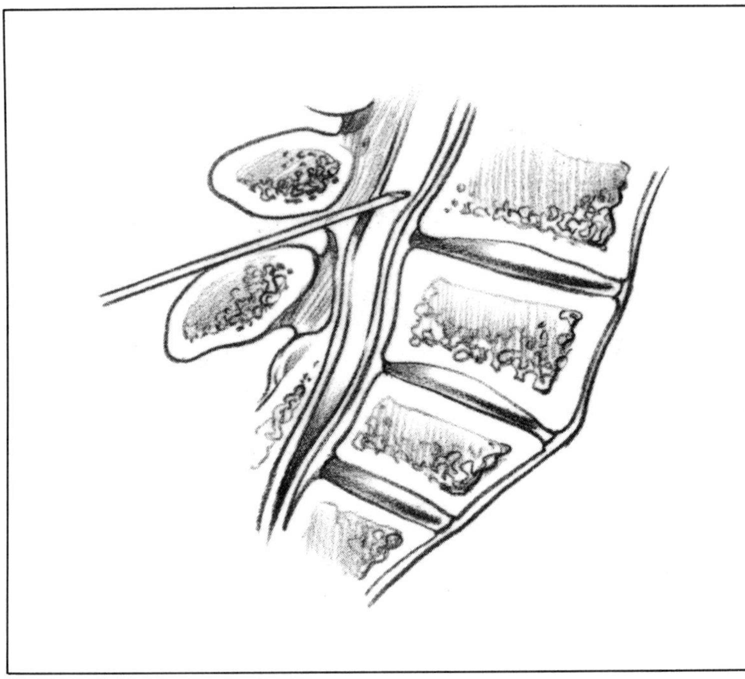

Figure 58-3 The needle that returns CSF is in the dural arachnoid. You may have to create negative pressure by attaching a syringe in order to achieve a free flow of fluid.

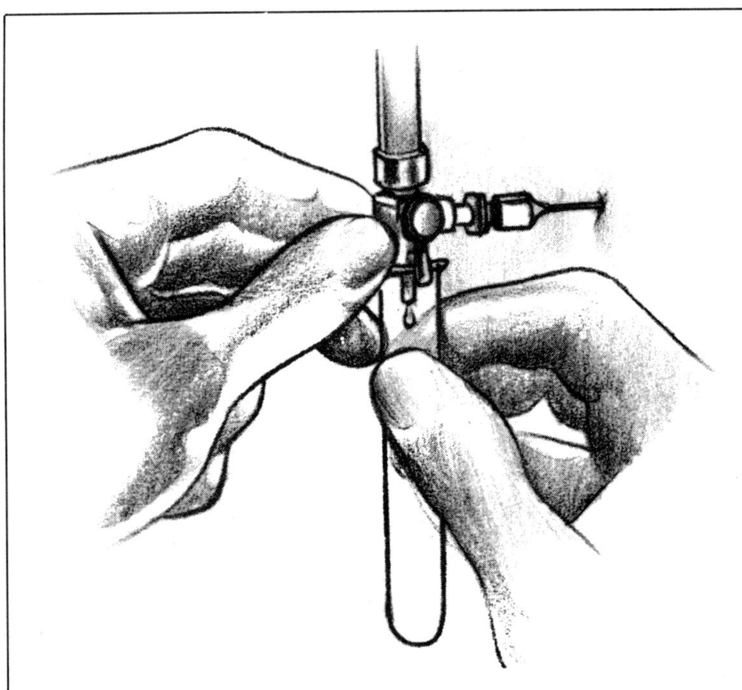

Figure 58-4 Attach a three-way stopcock and manometer to measure the CSF pressure.

TABLE 58-1

Cerebrospinal fluid findings

Condition	Appearance	Pressure (in mm H_2O)	Cells (per μl)	Protein	Misc. Cerebrospinal Fluid Findings
Normal lumbar tap	Clear & colorless	70-200	0-5	15-45 mg/dl	Glucose 50-70 mg/dl
Traumatic tap	Bloody; supernatant fluid clear	Normal	Red blood cells	4 mg/dl rise per 500 red cells	Bloody; supernatant fluid clear
Meningitis					
Acute Purulent	Clear, cloudy, xanthochromic; occasional clot formation	Greatly increased (250-700)	Polymorphonuclear cells, usually over 1000	Increased	Glucose decreased early; chlorides decreased late; organisms on smear and culture
Encephalitis	Clear & colorless	Normal	Normal or increased (mostly lymphocytes)	Normal or slightly increased	Serologic test of value in virus infections
Subdural hematoma	Classically yellow, but often clear & colorless	Usually increased	Normal	Normal or slightly increased	
Cerebral hemorrhage					
Ventricular Subarachnoid	Bloody; supernatant fluid yellow	Slightly increased	Red blood cells	Normal or slightly increased	Blood equal in all 3 specimens

ceptibility studies; and the third for CBC and differential (Figure 58-4). Other less common tests on CSF are fungal culture, culture and smear for acid-fast bacillus, VDRL, and cytology studies.

7. Measure the CSF pressure again.
8. Replace the stylet, and withdraw the needle.
9. Dress the puncture site with an adhesive strip.

Complications

In order of frequency, the complications that can occur following a lumbar puncture are as follows:

- Postpuncture headache, which occurs in one third of adults. Keeping all patients supine for 24 hours does not prevent headaches, but bed rest may prevent excess leakage of CSF from the puncture site.
- Blood-stained CSF from overadvancement of the needle with penetration of the venous plexus on the anterior aspect of the spinal canal. Such bleeding can cause irritation of spinal nerve roots with pain in the lower back and legs.
- Herniation of brain substance due to abnormally high intracranial pressure.
- Infection. A contaminated needle can introduce infection and cause bacterial meningitis.

Suggested Readings

Carbaat PAT, Van Crevel H: Lumbar puncture headache: Controlled study on the preventive effect of 24 hours' bed rest. *Lancet* 1981;2:1133-1135.

Evans CH: *Spinal Anesthesia.* New York, Paul B. Hoeber Inc, 1929.

Lee JA, Atkinson RS: *Sir Robert Macintosh's Lumbar Puncture and Spinal Analgesia,* ed 4. Edinburgh, Churchill Livingstone Inc, 1978.

Rodnitzky RL: *Van Allen's Pictorial Manual of Neurologic Tests,* ed 3. Chicago, Year Book Pubs Inc, 1988.

59

Lumbar Puncture in Infants and Children

George C. Xakellis, MD

Indications

- Symptoms of meningitis, which include seizures, intractable vomiting, unexplained fever, headache, stiff neck, positive Kernig's and Brudzinski's signs
- Suspicion of leukemia or CNS malignancy
- Instillation of therapeutic agents (chemotherapy, for example)

Contraindications

- Raised intracranial pressure, especially resulting from a space-occupying lesion. A possibly fatal cerebellar pressure cone or herniation of brain substance through the tentorial falx might result.
- Infection of the neighboring skin.
- Blood dyscrasias and full anticoagulant treatment. Intradural and extradural bleeding may occur.
- Stiff and unyielding back, from any cause.

Materials

- Sterile gloves and towels
- Antiseptic solution containing iodine, such as povidone-iodine (Betadine)
- 70% alcohol solution
- Gauze pads, 2 × 2 in.
- Spinal needle (22–25 gauge, 1½ in., with stylet)
- Manometer with three-way stopcock
- 0.5–1.0 mL 1% lidocaine HCl (Xylocaine HCl) and 2-mL syringe with 25-gauge needle
- Three sterile test tubes
- Adhesive strip

Preparation

1. Have the patient lie on one side.
2. With the help of an assistant, position the patient so that the lumbar vertebrae are flexed on each other as far as possible, the ligamenta flava are stretched, and the interlaminar spaces are increased. This will expand the target area and help ensure the success of the procedure, which is often determined by the ability to get the patient into the proper position.
3. The assistant should place one arm behind the patient's knees and one arm around the back of the patient's neck; he or she then flexes the patient's knees upward toward the chest and curls the patient's shoulders downward toward the umbilicus. With a small child, the assistant's arms will cradle the child (Figure 59-1).

Caution: Be careful that your assistant's head or breath does not contaminate the sterile field during the procedure.

4. Identify the site for puncture. At birth the spinal cord extends down to the body of the third lumbar vertebra, so in newborns the site of puncture should be the L3-4 interspace or below. During the first year of life the infant's vertebral column grows more rapidly than the spinal cord, and by about 1 year of age the spinal cord extends to only the L1-2 interspace, the adult position. In children older than 1 year, it is recommended but not absolutely necessary to perform the lumbar puncture at or below the L3-4 interspace. Find this interspace by drawing an imaginary line between the highest points of the patient's iliac crests (Figure 59-2).

Figure 59-1

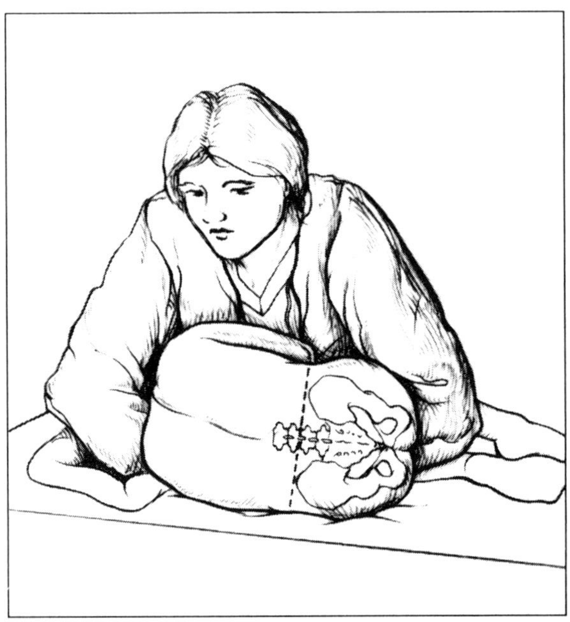

Figure 59-2

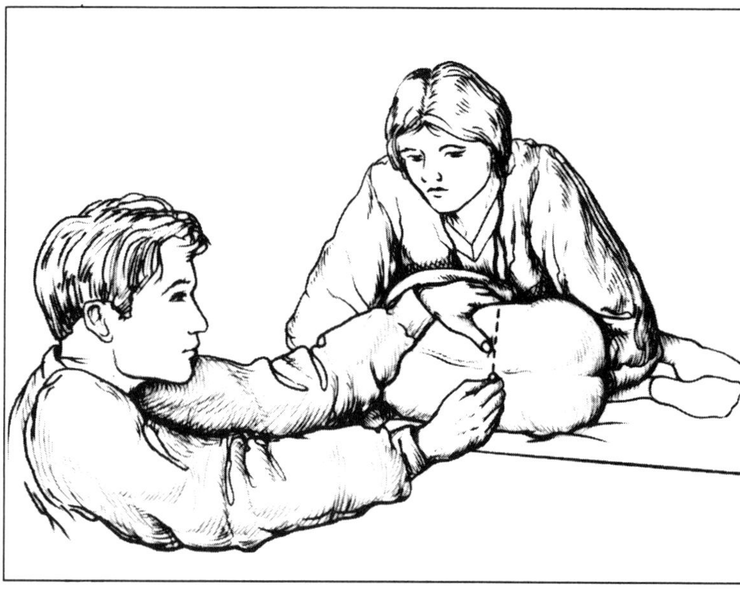

5. Observe strict antiseptic technique. Using gauze pads, first scrub the back with antiseptic, then with alcohol. Cleanse the puncture site first, then, using concentric circles, cleanse the area surrounding the puncture site.
6. Drape the patient's back with sterile towels.
7. In most infants the injection of anesthetic is as disturbing as the actual lumbar puncture and can be omitted. In older children, infiltrate the skin and subcutaneous tissue with 1% lidocaine HCl using a 2-mL syringe and a 25-gauge needle.

PROCEDURE

1. Place the needle on the skin at the L3-4 interspace in the midline. Line up your eye behind the hub of the needle, looking down the shaft. Keep the bevel facing cephalad.
2. Direct the needle slightly cephalad, toward the umbilicus. Advance it cautiously, either in millimeter steps or continuously, in the median plane.
3. You will feel a drop in resistance as the needle penetrates the dura (Figure 59-3). You will sometimes get the sensation that the needle is "popping" through the dura although this is seldom the case with infants.
4. Once the needle point penetrates the dura, remove the stylet. CSF should appear.
5. Check for free flow of fluid. If necessary, rotate, fractionally advance, or withdraw the needle.
6. Once free-flowing fluid appears, attach a three-way stopcock and

Figure 59-3

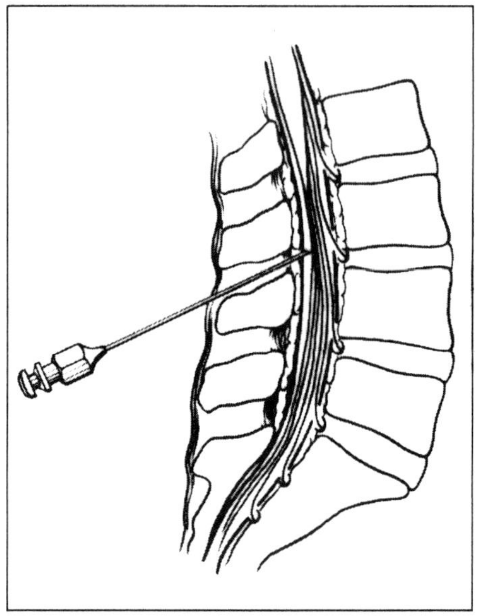

manometer to measure the CSF pressure. Unfortunately, these measurements are not clinically useful if the child is struggling. Then allow 0.5–1.0 mL CSF to drip into each of three sterile test tubes—the first for glucose and protein measurements; the second for Gram's stain, culture, and susceptibility studies; and the third for CBC and differential (Figure 59-4). Other less common tests on CSF are fungal culture, culture and smear for acid-fast bacillus, VDRL, and cytology studies

Figure 59-4

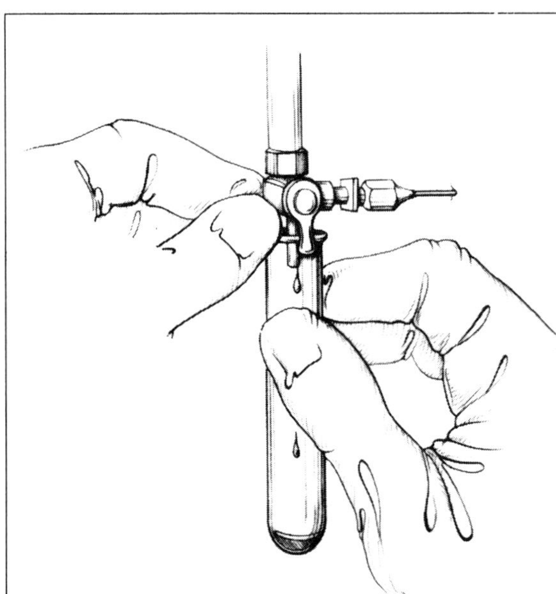

7. Measure the CSF pressure again.
8. Replace the stylet and withdraw the needle.
9. Dress the puncture site with an adhesive strip.

Complications

- Postpuncture headache, which occurs in one third of adults. It may also occur in children and may be relieved by bed rest.
- Blood-stained CSF from overadvancement of the needle with penetration of the venous plexus on the anterior aspect of the spinal canal. Such bleeding can cause irritation of spinal nerve roots with pain in the lower back and legs.
- Herniation of brain substance due to abnormally high intracranial pressure.
- Infection. A contaminated needle can introduce infection and cause bacterial meningitis.

Suggested Readings

Carbaat PAT, Van Crevel H: Lumbar puncture headache: Controlled study on the preventive effect of 24 hours' bed rest. *Lancet* 1981;2:1133-1135.

Custer JR: Special procedures, in Hoekelman RA, Blatman S, Friedman SB, et al (eds): *Primary Pediatric Care*. St. Louis, CV Mosby Co, 1987, pp 1659-1678.

Fingler RC: Pediatric regional anesthesia, in Gregory GA (ed): *Pediatric Anesthesia*. New York, Churchill Livingstone, 1983, pp 481-518.

Schreiner RL, Stevens DC, Jose JH, et al: Infant lumbar puncture: A teaching simulator. *Clin Pediatr* 1981;20(4):298-299.

60

Patient-Controlled Analgesia

George C. Xakellis, MD

Patient-controlled analgesia (PCA) is a relatively new method of pain control in which IV narcotic analgesic is delivered to the patient on demand. To receive a dose of narcotic analgesic, the patient pushes a button, and an electronic infusion pump delivers a prescribed dose into his or her IV line.

The patient is free to push the button as often as desired, but administration of the analgesic is usually limited to one dose during a specified amount of time—10 minutes, for example.

Indications

- Control of postoperative pain
- Control of other types of acute pain

Relative Contraindications

- Marginal respiratory status
- Significant mental status impairment
- Hypovolemia
- Poor patient understanding of the technique
- Patient history of drug abuse
- Untrained nursing personnel

Theoretical Basis for PCA

Among the assumptions to be made regarding PCA are these:

- Patients vary widely in the amount of analgesic required for adequate pain control.
- Predicting an adequate analgesic dose and dosing schedule for an individual is extremely difficult.

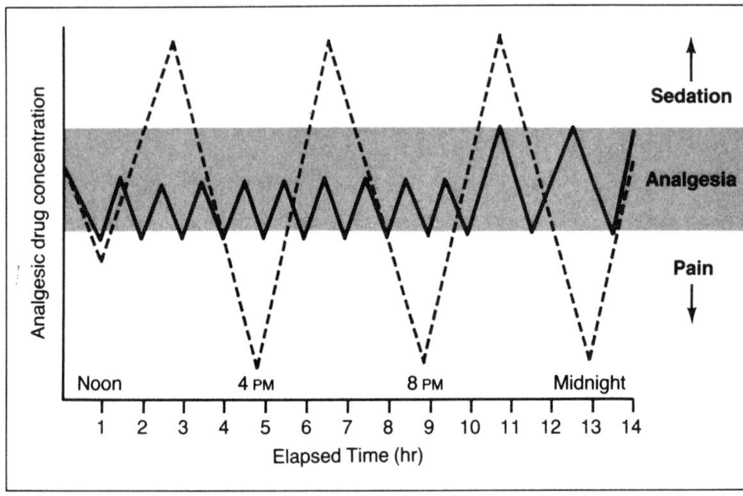

Figure 60-1 The theoretical relationship among dosing interval, analgesic drug concentration, and clinical effects is shown in this graph, which compares a system of patient-controlled analgesia (solid lines) with conventional IM therapy (dashed lines). Conventional therapy often leads to an initial overshooting of the therapeutic range and subsequent sedation; this is followed by a drop in serum levels below the therapeutic level and a worsening of pain.

- Normal analgesic dosing schedules of IM injections every three hours often lead to an initial overshooting of the therapeutic range, causing unnecessary sedation. This is followed by a drop in serum levels below the therapeutic level and a worsening of pain (Figure 60-1).
- With proper instruction, patients can monitor their pain level and self-administer the analgesic as needed.
- Technology is available that will not only deliver a metered dose but also define a maximum dosing frequency and thereby minimize the risk of accidental overdose.

Potential benefits of the procedure are as follows:

- The patient may improve pain control and require less narcotic analgesic.
- The postoperative patient may become mobile more rapidly.
- Self-control over the analgesic dosing schedule may increase the patient's satisfaction with his care.

Materials

- An infusion pump, with the following features:[1]

1. Computerized controls to set the infusion rate, the size of the analgesic bolus, and the minimum time interval between boluses.
2. Computerized record-keeping software that records the number of doses requested, the number of doses given, and the total amount of analgesic administered.
3. A patient-operated, push-button control to deliver the analgesic.

- A 30–60-mL syringe of analgesic such as morphine in a concentration of 1 mg/mL

[1] Such units are available from several manufacturers.

- IV tubing to attach the infusion pump to the patient's maintenance IV line
- A one-way valve on the IV tubing to prevent a backflow of analgesic into the maintenance IV bag

PROCEDURE

The patient self-medicates within the parameters programmed into the infusion pump by pushing the button each time he wants pain relief.

- Instruct nurses in the theory underlying the use of PCA before implementing the procedure.
- Have the nursing staff practice using the equipment, placing the analgesic-filled syringe into the infusion pump, and programming the dosing schedule.
- Instruct the patient in the theory of PCA and the operation of the device before surgery.
- Give an initial dose of narcotic analgesic in the recovery room to start to establish adequate pain control. Then order the PCA narcotic. A typical order is a 60-mL syringe with morphine in a 1 mg/mL concentration. Specify the amount to be delivered with each patient request, such as 1 mg, and the minimum time interval between doses, such as 10 minutes. Some systems also allow for the specification of a basal infusion rate, such as 1 mg/hr, in addition to the patient-controlled boluses.
- Have the nurse program the infuser. Have a second nurse double-check the programming.
- Monitor respiratory rate and pain control frequently during the first several postoperative hours. Adjust the analgesic dose as necessary. Continue to monitor the patient's respiratory status.
- Expect the patient's use of analgesic to be highest in the initial postoperative period and then gradually to decrease.

Complications

- Nausea and vomiting.
- Respiratory depression, excessive sedation, or both. These may be due to incorrect programming of the infusion pump or overestimation of the analgesic dose required for pain control.
- Inadequate pain relief.

Suggested Readings

White PF: Patient-controlled analgesia: A new approach to the management of postoperative pain. *Semin Anesthes* 1985;4:255-266.

White PF: Use of patient-controlled analgesia for management of acute pain. *JAMA* 1988;259:243-247.

XI

BEHAVIORAL MEDICINE PROCEDURES

61

Progressive Muscle Relaxation

Georgianna S. Hoffmann, RN, MA, CS

Helping patients learn relaxation techniques to aid stress reduction and management is based on the concept of the mind–body connection: Whatever relaxes the musculature produces mental relaxation and vice versa. Since the relaxation response counteracts the stress response, it is impossible to be both relaxed and tense at the same time. Further, the relaxation response can reduce existing distress and eventually ameliorate its effect. Progressive muscle relaxation is a simple and effective way to help patients learn how to relax.

Indications

- Chronic tension headaches or muscular pain apparently unrelated to organic causes
- Migraine
- Feelings of hostility and of being driven by pressures of time (typical of a type A personality)
- Feelings of being overwhelmed by the stresses of daily living
- Sleep problems
- Panic disorder
- Traumatic neurosis

Contraindications

- A tenuous hold on reality
- Active psychosis

Materials

- A recliner with head and foot rests is ideal. The patient can also lie on a couch or on a pad on the floor with a pillow under his or her head and knees. Enhance comfort in any way possible.

- Soft lighting and a quiet atmosphere are helpful, along with no telephones or interruptions. Restful, soft background music is optional.
- The relaxation script (see Procedure).

Preparation

- Whenever possible, include the patient's spouse, partner, or other family member in the training. This can provide support for practice at home. If family members are not supportive, they may resent the time required for practice and sabotage the process.
- Discuss the mind–body connection.
- Describe the relaxed state as the middle ground between full waking consciousness and sleep. Explain that the goal is to learn to identify the feeling of hovering comfortably there, as well as to find the most efficient way for this particular patient to reach the relaxed state.
- Emphasize the importance of a comfortable, quiet, interruption-free environment for practice.
- Have the patient loosen any constricting clothing or shoes, settle back comfortably, and close his eyes.
- Have him stretch out his arms comfortably at his side, stretch out his legs, and keep his ankles uncrossed.
- Be sure you are seated comfortably, too. Take a few deep, slow breaths before you begin. Your own level of relaxation will be communicated as you read the script. Attending to your own relaxation level will benefit both the patient and you: Read the script very slowly in a calm hypnotic voice. Breathe deeply and slowly yourself when you instruct the patient or patients to do so.

PROCEDURE

SCRIPT[1]

1. Now I'd like you to close your eyes and settle back as comfortably as you can. Let yourself relax to the best of your ability. Take a deep breath, and let it out very slowly. And now take another deep breath, and let it out very slowly and completely.
2. Now, as you relax like that, clench your *right fist* very tightly. Clench it even tighter, and study the tension as you do so. Keep it clenched, and feel the tension in your *right fist, hand,* and *forearm.* (Pause.) Now relax. Let the fingers of your *right hand* become loose, and let your hand open into a resting position. (Pause.) Now, sense the contrast in your feeling. Let yourself go, and try to become more

[1]Adapted with permission from Wolpe J, Lazarus A: *Behavior Therapy Techniques.* Oxford, Pergamon Press, 1966.

relaxed all over. Once more, clench your *right fist* very tightly, hold it, and notice the tension again. (Pause.) Now let go and relax. Let your fingers straighten out, and notice the difference once more.

3. Now repeat that with your *left fist.* Clench your *left fist* very tightly, while the rest of your body relaxes. Clench your fist as tightly as you can, and feel the tension in your *left hand* and *forearm.* (Pause.) And now relax. Let go of the tension, let your fingers relax, and again enjoy the contrast. (Pause.) Repeat that once more. Clench your *left fist* tightly, and notice the tension. (Pause.) Now do the opposite of tension; relax and feel the difference. Continue relaxing like that for awhile, and as you do, take a deep breath, and let it out very slowly.

4. Now clench *both fists*. Notice the tension in your *hands* and in your *forearms,* and study the feeling of that tension. (Pause.) Now relax *both hands* and *arms,* straighten out your fingers, and feel the relaxation flow into your hands. Continue relaxing your hands and forearms more and more. (Pause.)

5. Now bend your elbows, bring your hands up toward your shoulders, and tense your *biceps*. Tense your *biceps* harder, and study the feelings of tension. (Pause.) All right, now straighten out your arms, put your hands back down, let your arms relax, and feel that difference again. (Pause.) Let the relaxation develop all over your body. (Pause.) Once more, bring your hands up, tense your *biceps* again, hold the tension, and observe it carefully. Now straighten your arms again, and relax to the best of your ability. Take a deep breath, and let it out very slowly and completely. Each time, pay close attention to your feelings. When you tense up and when you relax, notice the difference. (Pause.)

6. Now hold both arms out straight in front of you, and tighten them so that you feel most of the tension in the *triceps* along the *back* of your arms. Stretch your arms, and concentrate on the tension in your *triceps.* (Pause.) And now relax, put your arms back down in a comfortable position, and let the relaxation proceed on its own. Your arms should feel comfortably heavy as you let them relax. (Pause.) Straighten your arms once more so that you feel tension in the *triceps,* hold the position tightly, feel the tension. Now relax. (Pause.) Let your arms go down to a resting position, and concentrate on pure relaxation in your arms without any tension. Let your arms relax very comfortably, and then let them relax further and further. Continue relaxing your arms even more; when they seem fully relaxed, try to go an extra bit further. Let yourself achieve deeper and deeper levels of relaxation. (Pause.)

7. Now we are going to attend to your *facial area,* as well as your *neck, shoulders,* and *upper back.* Let all of your muscles go loose and heavy. Let yourself be quiet and comfortable. Now I'd like you to wrinkle up your *forehead,* wrinkle it still tighter, and hold the tension. (Pause.) Now relax. Stop wrinkling your *forehead,* and let it smooth out. Picture your entire *forehead* and *scalp* becoming smoother and smoother as the relaxation increases. (Pause.) Now frown, crease your brows, and study the tension. (Pause.) Let go of the tension again, and smooth out your *forehead* once more. Let it become smoother and smoother, and notice the contrast. (Pause.) Now close your eyes tighter and tighter, and feel the tension as you squeeze them together. (Pause.) Now relax your eyes, and let them be closed gently and comfortably. Notice the relaxation as it develops in your *eyes* and *forehead* and *scalp*. (Pause.) Take a deep breath, and let it out very slowly.

8. Now clench your *jaws,* bite your teeth together, and study the tension throughout your *jaws.* (Pause.) Now relax your *jaws,* and let your lips part slightly as you feel the relaxation develop. (Pause.) Now again, clench your *jaws,* bite your teeth together, and study the tension throughout your *jaws*. (Pause.) Now relax. Let your *lips* part slightly, and appreciate the relaxation. (Pause.) Now press your *tongue* hard against the roof of your *mouth*, and look for the tension as you do this. (Pause.) All right, let your *tongue* return to a relaxed and comfortable position, and let your *mouth* and *jaws* relax as you do this. (Pause.) Now purse your *lips,* pressing them together tighter and tighter. (Pause.) Now relax your *lips,* and note the contrast between tension and relaxation. Feel the relaxation all over your *face,* all over your *forehead* and *scalp,* your *eyes, jaws, lips, tongue,* and *throat.* The relaxation progresses further and further as you breathe deeply and slowly. (Pause.)

9. Now we will attend to your *neck* muscles. Press your *head* back as far as it can go, and feel the tension in your *neck*. Roll your *head* to the right, and feel the tension shift. (Pause.) Now roll it to the left, and feel the tension shift again. (Pause.) Bring your *head* back to the center position, and then bring it forward, pressing your chin against your chest. Now let your *head* return to a comfortable position. Let the relaxation develop and study the feelings. (Pause.)

10. Now shrug your *shoulders* up, bring them up as close to your ears as you can get them, hold the tension, and study it. (Pause.) Now, let your *shoulders* relax, and appreciate the difference. Shrug your *shoulders* up again, then bring them forward as far as you can and back as far as you can. Feel the tension in your *shoulders* and *upper back.* (Pause.) Now drop your *shoulders* and relax. Let the relaxation spread deep into your *shoulders,* right into your *back* muscles. Relax your *neck* and *throat,* your *jaws* and other *facial areas* as the pure relaxation takes over and grows deeper, and deeper, and even deeper. (Pause.)

11. Continue to relax your *entire body* to the best of your ability. Feel that comfortable heaviness that accompanies relaxation. Breathe easily and freely, in and out. Notice how the relaxation increases as you exhale. As you breathe out, feel the relaxation develop. Now breathe right in, and fill your *lungs;* inhale deeply and hold your breath. Study the tension. (Pause.) Now exhale, let the walls of your *chest* grow loose, and push the air out automatically. Continue relaxing and breathe freely and gently. Feel the relaxation and enjoy it. (Pause.) With the rest of your body as relaxed as possible, fill your *lungs* again, breathe in deeply, and hold it again. That's fine. Breathe out now, and appreciate the relief. Let yourself breathe normally. (Pause.) Continue relaxing your *chest,* and let the relaxation spread to your *back, shoulders, neck,* and *arms.* Just let go and enjoy the relaxation. (Pause.)

12. Now pay attention to your abdominal muscles, your stomach area. Tighten your *stomach muscles,* and make your abdomen hard. Notice the tension. (Pause.) Now let go of all the tension and relax. Loosen the muscles, and notice the contrast. (Pause.) Once more, press and tighten your *stomach muscles,* hold the tension, and study it. (Pause.) Now relax and notice the general feeling of well-being that comes with relaxing your *stomach.* (Pause.) Now draw your *stomach* in, and feel the tension this way. (Pause.) Now relax again. Let your *stomach* out, and continue breathing normally and easily. Feel the gentle massaging action of your breathing all over your *chest* and *stomach*. (Pause.) Now pull your *stomach* in again, and hold the tension. Now push your *stomach* out, tense it, and hold that tension. (Pause.) Once more, pull your *stomach* in, and feel the tension. Now relax your *stomach* fully. Let the tension dissolve. Let the relaxation develop, both in your *lungs* and in your *stomach.* Notice how this relaxes your *chest* and *stomach* more and more. Try to let go of all contraction, all muscle tightness, anywhere in your body. (Pause.) Take a deep breath, and let it out slowly and gently. (Pause.)

13. Now direct your attention to your *lower back*. Arch your *back,* make your *lower back* quite hollow, and feel the tension as you do this. Try to keep the rest of your body as relaxed as possible. Try to localize the tension throughout your *lower back.* (Pause.) Relax again, and let yourself relax further and further. Relax your *lower back,* relax your *upper back* (pause), and spread the relaxation to your *stomach, chest, shoulders, arms, neck,* and *facial areas.* Feel all of these parts relaxing further and further, and even further, as you relax more and more deeply. (Pause.) Take a deep breath, and let it out very slowly and completely. If there is any tension remaining in your body, try to let go of it and relax even further. (Pause.)

14. Now attend to the lower part of your body. Flex your *buttocks* and *thighs.* Squeeze your *buttocks* together, and flex your *thighs* by pressing down on your heels as hard as you can. (Pause.) Now relax and notice the difference. (Pause.) Now straighten your *legs,* tighten your *thigh muscles,* and hold the tension. (Pause.) Now press your *feet* and *toes* downward, away from your face, so that you feel the tension in your *shins.* (Pause.) Now bring your *toes* straight up toward your face, and hold the tension. (Pause.) Now relax again, and keep relaxing for a while. (Pause.) Take a deep breath, and let it out very slowly.

15. Now let yourself relax even more *all over your body.* Relax your *feet, ankles, calves* and *shins, knees, thighs, buttocks,* and *hips.* Feel the heaviness of your lower body, as you relax still further. Now spread the relaxation to your *stomach, waist,* and *lower back.* Let go more and more. Feel the relaxation spreading all over your body. Let it proceed to your *upper back, chest, shoulders,* and *arms* and right down to the tips of your *fingers.* Keep relaxing more and more deeply. Make sure that no tension has crept into your *throat.* Relax your *neck,* your *jaws,* and all of your *facial muscles.* Keep relaxing your whole body like that for awhile, and enjoy the relaxation. (Pause.)

16. Now you can become twice as relaxed as you are merely by taking in a really deep breath and exhaling slowly. Breathe in deeply, and feel yourself becoming heavier and heavier. Take in a long deep breath, and let it out very slowly. Feel how heavy and relaxed you have become. Now you can say to yourself, "I am very much at rest." In a state of perfect relaxation you should feel unwilling to move a single muscle in your body. Think about the effort it would take to raise your right arm. As you think about raising your right arm, see if you can notice any tension that might have crept into your shoulder and your arm. Now you decide not to lift the arm, but to continue relaxing instead. Observe the relief and the disappearance of the tension. Just go on relaxing like that for as long as you like.

17. When you want to get up, count backward from four to one. Your eyes will open at the count of one, and you will feel fine—relaxed, refreshed, wide-awake, and calm.

Follow-up Care

- Give the patient a copy of the script, and advise practicing daily or at least three times a week. Regular practice is necessary to learn relaxation skills.
- Arranging for a family member or friend to read the script at first can help the learning procedure, and help both people relax.
- See the patient after one week to review experiences with the practice sessions and find out if he has any problems—which often involve finding the time to do the practice.
- Occasionally, a patient who has carried a great deal of muscle tension without knowing it may temporarily experience pain as he begins to learn relaxation skills. Encourage him to continue practicing until the pain is gone.
- At the close of the teaching session in your office, be sure the patient is fully alert and able to function safely before he leaves. Emphasize the importance of this caution each time the patient practices, since deep relaxation produces an altered state of consciousness.

Suggested Readings

Bernstein DA, Borkovec TD: *Progressive Relaxation Training: A Manual for the Helping Professions*. Champaign, Ill, Research Press, 1973.

Brallier L: *Successfully Managing Stress*. Los Altos, Calif, National Nursing Review, 1982.

Davis M, McKay M, Eshelman E: *The Relaxation and Stress Reduction Workbook*, ed 2. Oakland, Calif, New Harbinger Publications, 1982.

Sehnert KW: *Stress/Unstress: How You Can Control Stress at Home and on the Job*. Minneapolis, Augsburg Publishing House, 1981.

Stress Without Distress: A Guide to Self-Understanding and Prevention of Stress-Related Illness and Premature Death. Bozeman, Mont, Montana State University, 1981.

Tapes

Halpern S: *Spectrum Suite.* Halpern Sound, Belmont, Calif.

Miller E, Halpern S: *Letting Go of Stress*. Halpern Sound, *Suite.* Halpern Sound, Belmont, Calif.

62

Hypnosis in Office Practice

Leslie E. Weber, MD

Hypnosis in various forms has been used through the ages for many purposes. From time to time it has fallen into disfavor, but in recent years it has regained credibility and is now recognized as a valuable tool for a variety of problems.

Patients seen in primary care practice often have a significant emotional component in their presenting problems, of course, and many physical ailments have emotional elements. Used effectively, hypnosis can treat many such conditions.

Hypnosis techniques, now taught in many seminars and continuing medical education courses, are not difficult to learn. It's the application of the techniques that requires the greatest skill. (For more information, see the hypnosis societies listed on page 418.)

Characteristics of Hypnosis

- Hypnosis can be defined as "A state of altered awareness, usually but not always involving physical relaxation, in which the individual is able to accept suggestion to maximize performance in certain areas." The individual's attention is focused on potent internal images to the exclusion of the external environment.
- Hypnosis is as effective as many therapeutic agents, and the patient learns to have control at all times. The greatest advantage is that the patient may induce the trance state whenever he or she needs it, with no side effects, a claim that cannot be made for any medication.
- Using hypnosis effectively depends on the patient's ability to master the technique of self-hypnosis; maximum effectiveness comes from regular and frequent use and his or her learning to apply it appropriately.

Who Can Be Hypnotized

There are three levels of hypnosis. Some 95% of individuals can be hypnotized, and more than 50% can reach a therapeutic level at which most goals can be reached. About 20% will reach a trance state deep enough to attain major analgesia. The remainder attain a superficial level where they can get minimal but useful benefit in relaxation.

Indications

In the primary care setting, hypnosis is used mainly to control anxiety, as in these applications:

- Improving communication between physician and patients.
- Enabling patients to contribute to their own healing.
- Reducing time and morbidity in dealing with emergencies.
- Helping to implement a treatment of choice.
- Providing quick and easy self-relaxation.

Other important uses may include treating

- Habit and behavior problems, such as smoking, nail-biting, and eating disorders.
- Psychophysiologic disorders such as acute anxiety states, phobias, panic disorders, temporomandibular joint syndrome, and migraine.
- Acute and chronic pain.
- Various situations in obstetrics and pediatrics.

Contraindications

Do not use hypnosis when

- It would physically endanger the patient.
- Its only purpose is entertainment or curiosity.
- It would aggravate existing emotional problems or create new ones.
- Another mode of therapy would be more appropriate.
- Secondary gain is a motive, possibly inhibiting or deterring the patient's response to hypnotherapy.
- The diagnosis is incorrect, and a treatment other than hypnosis is warranted.
- The patient has a psychotic illness.

Materials

Nothing special is required. A quiet room with comfortable chairs is helpful, and the session should be uninterrupted and unhurried.

Preparation

- Begin by assessing the patient's problem and familiarizing yourself with significant historical and physical findings.
- Give the patient a complete, simple explanation of hypnosis to preclude misconceptions. Explain what can and cannot be accomplished. Assure him that it will never cause him harm, embarrassment, or loss of dignity.

- Emphasize that the value of hypnosis is in his ability to become an effective self-hypnotist and that it will be most effective if he uses it when he needs it most.
- Become familiar with the patient's occupation, interests, hobbies. Imagery is important in inducing a hypnotic trance, and familiar reminders help stimulate the imagination.
- With the patient's help, outline treatment goals and estimate the time it might take. Most patients can become accomplished self-hypnotists in two or three sessions, with additional sessions sometimes needed to develop further understanding or reinforce techniques.

PROCEDURE

1. Have the patient stare at a small object or focus of light, for eye fixation. The target should be slightly above eye level, to induce eye muscle fatigue and enhance the desire to eventually let the eyelids close. (Some hypnotists begin with a brief suggestibility test, but most feel this is not time-effective.)
2. Arm levitation often helps. Suggest that the arm feels light and will float. Do so, as in all instructions, in a slow, monotonous voice.
3. Encourage the patient to focus on sensory perceptions such as temperature differences, visual images, odors, distinctive sounds. This helps him sense that what he is experiencing is real.
4. Direct the patient to focus on the automatic nature of his breathing. Suggest that breathing will coordinate with total body relaxation, beginning with the feet and going up the body toward the head. Continue commands in a slow repetitive voice to encourage relaxation.
5. Make use of imagery, of the "Imagine that you are . . ." variety. Encourage recall of pleasant feelings from the patient's past. Suggest that he may recreate them and enjoy them later.
6. After the patient achieves this relaxed state, use a deepening exercise to reinforce total relaxation. Suggestibility is most effective at this stage. Mental images experienced now will most likely remain in the patient's memory. Say something like "This will remain burned in your memory even after returning to full awareness." Since posthypnotic suggestion is strong, give directions for recall, and concentrate on the suggestions needed to alter the patient's behavior—and thus to effect the cure.
7. Before suggesting a return to full awareness, give a simple posthypnotic suggestion to later demonstrate the power of the technique, such as "You will have an itchy nose when I rub my hand." At the posthypnotic cue, the patient will usually follow the suggestion.
8. Tell the patient to induce self-hypnotic trances frequently; it gets easier with practice. Reassure him that he can induce a trance without your being there. Many patients respond to the invitation, "Take my voice with you."

9. Tell the patient that he should teach himself to recall these five messages during his self-induced trances:

- You will be relaxed and rested as though you just had a nap, but without lethargy.
- You will feel less pain and muscle tension.
- You will have heightened powers of concentration.
- You will feel very self-confident.
- You will be able to suppress negative thoughts and pessimism.

10. Assure the patient that self-inductions will become progressively easier, that he will gain confidence in the power of hypnosis to help solve his problems, and that no one can induce a trance in him except for therapeutic reasons. This last suggestion makes it impossible to induce a trance solely for entertainment.

11. Bring the patient out of his trance with a straightforward directive.

Follow-up Care

- Schedule a return visit in a few days to evaluate the self-hypnosis technique. Teach the patient a quick induction technique to be used any time to recall and reinforce suggestions for a specific need. Many patients respond to the idea of "turning on a switch," which enables them to induce a trance state in a minute or less. The trance state may be brief, but is enough for the patient to call up appropriate suggestions.
- If a patient has complex problems, you may want to schedule additional visits in order to provide the patient for detailed instruction about more specialized needs.
- Suggest that a patient return for reinforcing techniques or telephone any time he feels the need. Most patients, once they learn this relaxation device, will encounter new situations where hypnosis can help.

Suggested Readings

For general information, contact

The American Society of Clinical Hypnosis
2250 East Devon Ave.
Suite 336
Des Plaines, IL 60018

The Society for Clinical and Experimental Hypnosis
128-A Kings Park Dr.
Liverpool, NY 13090

Additional Readings

Ambrose G, Newbold G: *A Handbook of Medical Hypnosis.* London, Bailliere Tindall, 1980.

Crasilneck HB, Hall JA: *Clinical Hypnosis: Principles and Applications,* ed 2. New York, Grune & Stratton Inc, 1985.

Hall JA, Crasilneck HB: Hypnosis. *JAMA* 1978;239:760-761.

O'Hanlon WH: *Taproots: Underlying Principles of Milton Erickson's Therapy and Hypnosis.* New York, Norton, 1987.

Spiegel D: The use of hypnosis in controlling cancer pain. *CA* 1985;35:221-231.

Wain HJ (ed): *Hypnosis in Clinical Medicine.* Chicago, Year Book Medical Pubs, 1980.

Index

[*Note:* Entries with the letter "n" refer to footnotes on the page indicated.]

A

Abscess(es):
  incision/drainage of, 307–311
    antibiotics and, 307–308
    complications from, 310–311
    contraindications for, 307
    follow-up care for, 310
    indications for, 307
    materials for, 308
    procedure for, 308–310, 311
  from intraosseous infusion, 19
  microbiology of, 307–308
Acetic acid, for androscopy, 223, 224
Acid-base disturbance, arterial puncture for, 103
Acute otitis media (AOM), cerumen removal and, 361
AIDS, instrument sterilization and, 125
Air embolism:
  from internal jugular vein cannulation, 48
  from IV, 7
Airway:
  control of, tactile orotracheal intubation for, 100
  obstruction of, in child, 41–44
  trauma to, from tactile orotracheal intubation, 102
Aluminum acetate (Domeboro), for paronychia, 313
American Academy of Family Physicians, 57
American Academy of Pediatrics, 41, 201
American Cancer Society, 120
American Heart Association, 45, 54, 62
Analgesic, patient-controlled (PCA), 401–403
Anaprox. *See* Naproxen sodium
Androscopy, 223–225
  follow-up care for, 225
  indications for, 223
  materials for, 223–224
  procedure for, 224–225
Anesthesia, 5, 12, 18, 46, 54, 69, 80, 91, 92, 96, 158, 175, 178–179, 197, 231, 243, 255, 301, 308–309, 327, 382, 397. *See also* Bupivacaine; Chloroprocaine; Cocaine; Ethyl chloride spray; Lidocaine; Mepivacaine; Procaine
  administration of, 269–282
  agents for, 269
  doses of, 270
  epinephrine and, 269–270. *See also* Epinephrine
  forms of, 269
  local,
    digital, 271–272, 320
    indications for, 270
    materials for, 270
    procedure for, 270–271
  precautions for, 269–270
  regional,
    for ankle blocks, 278, 280–281
    indications for, 271
    for infraorbital nerve block, 275–276, 278
    for intercostal nerve block, 276–277, 279
    with IV, 281–282
    materials for, 271
    metacarpal/metatarsal, 272
    procedure for, 271
    for supraorbital nerve block, 275, 277
    for wrist blocks, 273–274, 276
  toxicity from, 168, 172, 269
Angina, exercise testing and, 57
Angioplasty, exercise testing and, 58
Ankle:
  anesthesia for, 278, 280–281
  aspiration/injection of, 160
  compressive splinting for, 181
Antecubital veins, IV in, 10
Anterior epistaxis, 373
Antibiotics, for abscesses, 307–308
Anxiety, hypnosis for, 416
AOM. *See* Acute otitis media
Arterial puncture:
  for blood gas specimens, 103–107
  complications from, 106

Arterial puncture (*Continued*)
contraindications for, 103
indications for, 103
materials for, 103
preparation for, 104
procedure for, 105–106
Arterial thrombosis, from arterial puncture, 106
Ascites, paracentesis for, 133, 138
Asphyxia, from cricothyroidotomy, 81
Aspiration:
of breast, 237–241
from cricothyroidotomy, 81
endotracheal intubation for, 73
foreign body, death among children from, 41
from gastric intubation, 116–117
of joints, 157–165
for priapism treatment, 219–221
Atrium, right, perforation of, 49
Atrophic vaginitis, 260

B

Bacitracin, for peritoneal lavage, 133
Bacterial infections, Wood's light examination for, 346–347
Barium enema, for rubber band ligation of hemorrhoids, 128
Behavior problems, hypnosis for, 416
Behavioral medicine procedures, 407–419
hypnosis, 415–419
progressive muscle relaxation, 407–413
Beta-blockers, exercise testing and, 60
Beta$_2$-adrenergic inhalational agent, for spirometry, 86
Biopsy:
for breast tumor evaluation, 237
endometrial, 243–247, 261–266
punch, 283–286
of uterine cervix, 249–252
Bisacodyl suppository:
for constipation, 144
for flexible fiberoptic sigmoidoscopy, 121
Biting injury, from tactile orotracheal intubation, 102
Bivalving of glans, from newborn circumcision, 209
Black light. *See* Wood's light
Bleeding:
from biopsy of uterine cervix, 252
from fecal impaction removal, 143
from incision/drainage of abscesses, 311
from IUD insertion, 230–231, 235
from lumbar puncture, 394, 399
from paracentesis, 138
Blood gas specimens, arterial puncture for, 103–107
Blood pressure irregularities, from priapism treatment, 222
Blood transfusion, through intraosseous infusion, 15
Body composition, skinfold measurements for, 145
Body fat measurements:
guidelines for evaluating, 145
for men, 148
for women, 147
Bone marrow infusion. *See* Intraosseous infusion
Borg Scale of Perceived Exertion, 62
Bowel perforation, from paracentesis, 138
Bowenoid papulosis, androscopy and, 223
Brain herniation, from lumbar puncture, 394, 399
Breast, fine-needle aspiration of, 237–241
complications from, 241
indications for, 237
limiting factors for, 238
materials for, 238
procedure for, 238–241
Bronchitis, laryngoscopy for, 353
Bronchus, right main-stem, intubation of, 102
Bupivacaine (Marcaine, Sensorcaine), 269
maximum recommended doses of, 270
in trigger points, 167

C

Calan. *See* Verapamil
Cancer:
breast, 237–241
cervical, 249, 250
colorectal, 119–125
uterine, 243–247
Cannulation:
of femoral vein, 21–26
of internal jugular vein, 45–49
Carbocaine. *See* Mepivacaine
Carbon dioxide laser fulguration, for HPV treatment, 225
Cardiopulmonary arrest, from endotracheal intubation, 77
Cardiopulmonary resuscitation (CPR):
for adult, 27–31, 34
for child, 33–39
complications from, 31
endotracheal intubation and, 73–78
gastric intubation and, 111
for infant, 33–39
interruption of, from endotracheal intubation, 77
personnel for, 27
Cardiovascular procedures, 3–63
airway obstruction, in child, 41–44
CPR, in adult, 27–31, 34
CPR, in child, 33–39
defibrillation, 51–55
exercise treadmill testing, 57–63
femoral vein cannulation, 21–26
internal jugular vein cannulation, 45–49
IV, in adult, 3–7
IV, in newborn, 9–13
Cardioversion, electrical, 54
Cardizem. *See* Diltiazem
Catheter:
for central venous cannulation, 21
for IV in adult, 3–7
Swan-Ganz, 21, 45
wire-guided (Seldinger), 21–25
Catheter fragment embolism, from IV, 7

Catheterization:
  of internal jugular vein, 45–49
  urinary, 211–217
Cellulitis:
  from intraosseous infusion, 19
  from IV, 7
  from needle thoracentesis, 96
Cerebrospinal fluid (CSF), 390, 391, 392, 393, 394, 397, 398
Cerumen. *See* Earwax
Ceruminolytics, for earwax softening, 362
Cervical lymphadenopathy, laryngoscopy for, 353
Cervix, biopsy of, 249–252
Chest:
  injuries to, chest tube insertion for, 89–97
  pain in,
    anesthesia for, 276–277, 279
    exercise treadmill testing for, 57
    from fecal impaction removal, 221
  tube insertion into, 89–97
    complications from, 96–97
    contraindications for, 90
    follow-up care, 95
    indications for, 89–90
    materials for, 90
    needle thoracentesis and, 90–91, 96
    procedure for, 92–95
    removal and, 96
Child. *See also* Infant; Newborn
  airway obstruction in, 41–44
  clavicular fracture immobilization for, 187, 192
  CPR for, 33–39
  cricothyroidotomy in, 79n
  lumbar puncture in, 395–399
  suprapubic bladder tap for, 197–199
Chloroprocaine (Nesacaine), 269
Circumcision:
  arguments for and against, 201
  complications from, 209
  contraindications for, 201–202
  follow-up care for, 208–209
  materials for, 202
  procedure for, 202–208
Clavicular fracture:
  immobilization of, 185–194
    for child, 187, 192
    contraindications for, 188
    follow-up care for, 192–193
    indications for, 187
    materials for, 188
    for newborns, 187
    procedures for, 188–192
  incidence of, 185
  types of, 185–187
Cocaine, 173, 375
Colorectal cancer:
  detection of, 119
  flexible fiberoptic sigmoidoscopy for, 119–125
Colposcope, for androscopy, 224
Colposcopy, with guided biopsy, 249
Compressive ankle splinting, 181–184
  contraindication for, 181
  follow-up care for, 183–184
  indications for, 181
  materials for, 181
  procedure for, 181–183
Conjunctiva, foreign bodies in, 381, 382, 383–384, 385
Connective tissue procedures. *See* Musculoskeletal/connective tissue procedures
Constipation:
  fecal impaction and, 141
  treatment of, 143–144
Cornea, foreign bodies in, 382, 383, 384–385
Coronary bypass, exercise testing and, 58
Cortex, small needle-hole defect in, 19
Corticosteroids, joint injection of, 157, 162, 163
Cotton-ball wick, for cryotherapy, 292, 293, 294–295
Cotton wick insertion, for ingrown toenail, 319, 320–323
CPR. *See* Cardiopulmonary resuscitation
Cramps, from endometrial biopsy, 245
Cricothyroidotomy, 79–83, 99
  in adult,
    complications from, 81, 83
    procedures for, 80–81, 82, 83
  in child, 79n
  indications for, 79
  materials for, 79–80
Cryoprobe gun, for cryotherapy, 292, 293, 295, 296–297
Cryotherapy:
  approaches of, 291
  contraindications for, 292
  for HPV treatment, 225
  indications for, 291
  materials for, 292
  preparation for, 294
  procedure for, 294–298
  for skin lesions, 291–298
  techniques for, 292, 293
Culdocentesis, 253–256
  complications from, 256
  contraindications for, 253
  indications for, 253
  interpretation of, 255–256
  materials for, 254
  procedure for, 254–255
Cu-7 IUD, 229, 237
Cutaneous abscesses, incision/drainage of, 307–311
Cyst:
  breast, 237
  ovarian, 253
  skin, 287–289
Cystitis, from urinary catheterization, 211

D

Defibrillation, electrical, 51–55
  cardioversion and, 54
  contraindication for, 53
  indications for, 53
  materials for, 53

Defibrillation, electrical (*Continued*)
  paddle placement for, 52–53
  procedure for, 53–54
  transthoracic resistance and, 51
Delivery, without episiotomy, 257–260
  complications from, 260
  contraindications for, 258
  follow-up care for, 260
  indications for, 258
  preparation for, 258
  procedure for, 258–259
Dermatology procedures, 269–349
  cryotherapy for skin lesions, 291–298
  cutaneous abscess incision/drainage, 307–311
  electrocoagulation, 337–343
  fishhook removal, 331–335
  ingrown toenail treatment, 319–325
  local anesthesia administration, 269–282
  paronychia, 313–317
  punch biopsy of skin, 283–286
  ring removal from swollen finger, 327–330
  simple laceration repair, 299–306
  skin cyst removal, 287–289
  Wood's light examination, 345–349
Diazepam (Valium):
  for anesthesia toxicity, 269
  for cardioversion, 54
  as cause of priapism, 219
  for gastric intubation, 114
Digoxin (Lanoxin), exercise testing and, 60
Diltiazem (Cardizem), exercise testing and, 60
Diuretics, exercise testing and, 60
Dobutamine (Dobutrex), through intraosseous infusion, 15
Docusate sodium, for constipation, 143
Domeboro. *See* Aluminum acetate
Dopamine (Dopastat, Intropin), through intraosseous infusion, 15
Dorsal neurovascular bundle damage, from priapism treatment, 222
Drainage of cutaneous abscesses, 307–311
Drug overdose, gastric intubation for, 111
Dysmenorrhea, Progestasert IUD for, 230
Dysphagia, laryngoscopy for, 353
Dysrhythmia:
  exercise testing and, 58, 59
  from gastric intubation, 117

E

Ear perforation, tympanometry for, 367
Earache, laryngoscopy for, 353
Ear/nose/throat procedures, 353–377
  impacted earwax removal, 361–365
  laryngoscopy, 353–360
  posterior epistaxis control, 373–377
  tympanometry, 367–371
Earwax removal, 361–365
  agents for, 362
  contraindications for, 361–362
  follow-up care for, 364–365
  materials for, 362
  procedure for, 363–364, 365
ECG. *See* Electrocardiogram
Ectopic pregnancy:
  culdocentesis and, 253, 255–256
  incidence of, 229
  IUD insertion and, 229, 234
Edema:
  cricothyroidotomy for, 79
  of perineum, 260
Elbow, aspiration/injection of, 162
Electrocardiogram (ECG), exercise testing and, 58, 61, 63
Electrocoagulation, 337–343
  complications from, 342–343
  contraindications for, 337–339
  follow-up care for, 342
  materials for, 339
  procedure for, 340–342
  techniques of, 337
  unit for, 339
Electrodesiccation, 337, 338
Electrofulguration, 337, 338, 341, 342
Embolism:
  air, 7, 48
  catheter fragment, 7
Empyema, from chest tube insertion, 97
Endobronchial intubation, from endotracheal intubation, 77
Endocrinopathy, trigger point injection and, 168
Endometrial biopsy, 243–247
  complications from, 245
  contraindications for, 243
  indications for, 243
  materials for, 244
  minimally invasive, 261–266
    contraindications for, 262
    follow-up care for, 264
    indications for, 261–262
    materials for, 262
    preparation for, 262
    procedure for, 262–264, 265
  procedure for, 244–245, 246–247
Endotracheal intubation, 73–78, 99
  complications from, 77
  contraindications for, 73
  indications for, 73
  materials for, 73–74
  procedure for, 74–77
Enema:
  barium, 128
  mineral oil, 142
  sodium phosphate, 121, 128
Epididymitis, from urinary catheterization, 211
Epinephrine:
  anesthesia and, 203, 231, 270, 271–282
  contaminated wounds and, 302
  -saline, for priapism treatment, 221
  toxicity from, 269
  usefulness of, 269

Episiotomy:
  benefits of, 257
  complications from, 257–258
  delivery without, 257–260
  risks of, 257
Erythrasma, Wood's light examination for, 346–347
Erythromycin, for erythrasma, 347
Esophagus:
  intubation of, from tactile orotracheal intubation, 102
  laceration of, from cricothyroidotomy, 81
Ethyl chloride spray:
  for incision/drainage of abscesses, 308
  for trigger point injection, 170, 172
Exercise treadmill testing, 57–63
  contraindications for, 58–59
  equipment costs for, 57
  follow-up care for, 63
  indications for, 57–58
  materials for, 59–60
  personnel for, 60
  preparation for, 60
  procedure for, 61–63
  protocols for, 59
Expulsion, of IUD, 235
Extraoral approach, to TMJ dislocation management, 175, 177
Eye, removal of foreign bodies from, 381–386
  examination for, 382–384
  follow-up care for, 385
  materials for, 381–382
  preparation for, 382
  techniques for, 381
Eyelid, anesthesia of, 275–276, 277, 278

F

Face:
  anesthesia of, 275–276, 278
  lesions on, 310
Fecal impaction:
  diagnosis of, 142
  digital removal of, 141–144
    complications from, 143
    contraindications for, 142
    follow-up care for, 143–144
    indications for, 142
    materials for, 143
    preparation for, 142
    procedure for, 143
  etiology of, 141
Females:
  body fat measurements for, 147
  chronic pelvic pain in, 167
  culdocentesis for, 253–256
  delivery without episiotomy for, 257–260
  endometrial biopsy for, 243–247
    minimally invasive, 261–266
  fine-needle aspiration of breast for, 237–241
  IUD insertion in, 229–236
  pregnancy in, 235, 253, 319
  urinary catheterization for, 213–214
  uterine cervix biopsy for, 249–252
Femoral vein cannulation, 21–26
  complications from, 22
  indications for, 21–22
  materials for, 23
  procedure for, 23–25
  site selection for, 22
Fetal trauma, from delivery without episiotomy, 260
FEV_1 (forced expiratory volume in one second), 85, 86–88
Fibroadenoma, fine-needle aspiration for, 237
Fibromyalgia (myofascial syndrome), trigger point injection for, 167
Figure-of-8, clavicular fracture immobilization, 189–192
Fine-needle aspiration, of breast, 237–241
Finger:
  anesthesia of, 271–272, 320
  aspiration/injection of, 161
  swollen, removal of ring from, 327–330
    indication for, 327
    material for, 327
    procedure for, 327–329, 330
Fishhook removal, 331–335
  complications from, 334
  contraindications for, 331
  follow-up care for, 334
  indication for, 331
  materials for, 331
  procedures for, 331–335
Flexible fiberoptic nasopharyngolaryngoscope, 353, 354–356, 357
Flexible fiberoptic sigmoidoscopy, 119–125
Fluid:
  collection,
    peritoneal, 253
    pulmonary, 67–71
  studies, synovial, 163, 164
Fluorescein strips, for eye examination, 382
Foot, compressive splinting for, 181
Forehead, anesthesia of, 275, 277
Foreign body:
  aspiration, death among children from, 41
  removal, from eye, 381–386
Fournier's syndrome, from newborn circumcision, 209
Fungal infections, Wood's light examination for, 345–346
FVC (forced vital capacity), 85, 86, 88

G

Gas exchange disturbance, arterial puncture for, 103
Gastric bleeding, gastric intubation for, 111
Gastric distention, from CPR, 31
Gastric intubation, 111–117
  complications from, 116–117
  contraindications for, 112
  indications for, 111
  materials for, 112
  procedure for, 113–116

Gastrointestinal procedures, 111–153
flexible fiberoptic sigmoidoscopy, 119–125
gastric intubation, 111–117
intraosseous infusion, 15–20
paracentesis, peritoneal lavage and, 133–139
rubber band ligation of hemorrhoids, 127–131
skinfold measurements, 145–153
Genital warts, male, examination for, 223–225
Genitourinary procedures, 197–225
circumcision in newborn, 201–209
digital removal of fecal impaction, 141–144
male genital warts examination, 223–225
priapism treatment, 219–222
suprapubic bladder tap in child, 197–199
urinary catheterization, 211–217
Glans, bivalving of, 209
Glucose:
for peritoneal lavage, 133
through intraosseous infusion, 15
Glycerin suppository, for constipation, 143
Gomco clamp, for circumcision in newborn, 202–209
Gynecology procedures, 229–266. *See also* Obstetrics procedures
biopsy of uterine cervix, 249–252
culdocentesis, 253–256
endometrial biopsy, 243–247
endometrial sampling, minimally invasive, 261–266
fine-needle aspiration of breast, 237–241
IUD insertion, 229–236

H

Hair, around lacerations, 301
Hand, IV in dorsum of, 10–11
Headache:
chronic, progressive muscle relaxation for, 407
from lumbar puncture, 394, 399
Heimlich maneuver, for airway obstruction in child, 41–43
Hemarthrosis, synovial effusion versus, 157
Hematemesis, from gastric intubation, 117
Hematoma:
from arterial puncture, 106
from cricothyroidotomy, 81
from fine-needle aspiration of breast, 241
from internal jugular vein cannulation, 48
from IV, 7
from needle thoracentesis, 96
from priapism treatment, 222
from trigger point injection, 172
Hemoperitoneum, culdocentesis for, 253
Hemorrhage:
from cricothyroidotomy, 81
from newborn circumcision, 209
Hemorrhoidectomy, 131
Hemorrhoids, rubber band ligation of, 127–131
complications from, 129, 131
contraindications for, 128
follow-up care for, 131
indications for, 127
materials for, 128
procedure for, 128–129, 130
Hemothorax:
chest tube insertion for, 89
from CPR, 31
Heparin:
for blood gas specimen, 104, 105, 106
joint aspiration and, 162
for peritoneal lavage, 133
Hepatitis, instrument sterilization and, 125
Herpetic whitlow, paronychia versus, 313
Hippocrates, 127
Hoarseness, laryngoscopy for, 353
Hormone replacement therapy, endometrial biopsy and, 243
Human chorionic gonadotropin pregnancy test, 253
Human papillomavirus (HPV) infection:
examination for, 223–225
transmission of, 223
treatment of, 225
Hyfrecator, 339
Hypertension, exercise treadmill testing for, 58
Hypnosis, 415–419
characteristics of, 415
contraindications for, 416
follow-up care for, 418
indications for, 416
materials for, 416
preparation for, 416–417
procedure for, 417–418
self-induced, 417–418
usefulness of, 415–416
Hypoxia, from tactile orotracheal intubation, 102

I

Impacted earwax removal, 361–365
Incision of cutaneous abscesses, 307–311
Infant. *See also* Child; Newborn
airway obstruction in, 43–44
CPR for, 33–39
lumbar puncture in, 395–399
suprapubic bladder tap for, 197–199
Infection:
from arterial puncture, 106
from endometrial biopsy, 245
from fine-needle aspiration of breast, 241
from IUD insertion, 234
from lumbar puncture, 394, 399
from newborn circumcision, 209
from trigger point injection, 172
Wood's light examination for, 345–347
Infertility, endometrial biopsy for, 243, 261
Inflammatory joint disease, aspiration for, 157
Infraorbital nerve block, anesthesia of, 275–276, 278
Ingrown toenail:
prevention of, 324–325
treatment of, 319–325
contraindications for, 319
guidelines for, 319

indication for, 319
materials for, 319–320
procedure for, 320–324
Injection of joints, 157–165
Intercostal:
artery damage, from chest tube insertion, 96
myalgia, from chest tube insertion, 96
nerve block, anesthesia of, 276–277, 279
damage to, from chest tube insertion, 96
vein damage, from chest tube insertion, 96
Internal jugular vein catheterization, 45–49
complications from, 48–49
contraindications for, 45–46
follow-up care for, 49
indications for, 45
materials for, 46
preparation for, 46
procedure for, 46–48
Intraoral approach, to TMJ dislocation management, 175, 177–178
Intraosseus infusion, 15–20
complications from, 19
contraindication for, 16
drugs administered by, 15
follow-up care for, 19
indications for, 15–16
IV access versus, 15
materials for, 16
procedure for, 16–19
Intrathoracic organ damage, from chest tube insertion, 97
Intrauterine device (IUD) insertion, 229–236
candidates for, 230
complications from, 234–235
contraindications for, 229–230
follow-up care for, 235
materials for, 230
preparation for, 231
procedure for, 231–234
removal and, 236
timing of, 230–231
Intravenous (IV) access:
in adult, 3–7
complications from, 6–7
long-term, 4
materials for, 3
preparation for, 4–5
procedure for, 5–6
short-term, 4
site selection for, 3–4
to internal jugular vein, 45–49
intraosseous infusion versus, 15
in newborn, 9–13
materials for, 9–10
positions for, 10–11
procedure for, 12
site selection for, 10
patient-controlled analgesic using, 401–403
regional anesthesia with, 281–282
Intropin. *See* Dopamine
Intubation:
endobronchial, 77
endotracheal, 73–78, 99
esophageal, 102
gastric, 111–117
piriform recess, 102
of right main-stem bronchus, 102
tactile orotracheal, 99–102
tracheal, 117
Irrigation:
for impacted cerumen, 363–364
for priapism treatment, 219–222
Ischemia:
exercise treadmill testing for, 57–58
priapism and, 220
silent, 58
Isoptin. *See* Verapamil
IUD. *See* Intrauterine device
IV. *See* Intravenous access

J

Jet-trigger point injection, needle versus, 167
Joints, aspiration/injection of, 157–165. *See also* specific joints
complications from, 163
contraindications for, 157
indications for, 157
materials for, 158
preparation for, 158
procedure for, 155–159
Jugular vein, internal, cannulation of, 45–49

K

Kanamycin sulfate (Kanatrex, Klebcil), for peritoneal lavage, 133
Kegel exercises, 260
Kenny-Howard sling, for clavicular fracture immobilization, 192, 193
Kinking, from gastric intubation, 117
Knee, aspiration/injection of, 159

L

Lacerations, repair of simple, 299–306
contraindications for, 299–300
follow-up care for, 305–306
indications for, 299
materials for, 300
preparation for, 300–301
procedure for, 301–305
Lanoxin. *See* Digoxin
Laparotomy, paracentesis and, 133, 135, 138
Laryngeal mirrors, 353, 358–359
Laryngeal telescope, 353, 356, 358
Laryngoscopy, 99, 100, 353–360
equipment for, 353
indications for, 353

Laryngoscopy (*Continued*)
materials for, 354, 356, 358
procedures for, 354–359
usefulness of, 353
Larynx, fractured, cricothyroidotomy for, 79
Lavage:
gastric intubation for, 111
peritoneal, 133–139
Lesion(s):
biopsy of, 224–225
skin, 291–298
Leukemia, as cause of priapism, 219, 220
Lidocaine (Xylocaine), 269, 270, 271–282
for cardiovascular procedures, 23
for dermatology procedures, 284, 288, 301, 302, 308–309, 314, 332, 340
for gastrointestinal procedures, 18, 134
for genitourinary procedures, 220, 228
for gynecology procedures, 231, 238, 245, 250
maximum recommended doses of, 270
for musculoskeletal/connective tissue procedures, 158, 167, 170, 171, 172, 178, 188
for neurology procedures, 397
newborn IV access and, 12
pregnancy and, 319
for pulmonary procedures, 69, 91, 105
toxicity from 168, 172
without epinephrine. *See also* Epinephrine
for circumcision in newborn, 203
Ligation, of hemorrhoids, 127–133
Lip, anesthesia of, 275–276, 278
Lippes Loop IUD, 229, 235
Local anesthesia. *See* Anesthesia
Lodging, from gastric intubation, 117
Lumbar puncture:
in adults, 389–394
complications from, 394
contraindications for, 389
indications for, 389
materials for, 389–390
preparation for, 390–391
procedure for, 391–394
in child, 395–399
complications from, 399
contraindications for, 395
indications for, 395
materials for, 395
preparation for, 395–397
procedure for, 397–398
Lung. *See also* Pulmonary procedures
contusions of, from CPR, 31
disease of, spirometry for, 85. *See also* Pulmonary disease
puncture of, from internal jugular vein cannulation, 49

M

Magnesium hydroxide, for constipation, 144
Males:
body fat measurements for, 148
circumcision in newborn, 201–209
genital warts in, 223–225
priapism in, 219–222
urinary catheterization for, 214–215
Malnourishment, skinfold measurements and, 147
Mammary artery laceration, from needle thoracentesis, 96
Mammography, for breast tumor evaluation, 237
Marcaine. *See* Bupivacaine
Median nerve, anesthesia of, 273–274, 275
Men. *See* Males
Menses, heavy, Progestasert IUD for, 230
Menstrual disorders, endometrial biopsy for, 243
Mepivacaine (Carbocaine), 269
maximum recommended doses of, 270
Metabolic energy equivalents (METs), 59
Metacarpal/metatarsal anesthesia of, 272
MI. *See* Myocardial infarction
Migraine, progressive muscle relaxation for, 407
Mineral oil enema, for fecal impaction, 142
Minimally invasive endometrial sampling, 261–266
Morphine, for patient-controlled analgesia, 403
Motor vehicle accident (MVA), deaths from, 89
Muscle spasm, trigger point injection for, 167
Musculoskeletal/connective tissue procedures, 153–190
aspiration/injection of joints, 157–165
clavicular fracture immobilization, 185–194
compressive ankle splinting, 181–184
TMJ dislocation management, 175–180
trigger point injection, 167–173
Myalgia, intercostal, from chest tube insertion, 96
Myocardial infarction (MI), exercise testing and, 57, 58

N

Nail plate avulsion with phenolization, for ingrown toenail, 319, 320, 322, 323–324
Naproxen (Naprosyn), for IUD insertion, 231
Naproxen sodium (Anaprox), for IUD insertion, 231
Nasal approach, for gastric intubation, 113–114, 115–116
Nasal drainage, laryngoscopy for, 353
Nasopharyngolaryngoscope, flexible fiberoptic, 353, 354–356, 357
Needle:
fine-, for aspiration of breast, 237–241
-hole defect, from intraosseous infusion, 19
standard hypodermic, for intraosseous infusion, 18
thoracentesis with, 90–91, 96
trephine bone, for intraosseous infusion, 18–19
-trigger point injection, jet- versus, 167
Nesacaine. *See* Chloroprocaine
Neurology procedures, 389–403
lumbar puncture, in adults, 389–394
lumbar puncture, in child, 395–399
patient-controlled analgesia (PCA), 401–403
Newborn. *See also* Child; Infant
circumcision in, 201–209
clavicular fracture immobilization for, 187
IV access in, 9–13

Nitrogen spray, for cryotherapy, 292, 293, 295, 296
Normal saline (NaCl), for diagnostic tap, 133
Nose, anesthesia of, 275–276, 278
Nosebleeds, control of, 373–377
Novocain. *See* Procaine

O

Obesity, skinfold measurements and, 145
Obstetrics procedures. *See also* Gynecology procedures
  delivery without episiotomy, 257–260
Oral approach, for gastric intubation, 114–115
Oropharyngeal bleeding, cricothyroidotomy for, 79
Orotracheal intubation, tactile, 99–102
Ossicular chain disruptions, tympanometry for, 367
Osteomyelitis, from intraosseous infusion, 19
Otitis media:
  acute, (AOM), 361
  unilateral serous, 353
Ovarian cysts, culdocentesis and, 253

P

Pacemaker:
  electrocoagulation and, 343
  femoral vein cannulation and, 21
  internal jugular vein cannulation and, 45
Pain:
  chest, 57, 143, 276–277, 279
  chronic, hypnosis for, 416
  from endometrial biopsy, 245
  patient-controlled analgesia for, 401–403
  pelvic, trigger point injection for, 167
  from rib fractures, anesthesia for, 276–277, 279
  from rubber band ligation of hemorrhoids, 129, 131
  throat, laryngoscopy for, 353
Palpitations, exercise-related, exercise treadmill testing for, 58
Pancreatitis:
  paracentesis/peritoneal lavage and, 133
  testing for, 138
Panic disorder, progressive muscle relaxation for, 407
Pap smear, abnormal, 249, 252
Papaverine, as cause of priapism, 219
Paracentesis:
  complications from, 138
  contraindications for, 133–134
  indications for, 133
  materials for, 134
  peritoneal lavage and, 133–139
  procedure for, 134–137
Paronychia, 313–317
  complications from, 316
  contraindications for, 313
  etiology of, 313
  follow-up care for, 315–316
  indication for, 313
  materials for, 313–314
  procedure for, 314–315, 316, 317
Patient-controlled analgesia (PCA), 401–403
  benefits of, 402
  complications from, 403
  contraindications for, 401
  indications for, 401
  materials for, 402–403
  procedure for, 403
  theoretical basis for, 401–402
Pelvic floor relaxation, from delivery without episiotomy, 260
Pelvic pain, trigger point injection for, 167
Penile warts, androscopy and, 223
Pentothal. *See* Thiopental sodium
Perineum:
  edema of, from delivery without episiotomy, 260
  laceration of, from delivery without episiotomy, 260
Peritoneum:
  fluid collection from, with culdocentesis, 253
  lavage of,
    electrolyte solution for, 133
    laboratory results from, 138
    paracentesis and, 133–139
    procedure for, 135–137
Peritonitis:
  paracentesis/peritoneal lavage and, 133
  testing for, 138
Peroneal nerves, anesthesia of, 278, 280, 281
Phenol:
  in nail plate avulsion, for ingrown toenail, 319, 320, 322, 323–324
  pregnancy and, 319
Phlebitis, from IV, 7
Pigmentary alterations, Wood's light examination for, 347
Piriform recess intubation, from tactile orotracheal intubation, 102
Plasma, through intraosseous infusion, 15
Plastibell method, of circumcision in newborn, 202
Pleural effusion, chest tube insertion for, 89
Pleural infection, from needle thoracentesis, 96
Pneumonia, laryngoscopy for, 353
Pneumothorace, from trigger point injection, 172
Pneumothorax:
  chest tube insertion and, 89, 97
  from CPR, 31
  from fine-needle aspiration of breast, 241
  from internal jugular vein cannulation, 48
  from needle thoracentesis, 96
Poisoning, gastric intubation for, 111
Porphyria, Wood's light examination for, 347
Posterior epistaxis, control of, 373–377
  complications from, 376
  contraindications for, 374
  materials for, 374–375
  procedure for, 375–376, 377
  vessels involved in, 374
Postmenopausal bleeding, endometrial biopsy for, 243
Pouch of Douglas, culdocentesis of, 253–256
Pregnancy:
  ectopic. *See* Ectopic pregnancy
  IUD and, 235

Pregnancy (*Continued*)
lidocaine and, 319
phenol and, 319
test, human chorionic gonadotropin, 253
Priapism:
etiology of, 219
ischemia and, 220
treatment of, 219–222
complications from, 222
indications for, 220
materials for, 220
procedure for, 220–222
Procaine (Novocain), 269
maximum recommended doses of, 270
trigger point injection and, 168
Progestasert IUD, 229, 230
Progesterone, in IUD, 229
Progressive muscle relaxation, 407–413
contraindications for, 407
follow-up care for, 412
indications for, 407
materials for, 407–408
preparation for, 408
procedure/script for, 408–412
Protocols, for exercise, 59
Pseudomonal infections, Wood's light examination for, 347
Psychophysiologic disorders, hypnosis for, 416
Psyllium hydrophilic mucilloid, for constipation, 143
Pulmonary disease:
arterial puncture for, 103
spirometry for, 85
Pulmonary fluid removal, thoracentesis for, 67–71
Pulmonary procedures, 67–107. *See also* Lung
arterial puncture, 103–107
chest tube insertion, 89–97
cricothyroidotomy, 79–83
endotracheal intubation, 73–78
spirometry, 85–88
tactile orotracheal intubation, 99–102
thoracentesis for fluid removal, 67–71
Pulmonary thromboembolism, from IV, 7
Pulse irregularities, from priapism treatment, 222
Punch biopsy, of skin, 283–286

R

Radial nerve, anesthesia of, 273, 274, 276
Reduction, for clavicular fracture immobilization, 188–189, 190
Regional anesthesia. *See* Anesthesia, regional
Relaxation, progressive muscle, 407–413
Respiratory depression, from patient-controlled analgesia, 403
Restenosis, exercise testing and, 58
Rib fractures:
from CPR, 31
pain from, anesthesia for, 276–277, 279
Right atrium, perforation of, from internal jugular vein cannulation, 49
Rigid sigmoidoscopy, for detection of colorectal cancer, 119, 120
Ring removal, from swollen finger, 327–330
Ringer's lactate, through intraosseous infusion, 15
Rubber band ligation, of hemorrhoids, 127–131

S

Saf-T-Coil IUD, 229
Saline:
-epinephrine, for priapism treatment, 221
in trigger points, 167
through intraosseous infusion, 15
Saphenous vein, IV in, 10
Scabies, Wood's light examination for, 348
Scalp:
anesthesia of, 275, 277
vein of, IV in, 10–11
Scrotal lacerations, from newborn circumcision, 209
Sedation, excessive, from patient-controlled analgesia, 403
Seldinger (wire-guided) catheter, 21–25
Sensorcaine. *See* Bupivacaine
Sepsis:
from intraosseous infusion, 19
from IV, 7
from urinary catheterization, 211
Septicemia, from newborn circumcision, 209
Sheldon method, of circumcision in newborn, 202
Shoulder, aspiration/injection of, 161
Sickle cell disease, as cause of priapism, 219, 220
Sigmoidoscopy:
flexible fiberoptic, 119–125
contraindications for, 120
indications for, 120
instrument for, 119, 125
materials for, 120–121
preparation for, 121
rigid, 119, 120
Simple lacerations, repair of, 299–306
Sinusitis, laryngoscopy for, 353
Skin, punch biopsy of, 283–286
complications from, 285–286
indication for, 283
materials for, 283
procedure for, 283–285
Skin cyst removal, 287–289
indications for, 287
materials for, 287
procedure for, 288–289
Skin lesions, cryotherapy for, 291–298
Skinfold measurements, 145–153
contraindications for, 146
indications for, 145
materials for, 146
procedure for, 146–152
site selection for, 146, 147–148
Sleep problems, progressive muscle relaxation for, 407
Sling, Kenny-Howard, 192, 193
Snellen's chart, 383

Sodium phosphate enema:
for flexible fiberoptic sigmoidoscopy, 121
for rubber band ligation of hemorrhoids, 128
Spirometry, 85–88
contraindications for, 85
follow-up care for, 88
indications for, 85
interpreting results from, 86–87
materials for, 85
procedure for, 86–88
Splenic rupture, paracentesis and, 133
Splinting, compressive ankle, 181–184
Stenosis, from cricothyroidotomy, 81
Stress:
progressive muscle relaxation for, 407–413
testing for. *See* Exercise treadmill testing
Subcutaneous emphysema, from chest tube insertion, 97
Sump tube (double lumen), for gastric intubation, 112
Suppository:
bisacodyl, 121, 144
glycerin, 143
Supraorbital nerve block, anesthesia of, 275, 277
Suprapubic bladder tap, for child, 197–199
indication for, 197
materials for, 197
procedure for, 197–199
Sural nerve, anesthesia of, 280, 281
Swan-Ganz catheter:
femoral vein cannulation and, 21
internal jugular vein cannulation and, 45
Swollen finger, removal of ring from, 327–330
Swollen joints, aspiration for, 157
Synovial effusion, hemarthrosis versus, 157
Synovial fluid studies, 163, 164

T

Tachydysrhythmias, electrical cardioversion for, 54–55
Tactile orotracheal intubation, 99–102
complications from, 102
contraindications for, 100
indications for, 100
materials for, 100
procedure for, 100–102
Tatum-T, IUD, 229
Teeth fractures, from endotracheal intubation, 77
Temporomandibular joint. *See* TMJ
Tetanus prophylactic treatment, following fishhook removal, 334
Tetracycline, Wood's light examination and, 348
Thiopental sodium (Pentothal), through intraosseous infusion, 15
Thoracentesis:
materials for, 67
needle, 90–91, 96
procedure for, 68–71
for pulmonary fluid removal, 67–71
Throat pain, laryngoscopy for, 353
Thrombosis, from IV, 7
Tibial nerve, anesthesia of, 280–281
Tinea infections, Wood's light examination for, 345–346
TMJ dislocation management, 175–180
contraindication for, 176
indication for, 175
materials for, 176–177
procedure for, 177–179
symptoms of, 175
Toe, anesthesia of, 271–272, 320
Toenail, ingrown, 319–325
Toxic shock syndrome, from control of posterior epistaxis, 376
Toxicity, of anesthesia, 168, 172, 269
Trachea:
intubation of, from gastric intubation, 117
laceration of, from cricothyroidotomy, 81
Tracheostomy, 99
Traumatic neurosis, progressive muscle relaxation for, 407
Treadmill, for exercise testing, 57, 59–60
Trichloracetic acid (Tri-Chlor), for HPV treatment, 225
Trigger point(s):
injection of, 167–173
complications from, 172
contraindications for, 168
follow-up care for, 172
indications for, 167
jet versus needle, 167
materials for, 168
preparation for, 168–169
procedure for, 170–171
multiple, 168
Tumor, breast, evaluation of, 237
Tympanometry, 361, 367–371
contraindications for, 367
indications for, 367
interpretation of, 370–371
materials for, 368
procedure for, 368–369
usefulness of, 367
Type A personality, progressive muscle relaxation for, 407

U

Ulnar nerve, anesthesia of, 273, 274
Unilateral serous otitis media, laryngoscopy for, 353
University of Iowa Hospital, exercise treadmill testing at, 59
Urethral damage, from priapism treatment, 222
Urethral fistulas, from newborn circumcision, 209, 211
Urethral obstruction, urinary catheterization for, 211
Urinary calculi, from urinary catheterization, 211
Urinary catheterization, 211–217
complications from, 211, 216
contraindications for, 212
indwelling, indications for, 212
materials for, 212
postinsertion procedure, 215–216
preparation for, 212–213

Urinary catheterization (*Continued*)
  procedure for females, 213–214
  procedure for males, 214–215
  temporary, indications for, 211
Urinary retention, from priapism treatment, 222
Urine specimen:
  suprapubic bladder tap for, 197
  urinary catheterization for, 211
Uterine cancer, endometrial biopsy for, 243–247
Uterine cervix, biopsy of, 249–252
  colposcopy with, 249–251
  complications from, 252
  contraindication for, 249
  follow-up care for, 252
  indication for, 249
  materials for, 249
  procedure for, 249–252
Uterine perforation:
  from endometrial biopsy, 245
  from IUD insertion, 234–235

V

Valium. *See* Diazepam
Valsalva's maneuver, 129, 258
Vasculitis, as cause of priapism, 219
Vasodilators, exercise testing and, 60
Vasovagal syncope, from endometrial biopsy, 245
Ventricular fibrillation (VF), electrical defibrillation for, 51–55
Ventricular tachycardia, defibrillation for, 53
Verapamil (Calan, Isoptin), exercise testing and, 60
VF. *See* Ventricular fibrillation
Vocal cord spasm, from endotracheal intubation, 77
Vomiting:
  from endotracheal intubation, 77
  gastric intubation for, 111
  from patient-controlled analgesia, 403

W

Warts, male genital, 223–225
Wire-guided (Seldinger) catheter, 21-25
Women. *See* Females
Wood's light examination, 345–349
  for bacterial infections, 346–347
  for drug detection, 348
  of eye, 383
  for fungal infections, 345–346
  guide to, 346
  materials for, 348
  for pigmentary alterations, 347
  for porphyria, 347
  procedure for, 348
  for scabies, 348
  sources of error in, 348–349
Wrist:
  anesthesia of, 273–274, 276
  aspiration/injection of, 163

X

X-ray:
  cervical spine, tactile orotracheal intubation and, 99
  chest,
    chest tube insertion/removal and, 89, 90, 94, 96
    following internal jugular vein cannulation, 49
    thoracentesis and, 68
  for clavicular fracture immobilization, 193
Xylocaine. *See* Lidocaine